NATURAL
prescriptions
for women

NATURAL
prescriptions
for women

What to do—and ***when***
to do it—to solve more than
100 female health problems
—***Without Drugs***

By the Editors of

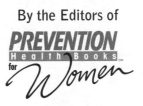

PREVENTION
Health Books
for *Women*

Rodale Press, Inc.
Emmaus, Pennsylvania

Copyright © 1998 by Rodale Press, Inc.
Illustrations copyright © 1998 by Karen Bell, Karen Kuchar, and Steven Stankiewicz

1. The chart "Asthma Emergencies and Your Menstrual Cycle" on page 165 was adapted from "Emergency Department Visits Based on Phase of Menstrual Cycle," which was originally published in *Glamour*. Copyright © 1997 by Typemasters Design. Reprinted by permission.
2. The RETHINK technique on page 381 was adapted from *Anger Management* by the Institute for Mental Health Initiatives. Reprinted with permission. Copyright © by the Institute for Mental Health Initiatives. Reprinted with permission.
3. The chart "A Day in the Life of Your Moods" on page 384 was adapted from "The Origin of Moods," which was originally published in *The Origin of Everyday Moods* by Robert E. Thayer, Ph.D. Copyright © 1996 by Oxford University Press, Inc. Used by permission of Oxford University Press, Inc.
4. The numbered criteria on page 399 were adapted from *The Case against Divorce* by Diane Medved, Ph.D. Copyright © 1989 by Diane Medved, Ph.D. Reprinted with permission.

Library of Congress Cataloging-in-Publication Data

Natural prescriptions for women : what to do—and when to do it—to solve more than 100
   female health problems—without drugs / by the editors of Prevention Health Books
   for women.
       p.   cm.
   Includes index.
   ISBN 0–87596–433–8   hardcover
     1. Women—Health and hygiene.   2. Women—Medical care.   3. Self-care, Health.
   4. Alternative medicine.   I. Prevention Health Books.
   RA778.N38   1998
   613'.04244—DC21   98–10112

Distributed in the book trade by St. Martin's Press

2   4   6   8   10   9   7   5   3   1   hardcover

Natural Prescriptions for Women Staff

MANAGING EDITOR: Sharon Faelten
EDITOR: Susan G. Berg
WRITERS: Michelle Bisson, Julie A. Evans, Gale Maleskey,
   Sara Altshul O'Donnell
ASSISTANT RESEARCH MANAGER: Anita C. Small
LEAD RESEARCHERS: Carol J. Gilmore, Shea Zukowski
EDITORIAL RESEARCHERS: Jennifer A. Barefoot, Elizabeth Brown,
   Susan Burdick, Lori Davis, Jennifer L. Kaas, Mary Kittel,
   Terry Sutton Kravitz, Nanci Kulig, Sandra Salera-Lloyd,
   Deanna Moyer, Deborah Pedron, Staci Ann Sander, Lorna S. Sapp,
   Teresa A. Yeykal
SENIOR COPY EDITORS: Amy K. Kovalski, Karen Neely
ART DIRECTOR: Darlene Schneck
COVER DESIGNER: Rich Kershner
INTERIOR DESIGNERS: Rich Kershner, Elizabeth Youngblood
ILLUSTRATORS: Karen Bell, Karen Kuchar, Steven Stankiewicz
LAYOUT DESIGNERS: Keith Biery, Donna G. Rossi
OFFICE MANAGER: Roberta Mulliner
OFFICE STAFF: Julie Kehs, Suzanne Lynch, Mary Lou Stephen
MARKETING MANAGER: Kristine Siessmayer
MANUFACTURING COORDINATOR: Patrick T. Smith

Rodale Health and Fitness Books

VICE-PRESIDENT AND EDITORIAL DIRECTOR: Debora T. Yost
EXECUTIVE EDITOR: Neil Wertheimer
DESIGN AND PRODUCTION DIRECTOR: Michael Ward
RESEARCH MANAGER: Ann Gossy Yermish
COPY MANAGER: Lisa D. Andruscavage
PRODUCTION MANAGER: Robert V. Anderson Jr.
STUDIO MANAGER: Leslie M. Keefe
BOOK MANUFACTURING DIRECTOR: Helen Clogston

MARY LAKE POLAN, M.D., PH.D.
Professor and chairman of the department of gynecology and obstetrics at Stanford University School of Medicine

ELIZABETH LEE VLIET, M.D.
Founder and medical director of HER Place: Health Enhancement and Renewal for Women and clinical associate professor in the department of family and community medicine at the University of Arizona College of Medicine in Tucson

LILA AMDURSKA WALLIS, M.D., M.A.C.P.
Clinical professor of medicine at Cornell University Medical College in New York City, past president of the American Medical Women's Association (AMWA), founding president of the National Council on Women's Health, director of continuing medical education programs for physicians, and master and laureate of the American College of Physicians

CARLA WOLPER, R.D.
Nutritionist and clinical coordinator at the Obesity Research Center at St. Luke's/Roosevelt Hospital Center in New York City and nutritionist at the Center for Women's Health at Columbia Presbyterian Eastside in New York City

Contents

INTRODUCTION
Programming Your Body to Heal Faster, with Nature xv

PART 1
Personal Prescriptions for Healing

CHAPTER 1

Prescriptions for Common Problems 3

ACHES AND PAINS
Fold and Hold to Feel Better Fast 4

BACK PAIN AND STIFFNESS
Relief Is As Close As Your Fridge 9

BAD BREATH
Nibble Your Garnish to Mellow Mouth Odor 19

BLOOD SUGAR PROBLEMS
A Turkey Sandwich Prevents Wooziness 21

BREAST DISCOMFORT
Temper Tenderness with Vitamin E 24

COFFEE NERVES
Snack While You Sip 28

COLDS AND FLU
Echinacea Eases Symptoms 30

COLD SORES AND CANKER SORES
Try a Little Tenderizer 34

CONJUNCTIVITIS
A Chamomile Compress Is Respite for Sore Eyes 39

CONSTIPATION
Psyllium Seed Gets Things Moving 43

Contents

COUGH, SORE THROAT, AND LARYNGITIS
Take Your Thyme 47

CUTS, SCRAPES, BRUISES, AND ABRASIONS
Calendula Speeds Healing 51

DANDRUFF AND SCALP PROBLEMS
Prone to Flaking? Relax 54

DIARRHEA
Raspberry Leaf Tea Reins In the Runs 57

DRY EYES
Increase Your Olive Oil Intake 60

DRY MOUTH
Lemon Gets the Juices Flowing 64

ENERGY SLUMP
Carbs and Caffeine — A Stimulating Combination 68

GAS
Chew Fennel Seeds for Speedy Relief 73

GUM DISEASE
Herbal Toothpaste Keeps Gums in the Pink 77

HEARTBURN
Timely Advice to Banish the Burn 84

HEMORRHOIDS
Take 'Em Lying Down 88

POST-WORKOUT SORENESS
Rub Out the Ache with Arnica 93

QUEASY STOMACH
Ginger Ale Douses Digestive Upset 103

SINUSITIS
Clear Congestion with Acupressure 106

SLEEP PROBLEMS
Use Your Imagination 112

STIFF JOINTS
Eating Fish Keeps You Flexible 118

TENSION HEADACHES AND MIGRAINES
Grab a Golf Ball and Roll Away Pain 122

TINNITUS
Ginkgo Biloba Turns Down the Sounds 130

URINARY TRACT INFECTIONS
Cranberry Juice — The Classic Cure 134

VAGINITIS
Homeopathic Remedies to the Rescue 139

VARICOSE VEINS
Bank On Bioflavonoids to Strengthen Veins. 142
YEAST INFECTIONS
A Yogurt Compress Ends the Itching 147

─── **CHAPTER 2** ───

Prescriptions for Fighting Disease. 152

ANEMIA
Enhance Iron Absorption with Orange Juice 153
ARTHRITIS
Nighttime Stretching Eases Morning Soreness 157
ASTHMA
Breathe Easy with Supplements. 164
CANCER PREVENTION
Why Tomatoes Are Terrific. 170
CHRONIC FATIGUE
Beef Up on B Vitamins. 174
DIABETES
A Meal Plan for Managing Blood Sugar. 181
FIBROMYALGIA
Deep Breathing Diminishes Pain. 187
FOOD ALLERGIES
Could Cosmetics Trigger Symptoms? 194
HEART DISEASE
Stress-Proof Your Heart with Yoga. 199
HIGH BLOOD PRESSURE
Celery Pares Points 204
HIGH CHOLESTEROL
Get Help from the Stinking Rose 209
IRRITABLE BOWEL SYNDROME
Soothe Spasms with Cramp Bark. 215
OSTEOPOROSIS
Bypass the Bone Robbers. 220
OVERWEIGHT
Water—The Best Diet Drink Around 226
POOR RESISTANCE
Boost Immunity with Herbs 231
REPETITIVE STRAIN INJURY
Change Positions to Outmaneuver Pain. 237

CHAPTER 3

Prescriptions for Hormonal and Reproductive Problems . . 245

BURNING MOUTH SYNDROME
Hot Peppers Fight Fire with Fire 246

DIFFICULTY CONCEIVING
A B Vitamin for Infertility 249

HOT FLASHES
Use Your Mind to Cool Your Body 254

LABOR PAIN
Exercises for an Easy Delivery 261

MENOPAUSE
Silence Symptoms with Soy 267

MENSTRUAL DISCOMFORTS
Relax Cramps with Aromatherapy Massage 273

MORNING SICKNESS
Treat Your Stomach Gingerly 282

POSTPARTUM DEPRESSION
Walk Away from the Blues 286

PREMENSTRUAL SYNDROME
Eat to Beat PMS 290

URINARY INCONTINENCE
The Kegel Cure 297

VAGINAL DRYNESS
Licorice Root Restores Moisture 303

CHAPTER 4

Prescriptions for Looking Your Best 310

AGE SPOTS
Protect Your Skin When Heading Outdoors 311

BLEMISHES
Zap Breakouts with Supplements 315

CELLULITE AND STRETCH MARKS
A Dual Strategy for Smoother Skin 320

DARK CIRCLES
Witch Hazel Works Wonders 323

DRY HAIR
Aromatherapy Oils Make Your Mane Manageable 327

EXPRESSION LINES
Fade 'Em with Fruit Acids 332

FINE HAIR
Choose the Kindest Cut 335

FRIZZY HAIR
Lather Up to Avoid "Bed Head". 341

MELASMA (MASK OF PREGNANCY)
To Save Face, Skip the Sun 345

OILY HAIR
Herbal Shampoo Cleanses Tresses Gently 348

PUFFY EYES
Reduce Swelling with Chamomile Tea Bags. 351

SENSITIVE SKIN
An Oatmeal Bath Soothes You All Over 354

SPLIT NAILS
Rehydrate with an Olive-Oil Soak 358

TROUBLE ZONES
Strength-Training Exercises to Trim and Tone 360

WRINKLES
Try Topical Vitamin C. 372

 CHAPTER 5 ---

Prescriptions for Emotional Health. 377

ANGER
Stop and Smell the Rose Oil. 378

BAD MOODS
Sack Sugary Foods 383

BOREDOM
Broaden Your Horizons 387

COMPUTER ANXIETY
Take a Child's Point of View. 391

DEPRESSION
St.-John's-Wort Beats the Blues 394

DIVORCE
Ground Rules for Emotional Survival 399

FORGETFULNESS
Sniff Rosemary Oil for Peak Mental Performance. 404

GUILT
The Cure for Do-It-All Syndrome 408

HOSTILITY
Walk Away When Tempers Flare 413

INHIBITED SEXUAL DESIRE
Make Time for Romance 415

INSECURITY AND LOW SELF-ESTEEM
A Positive Approach 421

MENTAL BLOCKS
Leapfrog to Achievement 423

NEGATIVE THINKING
Shed the "Poor Me" Attitude 426

NERVOUS TENSION
Relax from Head to Toe 429

OVERCONTROLLING TENDENCIES
Be an Advisor, Not a Critic 434

OVEREATING
Eat More Often, Not Less 436

POOR BODY IMAGE
Love What You See 441

WINTER DOLDRUMS
Lighten Up! 443

WORRY
Expect the Best 445

PART 2
Prescriptions for a Healthy Lifestyle

— CHAPTER 6 —

Prescriptions for Inactive Women 453

— CHAPTER 7 —

Prescriptions for Exercise Fanatics 461

— CHAPTER 8 —

Prescriptions for Chronic Dieters 468

— CHAPTER 9 —

Prescriptions for the Married and Harried 475

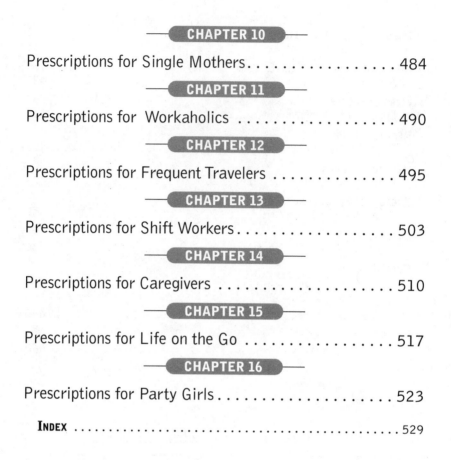

CHAPTER 10

Prescriptions for Single Mothers.................484

CHAPTER 11

Prescriptions for Workaholics 490

CHAPTER 12

Prescriptions for Frequent Travelers 495

CHAPTER 13

Prescriptions for Shift Workers..................503

CHAPTER 14

Prescriptions for Caregivers 510

CHAPTER 15

Prescriptions for Life on the Go 517

CHAPTER 16

Prescriptions for Party Girls....................523

INDEX 529

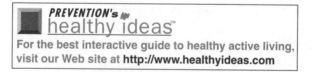

PROGRAMMING YOUR BODY

TO HEAL FASTER, WITH NATURE

You probably knew that jet lag, blood sugar problems, and menstrual cramps are affected by changes in body physiology over time. But did you know that asthma, arthritis, migraines, and a whole host of other health conditions also vary from day to day, month to month, season to season?

We know our bodies can and do change significantly from year to year. But evidently, our bodies change from hour to hour, day to night, week to week, month to month, and season to season. And that's enough to affect our health.

For years, botanists and biologists were the only people who paid attention to the study of daily rhythms on plants or animals. Now, scientists are taking a closer look at how daily, monthly, or seasonal changes affect not only animals, but people.

What's more, medicine is beginning to take these changes, called circadian rhythms, into account. Doctors notice that a host of conditions—from asthma and heartburn to arthritis and high blood pressure—fluctuate within the course of a day or month. If you have asthma, for example, and your triggers are molds, pollens, and cigarette smoke, you are more likely to have an attack in the morning. But if your asthma is triggered by dust mites, you are more prone to attacks in the middle of the night. Similarly, the pain of rheumatoid arthritis tends to be worse when you first awaken. But with osteoarthritis, you may feel fine in the morning but have pain later in the day.

Because of monthly fluctuations in the amount and type of female hormones released during the monthly menstrual cycle, chronobiological changes are most notable in women. In fact, according to a poll conducted for the American Medical Association, three out of four doctors surveyed agreed that the female reproductive system is influenced by chronobiology, the relationship between time and your health.

Many of the same physicians polled said that they give consideration to the body's natural rhythms when prescribing treatment. Synchronizing treatment with the chronobiological patterns of a specific condition, such as asthma or migraine headaches, is called chronotherapeutics.

Within the scientific community, there is a general trend toward taking a closer look at how the dimension of time can help people get the most benefit from their medications, says Timothy Monk, Ph.D., professor of psychiatry and director of the human chronobiology research program at the University of Pittsburgh School of Medicine. Doctors are starting to prescribe medication so that it is taken when the body can use it most efficiently. Doctors are also giving more consideration to the delivery of powerful drugs, such as those used in chemotherapy, so that they are administered at a time when they are less likely to be toxic to the body.

The idea is simple. By taking medication at the time when your body can make the most of it, you may benefit in three ways: The disease may be better managed. You will experience fewer side effects. And you might need less medication.

Growing evidence reveals that prescribing nondrug remedies at the right time of the day, month, or season can also go a long way toward relieving symptoms.

Modeled after the kinds of prescriptions that you are accustomed to receiving for medical treatments, the natural prescriptions you'll discover in this book are very specific. You'll find out what to do, when, how often, and for how long. Throughout, the focus is on *timing* your actions to glean the most benefit in the shortest period of time. As a quick reference aid, you'll find advice keyed to certain biological rhythms flagged with symbols. These handy icons spotlight remedies best used at certain times of the day or night, month, or season.

Sometimes all it takes is the right action at the right time to relieve the problem. A gentle stretch when you wake up in the morning. A cup of a healing herbal tea in the afternoon. A restorative food at dinnertime. A calming visualization at bedtime. The right supplement at the right time of the month. These natural prescriptions may ease your ills, often without drugs—or at least reduce your need for medication, if your doctor approves.

Part 1 of the book offers natural prescriptions for the health problems that most concern women. Chapter 1 presents self-care measures for everyday ailments—the kinds of things that we are all apt to encounter sooner or later, such as colds and heartburn. Chapter 2 has time-oriented advice for fighting disease, with timely tips on high cholesterol, diabetes, high blood pressure, and other preventable problems. Chapter 3 pays special attention to hormonal and reproductive problems experienced exclusively by women, such as menstrual discomforts and hot flashes. Chapter 4 features dozens of natural tips and techniques for looking your best.

Because our mental and spiritual well-being affects our physical health, chapter 5 offers nondrug tactics for emotional health. And of course, since so many ills can be traced to less-than-healthful lifestyles, part 2 features "prescriptions" for healing 11 potentially harmful lifestyles, such as inactivity, chronic dieting, and life on the go.

Natural is better. But timing is everything. You'll see.

Sharon Faelten

Sharon Faelten
Editor

Part 1

PERSONAL PRESCRIPTIONS FOR HEALING

Chapter 1

PRESCRIPTIONS

FOR COMMON PROBLEMS

It never fails. A woman can go for days, weeks, even months without even the slightest blip on her health screen. Then out of the blue, something goes wrong.

Chances are, it has happened to you. Ever wake up on a Saturday morning with a raging case of the flu? Or arrive home from work with a splitting headache? Or sprout a cold sore on the day of an important presentation?

Let's face it: There is never a good time to get sick. And no matter what the ailment, you want fast relief. You could head for the medicine chest and have your choice of pills and potions. But if you're like most people, you are just as likely to try a natural alternative. In fact, a study conducted at Harvard Medical School found that one-third of adult Americans use some kind of complementary and alternative medicine.

You might sip a cup of ginger tea to ease the nausea and achiness that often accompany the flu. Or you may swallow a capsule of feverfew—

a natural source of salicylic acid, the active ingredient in aspirin—to short-circuit a headache. Or you might try a daily dose of zinc to send that cold sore packing.

In the pages that follow, you will find these and dozens of other natural remedies for more than 30 everyday ailments. You can sample the healing powers of herbs, foods, and supplements as well as other nondrug therapies. Find the ones that work for you and make them part of your own treatment repertoire.

Keep in mind that how well a given remedy works may be influenced by *when* you use it. The icons that appear throughout this book show you at a glance what time of day (or month or year) a remedy works best. Refer to these to choose just the right "prescription" for your particular symptoms.

Aches and Pains

Modern life is a pain. And we mean literally, not figuratively. Nearly half of all Americans experience some type of pain within any two-week period, according to a national survey conducted by *Prevention* and *NBC Today— Weekend Edition*. About one-third of us take medication for relief. Another one-third turn to relaxation or stress-reduction techniques. And the final one-third simply grin and bear it, waiting for the pain to go away on its own.

Keep in mind that regardless of your approach, you hurt for a reason. Pain is a symptom. It tells you that your body has been injured, infected, or otherwise wronged. "Taking proper care of little aches and pains as they occur can mean that you'll have fewer big aches and pains down the road," notes Dale L. Anderson, M.D., clinical assistant professor at the University of Minnesota Medical School in Minneapolis and author of *Muscle Pain Relief in 90 Seconds*.

Rx

Prescriptions
FOR HEAD-TO-TOE HURTS

Pain affects each of us a little differently. So what makes one person feel better may have little benefit for someone else. Finding remedies that work for you may require a bit of trial and error. Try one of the following remedies tailored to your particular hurt.

❐ For migraines, including menstrual migraines, take 600 milligrams of magnesium glyconate every day. "Research has shown that people with low blood levels of magnesium are more likely to experience certain types of headache, such as migraine," says Alexander Mauskop, M.D., director of the New York Headache Center in New York City and author of *The Headache Alternative*. Among his own migraine-prone patients, about half report that their headaches significantly improve when they add magnesium supplements to their diets.

Dr. Mauskop suggests trying magnesium therapy for one month. If you notice a reduction in the frequency or severity of your headaches, you can safely continue taking the mineral in the same dose. If you develop diarrhea—a common side effect of ingesting large amounts of magnesium—Dr. Mauskop recommends dividing the dose so that you're taking 200 milligrams three times a day. "Some people may need magnesium injections because their bodies have a hard time absorbing the mineral in pill form," he adds. Check with your doctor to see if magnesium injections are for you.

Note: The recommended dosage of 600 milligrams exceeds the Daily Value for magnesium, which is 400 milligrams. If you decide to give supplements a try, and particularly if you have heart or kidney problems, you should be working with a doctor who is willing to monitor your progress.

❐ For pain in your neck, shoulders, and back, wear a bra that provides ample support and that has shoulder straps of at least one inch in width. A good-fitting undergarment may be all you need to ease your upper-body aches, says LaJean Lawson, Ph.D., adjunct professor of exercise science at Oregon State University in Corvallis and a consultant to the intimate-apparel industry. Large-breasted women, in particular, may suffer when they wear poorly designed bras with too-narrow straps that cut deeply into the shoulder muscles and impair blood flow.

Try switching from a "standard" bra to a sports bra, advises Dr. Lawson. Look for one made by Champion or Jogbra. If you're not satisfied with the selection of sports bras at your nearby mall, you may want to shop by catalog instead. Among the mail-order companies that offer sports bras in a variety of styles and sizes: Title 9, 5743 Landregan Street, Emeryville, CA 94608 (bras up to size 42DD, plus the size EE/F Sport top, available by special order); and Enell Company, P.O. Box 808, Haver, MT 59501 (bras up to size 52DDD, with crisscross back support).

❐ For pain in your lower back, lie on the floor or another hard surface, with a pillow placed under your knees so that they bend slightly. This position rests your iliopsoas, or marching muscles, as Dr. Anderson calls them. These muscles extend from your lower back around either side of your body to the thighbone, enabling you to lift your knees. When the iliopsoas go into spasm, they make your lower back ache.

❐ For pain in the ball of your foot or between your toes, lace your fingers between your toes and gently stretch your toes apart. "This self-massage technique keeps your toes flexible and stretches the connective tissue in your foot," explains Helen Drusine, a massage therapist who works with professional ballet and Broadway dancers in New York City. "It may even reduce your chances of developing bunions and soft corns between your toes." You

From Here to Serenity

Stress can transform a minor pain into a major one. Feeling harried and harassed not only wears you down but also turns up the volume on your body's pain messages. Over time, these factors conspire to worsen almost any health problem.

By practicing deep relaxation for as little as 10 minutes a day, you can switch off your body's response to stress and, with it, alter pain sensations, says Margaret Caudill, M.D., Ph.D., assistant clinical professor of medicine at Harvard Medical School, co-director of the Arnold Pain Center at Beth Israel Deaconess Medical Center in Boston and Lahey Hitchcock Clinic in Nashua, New Hampshire, and author of *Managing Pain Before It Manages You*. She recommends the following relaxation technique. It's best to do this wearing loose, comfortable clothing—but at the very least, open your belt and other tight, constricting garments.

1. Sit in a comfortable chair. Close your eyes and imagine

can use this technique whenever you like, but you'll find it especially soothing at the end of the day, after your feet have been confined inside shoes for hours.

Prescriptions
FOR ANYWHERE ACHES

Rx

Overuse and injury invariably produce pain. When your body takes a beating, try these remedies for relief.

❐ For muscle strain—which usually results from overuse or over-load—apply ice (wrapped in a towel) at least six times each day. At least three of those times should be in the evening. How long you leave the ice in place depends on the size of the muscle. Large muscles such as those in

TIME IT RIGHT

---

that your abdomen is a balloon. As you inhale, fill the balloon with air. As you exhale, allow the balloon to collapse.

2. Continue to focus on your breath coming in and going out.

3. As thoughts and worries pop into your mind, simply observe them and let them go. Then gently refocus on your breath. If you desire, repeat a soothing word such as *one*, *peace*, or *shalom*. This helps draw your attention away from distracting thoughts.

4. As you inhale, envision your breath filling the part of your body that hurts and bathing it with soothing warmth. Then as you exhale, imagine your breath carrying away pain.

5. Continue to belly-breathe for 10 to 20 minutes.

Dr. Caudill suggests practicing this relaxation technique for 10 to 20 minutes once or twice a day. You can do a shorter version whenever you have a few minutes during the day— whether you're on hold, stuck in traffic, or waiting in line at the supermarket.

the back and thighs require 20-minute treatments. Smaller muscles such as those in the elbows and calves require 10- to 15-minute treatments. For even smaller muscles such as those in the face, hands, and feet, 5 minutes should do. Continue applying ice until swelling subsides, bruising fades, and pain is reduced by half, advises David Troppy, D.C., a chiropractic sports physician in private practice in Napa, California. This could mean 5 days of ice treatments for minor muscle strain, 10 days for moderate strain.

A severe strain, or a muscle tear, will produce immediate and debilitating pain. You need to see your doctor right away for treatment.

TIME IT RIGHT

❒ For muscle pain often associated with a tender knot, use the Fold and Hold Method. Developed by Dr. Anderson, Fold and Hold involves relaxing the sore, tight muscle until you feel relief. Begin by "folding" your body over the tender spot in such a way that the pain decreases by at least 75 percent or disappears completely. The position may appear awkward and painful, but your body will ultimately feel good. "People seek out these positions instinctively, even while they're sleeping," notes Dr. Anderson. You'll know when you've found the right "hold" position, because the pain and any associated tender spot subsides. Hold for 90 seconds, then slowly release. Follow with a gentle stretch of the muscle the opposite way.

You can use the Fold and Hold Method for all the muscles in your body. If you develop pain in either hip, for instance, try raising your leg out to the side and resting the inside of your foot on a chair. Or you can lie on your back on a bed or the floor and slowly swing your leg out to the side. Your skin will fold at the site of the pain, and the tender spot will disappear. Hold the fold for 90 seconds. Either position shortens the muscle that connects your hip to your knee, thus allowing the muscle to relax and release the pain, says Dr. Anderson.

❒ For bruising or swelling, apply Arnica gel or oil to the affected area once a day for two or three days. Practitioners of homeopathy commonly prescribe Arnica for injuries. "The remedy works so well, in fact, that I have known it to convert people to homeopathy," says Judyth Reichenberg-Ullman, N.D., a naturopathic doctor with the Northwest Center for Homeopathic Medicine in Edmonds, Washington, and co-author of *Homeopathic Self-Care*.

You can buy Arnica gel or oil in health food stores. Simply apply the gel or oil to cover the affected area, suggests Dr. Reichenberg-Ullman. Avoid using Arnica on broken skin since it can cause a rash.

Medical **Alert**

Minor pain usually goes away on its own within a matter of days, even if you do nothing to treat it. You should see your doctor for pain that persists for more than a week, that recurs frequently, or that becomes more severe over time, says Dr. Anderson. And if your pain is associated with any kind of an injury—a blow to the head or a fall, for example—seek medical attention without delay.

Back Pain and Stiffness

If you're like most people, you don't give much thought to your back until it starts giving you trouble. Suddenly, all you have to do is twist to pick up a package or your toddler, and your back screams out for recognition. And the fact is that almost everyone has back pain at some point in her life, and chances increase as you get older.

Lower-back pain often results from strains or sprains in the muscles that connect bones and cartilage in your spine. Childbearing and child rearing also put a heavy load on women's backs. Even monthly hormonal changes can produce back pain and stiffness, possibly by loosening and weakening joint ligaments, according to Karen Rucker, M.D., chairman of the department of physical medicine and rehabilitation at Virginia Commonwealth University in Richmond. The sacroiliac joint, located where the pelvis connects to the tailbone, is commonly affected by the menstrual cycle.

MONTHLY

Back pain doesn't have to put a crimp in your life—if you follow these prescriptions for a pain-free back.

Prescriptions
FOR FAST RELIEF

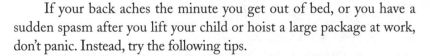

Rx

If your back aches the minute you get out of bed, or you have a sudden spasm after you lift your child or hoist a large package at work, don't panic. Instead, try the following tips.

❑ **Stop what you're doing.** Pain is your body's red light. If you hurt, take a break and try to figure out why the pain is occurring, says Bill Case,

P.T., president of Case Physical Therapy in Houston. You may be able to correct the problem and continue the activity in comfort.

❐ Once the pain eases up a bit, perform the following sequence of exercises to relax and stretch your back muscles, suggests Case.

LOWER BACK STRETCH

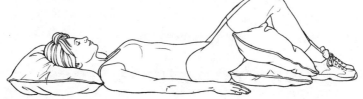

To stretch aching back muscles, lie on your back either on the floor or in bed. Place one or two pillows beneath your bent knees.

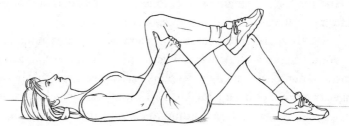

As the pain subsides, progress to this stretch: Lie on your back either on the floor or in bed. Clasp your hands behind one thigh and gently bring that knee toward your chest. Keep your other knee bent, with your foot on the floor. Hold for five seconds. Repeat five times, then switch legs.

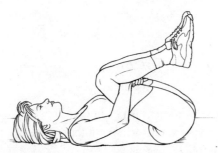

Once you can raise one knee comfortably, you can vary the stretch by gently pulling both knees toward your chest.

❏ Within the first 24 hours of a back injury, apply ice two or three times to relieve pain. Wrap an ice pack or a bag of frozen vegetables in a towel. Lie on your stomach with a pillow under your hips. Lay the ice on the affected part of your back for 10 to 15 minutes at a time, advises Case. Applying ice to strained muscles soothes inflammation and stops pain messages from going to the brain.

❏ For pain from a muscle spasm, apply a comfortably hot washcloth to the part of your back that hurts for up to 30 minutes at a time. To keep the cloth hot, resoak it in hot water every 3 minutes or so. Most of the time, back pain results from the contraction of specific muscle groups around a vertebra. In this case, heat relieves pain better by increasing blood flow to the area and relaxing the muscles involved, explains Paul Petit, D.C., a chiropractor in Poway, California.

❏ As the pain subsides, try taking a 20-minute bath in comfortably hot water. Repeat up to three times a day, says Dr. Petit.

❏ Stay in bed for no more than two days, even if your back still hurts. Lying around for too long will worsen your back pain and stiffen your joints, says John Dunn, M.D., of Washington Orthopedic Services in Seattle.

Prescriptions
FOR KEEPING YOUR BACK PAIN-FREE

EXERCISE
Rx

Once you have had back pain, there is a chance that you'll experience another episode. Here are some further suggestions on how to lessen lingering pain and keep it at bay when it is gone.

❏ Exercise in the morning. A hot shower first thing in the morning followed by a walk will limber up a stiff back, says Case. If you're not used to exercising, start with a 5-minute walk each day and work up to 30 minutes within four weeks.

❏ Walk every day, no matter how briefly, to strengthen your leg and buttock muscles. Those muscles support the lower back, so the stronger they are, the less stress you will place on your back, according to Case.

❒ Try swimming. Swimming strengthens your leg muscles without putting stress on your back, because you are practically weightless in a pool, notes Case.

TIME IT RIGHT

❒ Limber up your back muscles with 5 to 10 minutes of stretching at least once a day. Be sure to include the following stretch in your routine, advises Willibald Nagler, M.D., physiatrist in chief and professor of rehabilitation medicine at the New York Hospital/Cornell Medical Center in New York City.

SEATED STRETCH

Sit in a straight chair, with your feet flat on the floor. Inhale and put your fingertips on your shoulders so that your elbows are pointing outward at shoulder height. Keeping your fingertips in this position, slowly try to touch your elbows together in front of your chin while breathing out. Hold the stretch for five seconds, then relax. Repeat six times.

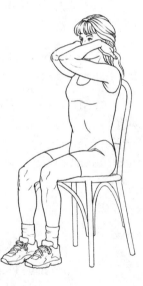

TIME IT RIGHT

❒ If you have a desk job, get up and walk around every 30 minutes. The longer you sit, the weaker your back muscles will become. The more you move, the stronger your spine, says Case.

TIME IT RIGHT

❒ Keep your back muscles loose and relaxed during the day with these simple two-minute exercises, suggests Dr. Nagler. Do them whenever time and space permit.

PELVIC TILT

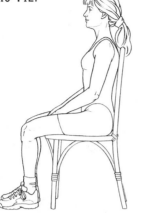
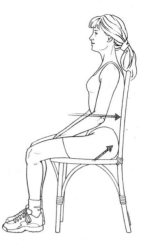

Sit in a straight chair with your feet flat on the floor. Relax against the back of your chair.

Pull in your abdominal muscles, squeeze your buttocks together, and try to push the small of your back into the back of your chair. Count to five and relax. Repeat 12 times.

CHAIR LIFT

For general strengthening, sit in a straight chair with armrests but without wheels. Plant your feet flat on the floor, then place your hands on the armrests and push up with your arms. Lift yourself off the seat until your arms are straight and your elbows are locked, as shown. Make sure that you don't shrug your shoulders. Hold for a count of six, then lower. Repeat six times.

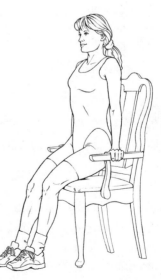

CURLUP

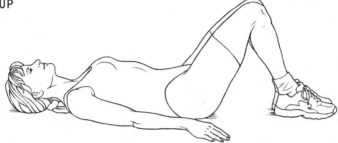

Lie on your back with your knees bent and your feet flat on the floor.

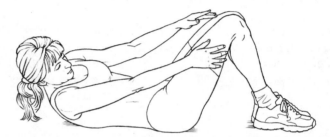

Tuck your chin into your chest and curl your body up to the count of six, bringing your left shoulder toward your right knee while breathing out. Your arms should reach toward your right knee. Then return your left shoulder and your head to the floor. Roll your head to the other side.

Inhale, then exhale as you repeat with your right shoulder. Do this six to eight times on each side.

Rx ——— *Prescriptions*
FOR IMPROVED BACK POSTURE

Slumping, twisting around, and other bad postural habits weaken the discs that support your spine, says Dr. Rucker. Chores such as working (or playing) at a computer for hours, hefting several bags of groceries in and out of your car, and cleaning the attic or basement can be murder on your back. The following prescriptions will take pressure and strain off your back when you sit or stand.

❐ Sit with your feet flat on the floor, advises Dr. Rucker. Refrain from crossing your legs, twisting your ankles around each other, sitting on your feet, sitting cross-legged, or sitting curled up in your chair with your legs out to the side or under you.

❐ If you spend long hours at a computer, consider investing in an ergonomically adjustable chair. This kind of chair can help minimize strain on your hips, knees, and back, says Dr. Rucker. Look for a model that allows you to adjust the height of the chair and the position of the back and armrests.

❐ If an adjustable chair isn't in your budget, look for a lumbar roll, a special lower-back pillow available in medical supply stores. Or place a rolled-up towel behind your lower back. Use one in the car, too, says Case.

❐ Consider wearing a sacroiliac belt, available at drugstores. This special device will support and stabilize your pelvis when you are doing housework or yard work that might put unusual demands on your back, Dr. Rucker says.

❐ Push, don't pull, your loads. For example, if you have a heavy box to move, push it. That way, your legs bear most of the weight, and you will give your back a break, explains Dr. Rucker.

❐ Every time you pass a mirror, check your posture. If you are slouching or slumping, pull back your shoulder blades to take the pressure off your lower back, says Case.

Prescription
for Strengthening Your Back
after Pregnancy

Rx

Pregnancy is one of the major causes of lower-back pain in women, says Loren Fishman, M.D., clinical assistant professor at Albert Einstein College of Medicine in New York City, physiatrist at Flushing Hospital Medical Center, and author of *Back Talk*. Especially in the second or third trimester, more than half of all pregnant women experience some lower-back pain.

To begin with, pregnant women gain most of their weight in the abdomen. To support the weight, they tend to arch their backs, which in turn puts added pressure on the spine. On top of that, the placenta releases relaxin, a hormone that relaxes ligaments in the back and pelvis so that the baby can emerge more easily. Relaxin causes back ligaments to weaken and stretch.

The 10-Second Refrigerator Stretch

Here's a quick stretch to relieve an achy, stiff back, says Willibald Nagler, M.D., physiatrist in chief and professor of rehabilitation medicine at the New York Hospital/Cornell Medical Center in New York City. (You can also do this stretch using a filing cabinet instead of a refrigerator.)

Stand in front of your refrigerator, about three feet away. Inhale and stretch your arms overhead. Bring your arms down in front of you until your wrists rest on top of the refrigerator (you should be bent forward at the waist). Then walk your feet forward until your legs are positioned directly under your hips, as shown. Let your feet point outward and your knees bend slightly.

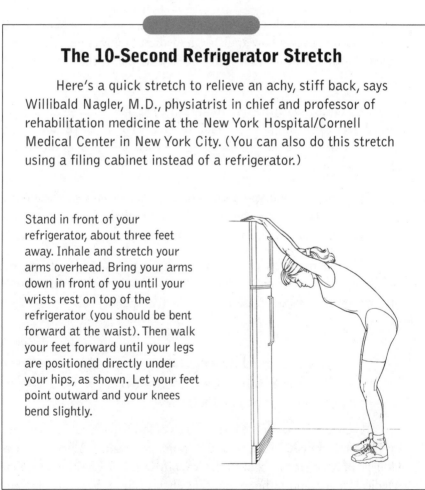

Luckily, what can be stretched and weakened can be toned and strengthened after your child is born. Once your doctor gives you the green light to exercise, one of the best ways you can relieve lower-back pain is to gently strengthen your abdominal muscles.

The post-pregnancy back curl on page 18 is different from the usual "cat" exercise, which is used to improve flexibility. In this version, the emphasis is on strengthening your abdominal muscles, points out Dr. Fishman.

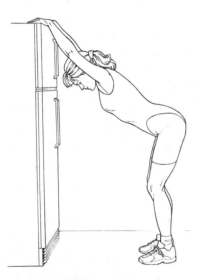

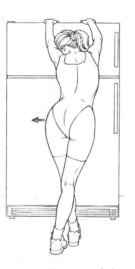

Exhale and flex your spine, lifting your hips so that your back is slightly bowed, as shown. Take five or six breaths, deepening the stretch with each exhalation. Increase the stretch by walking toward the refrigerator and lowering your arms.

To increase the area of the stretch, extend one leg across the midline of your body, crossing it behind the leg that supports you. Keep your heel flat on the ground. As you feel this stretch on one side of your body, slowly lean in the opposite direction.

POST-PREGNANCY BACK CURL

Kneel on all fours with your knees slightly
apart, your hands directly below your
shoulders, and your knees under your
hips. Slowly tighten your abdominal
muscles as you round your back
and tuck in your pelvis.
Hold for 15 to 20
seconds. Relax, then
repeat once more.

Rx

Prescription
FOR CARRYING AN INFANT OR TODDLER

Toddlers look so small, and strollers can be such a nuisance, that many women don't think twice before slinging a two-year-old onto their hips for a quick errand. But carrying a child who weighs more than 10 pounds can contribute to back strain. It is best if you use a carrier so that the child's weight is centered on your back, advises Dr. Fishman. Just as important, you should pick up your child so that you keep your spine straight and lift with your legs. In lifting and carrying with your arms, keep the child as close to your torso as possible.

LIFTING A CHILD

Bend at your knees and hold your child
close in front of you, as shown. Then as
you lift, keep your abdominal muscles
contracted to give your legs extra support.

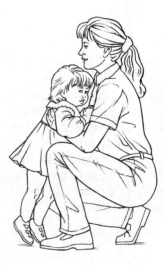

Medical **Alert**

See your doctor if your back pain lasts for more than a week or strikes intermittently every day, says Dr. Nagler. You should also see your doctor immediately if pain runs into your groin or if you experience numbness or weakness in your leg. These symptoms may be a sign of a more serious condition, such as sciatica or a kidney infection, he explains.

Bad Breath

To breathe is human, to breathe sweetly, divine—but at least once a day, most adults fall far short of divinity.

"Everybody wakes up with bad breath," says JoAnne Allen, D.D.S., a dentist in private practice in Albuquerque, New Mexico.

That's because saliva flow slows down as we sleep. That way, you don't drool all night. But without the buffering effect of saliva, your mouth has less defense against the acids created by festering foods or the dryness created by smoking or drinking alcohol. And bacteria thrive in a dry, acidic environment, says Flora Parsa Stay, D.D.S., a dentist in Oxnard, California, and author of *The Complete Book of Dental Remedies*.

Of course, bad breath doesn't occur only at night. Gum disease or other conditions can cause bad breath day or night. Same goes for eating garlic and onions. Their aromatic compounds actually enter your bloodstream and exit through your lungs, so that even if you brush and floss, you won't be able to rid your breath of their stink, says Heidi Hausauer, D.D.S., assistant clinical professor in the department of operative dentistry at the University of the Pacific in San Francisco and spokesman for the Academy of General Dentistry.

Many women experience dry mouth as they get older, and some say they have bad breath at menstruation, says Dr. Allen. But most of the time, bad breath occurs because food festers in the mouth and between the teeth.

Some mouthwashes can kill some of the bacteria that can cause bad breath, says Caren Barnes, a dental hygienist and professor of clinical dentistry at the University of Alabama School of Dentistry in Birmingham. But some people don't like the medicinal aroma they leave behind.

Rx ——— *Prescriptions*
TO SWEETEN BREATH FAST

To test your breath, nothing beats the old standby: Cover your nose and mouth with your hand, exhale, and smell your breath. If it needs sweetening, try these prescriptions.

❒ Drink a total of eight eight-ounce glasses of water a day, especially if you exercise. Acids from food—and bacteria that cause bad breath—thrive when the inside of your mouth is dry. So staying hydrated prevents bad breath, says Dr. Stay. To sweeten breath further, add a twist of lemon or lime to your water.

LIFETIME

❒ If you suffer from dry mouth around your period or at menopause, pay special attention to keeping salivary juices flowing with water, fruits, and, if you like, sugarless gum, says Dr. Allen.

❒ Cleanse your system with yogurt. Ten percent of bad breath is related to acid imbalances when you digest your food, says Dr. Stay. To help balance acids during digestion and to cut down on bad breath, have a cup of yogurt, or a glass of kefir or acidophilus milk (sweet-tasting, fermented milk products available in health food stores).

NIGHTTIME

❒ Brush and floss—especially at bedtime. Optimally, you should brush and floss after each meal. But if you can only brush and floss once a day, do so right before you go to bed to prevent bacteria from having a feast during the eight hours that you're sleeping, says Dr. Stay.

❒ Brush the back of your tongue. That's where most of the bacteria that cause bad breath thrive, says Dr. Hausauer.

❒ Always carry a toothbrush. Keep one in a plastic bag in your purse, the glove compartment of your car, and your office desk, says Dr. Allen. That way, you can always keep your mouth clean.

❒ If you can't spare the time to brush, use a balsa-wood wedge toothpick (such as Desert Essence, available in health food stores) to clean the area between the gum and the tooth. First, soften the toothpick by moistening it in your mouth. Then, firmly press the toothpick against the side of the tooth, above the gum line, and gently move it in and out between the teeth, says Dr. Stay.

❐ In a pinch, munch an apple, raw carrots, a sprig of parsley, or a stalk of celery to cleanse your breath after lunch, Dr. Stay says.

❐ If you don't finding chewing parsley convenient or attractive, try parsley capsules, such as BreathAsure (made from parsley and sunflower oil), says Dr. Hausauer. BreathAsure is available in drugstores and some supermarkets.

❐ Sip alfalfa tea after each meal, suggests Dr. Stay. Pour one cup of freshly boiled water over one heaping teaspoon alfalfa. Cover and steep the tea for five minutes; strain out the tea leaves and drink the remaining brew. If you prefer, alfalfa is also available in tablets or capsules (all forms are available in health food stores). Take as directed on the package.

❐ Ditch the cigarettes for good. Smoking causes bad breath, in part, because it slows down the flow of saliva in your mouth, says Dr. Allen.

Medical **Alert**

If you brush, floss, and brush your tongue, but you still have bad breath, see your dentist to make sure there's no underlying dental problem. Gum disease, tooth decay, and abscessed teeth can all cause bad breath, says Dr. Hausauer. Once your dentist rules out a dental problem, make an appointment with your physician. The reason is that bad breath can indicate an underlying condition such as diabetes, hiatal hernia, or pneumonia. Also, check your medications. Many drugs, such as heart medicines and anti-depressants, can cause a dry mouth, which can lead to bad breath because of reduced salivary flow.

Blood Sugar Problems

Most women need to eat something nutritious every four hours, says Nancy Clark, R.D., a nutritionist at Sports Medicine Brookline in Brookline, Massachusetts, and author of *Nancy Clark's Nutrition Guidebook*. For those who don't heed their bodies' call for food, trying to function is like trying to drive cross-country without refueling. You get only so far. A woman who skips breakfast; tries to get through the day subsisting on coffee, diet soda, and salad; and eats the bulk of her daily calories in the evening—as many women do—may experience faintness, inability to concentrate, and irritability during the day, symptoms associated with low blood sugar.

"Nutritionally speaking, low blood sugar is a sign that there is not enough gas in the tank," says Clark. "You're running on fumes."

Simply put, blood sugar is the usable fuel—or energy—created by the food you eat and then sent through your circulatory system to your vital organs and muscles. Digestive juices convert what you consume into glucose, a simple sugar absorbed into your bloodstream. So a certain amount of blood glucose, or blood sugar, is normal and necessary for optimum functioning.

Hypoglycemia refers to a very specific deficiency in blood sugar that is most often experienced by people who have problems making proper amounts of insulin, one of the endocrine hormones that control blood sugar. The most likely candidates for hypoglycemia are people with diabetes or a pre-diabetic condition known as phase I insulin release, says Elizabeth Livingston, M.D., assistant professor of obstetrics/gynecology in the department of maternal and fetal medicine at Duke University Medical Center in Durham, North Carolina.

Unless you have an endocrine- or hormone-deficiency problem, you don't have low blood sugar by medical definition, says Dr. Livingston. But if you have ever experienced that midmorning or midafternoon feeling of "I have to eat something now or I'll faint," you'll have no trouble recognizing that low-blood-sugar feeling. If you feel lousy when you skip meals and feel better when you refuel, that's reason enough to rethink your eating habits, she adds.

Rx ——— *Prescriptions*
FOR BLOOD SUGAR CONTROL

Usually, all you have to do to defeat the woozies is to change what you eat and when.

❏ Give yourself permission to eat, says Clark. "If you eat enough, you'll be more efficient, won't be hungry, and will be able to concentrate during the day."

❏ Focus on combinations of carbohydrates, modest amounts of protein, and a little bit of fat, says Dr. Livingston. A turkey sandwich is a perfect combination of all three: Bread is a carbohydrate and turkey contains protein and a little bit of fat. A dab of low-fat mayonnaise won't hurt.

❒ **Don't skimp, but don't overeat.** Aim for moderate-size meals of about 500 calories each and a snack of 200 to 300 calories. For example, you might have a plain bagel with two tablespoons peanut butter to start your morning, and eight ounces low-fat fruit yogurt a few hours later, suggests Clark.

Or shoot for three meals and three snacks, especially if you're pregnant, says Dr. Livingston. You could have a bagel with low-fat cream cheese for breakfast, for example, and a banana or glass of orange juice for a mid-morning pick-me-up two hours later.

You might need some time to adjust to frequent feedings, especially if you're used to living on salad all day and chowing down at dinner. But eating mini-meals throughout the day is a surefire way to keep your blood sugar levels stable, Dr. Livingston says.

❒ **Make smart food choices.** Eating all the time doesn't mean that you have a license to gain a large amount of weight, especially if you're pregnant, Dr. Livingston cautions. Overweight is a major risk factor for diabetes, so make sure that the food you eat is low in fat and sugar. You want to change your eating pattern but not increase your total calorie intake.

❒ **If you're going to exercise strenuously, snack first,** says Stanley Mirsky, M.D., associate clinical professor of metabolic diseases at Mount Sinai School of Medicine of the City University of New York in New York City and co-author of *Controlling Diabetes the Easy Way.* Vigorous activity quickly depletes the body of blood sugar, so it is wise to eat a carbohydrate snack beforehand—crackers or a piece of fruit, for example. Just be sure to wait at least 30 minutes after eating to begin your workout so that the food has a chance to digest.

❒ **If you're going to be active for a long period of time, take carbo-**hydrate foods with you and have a light snack every hour, says Dr. Mirsky.

❒ **Cut down on caffeine.** Coffee, tea, cola, chocolate, and cocoa may trigger hypoglycemic reactions in some people, says Dr. Mirsky. If you feel shaky or faint after consuming caffeine, cut down on all sources of caffeine and caffeine-related compounds. If you still have a low-blood-sugar reaction, cut out caffeine entirely.

Medical **Alert**

Unchecked, a serious episode of hypoglycemia in anyone with diabetes can lead to seizures or even a coma, says David Maggs, M.D., assistant professor of endocrinology at the Yale School of Medicine. Some symptoms of a hypoglycemic reaction include extreme irritability, tremors or shakiness, intense or inappropriate hunger, difficulty with speech, double vision, numbness, and extreme sleepiness. If you have been diagnosed with diabetes and are on insulin therapy, and you experience several or all of these symptoms, the problem can often be corrected by ingesting a quickly absorbed carbohydrate, such as juice, he says. If your symptoms persist or worsen, contact a physician immediately.

Breast Discomfort

Whoever wrote that "music has charms to soothe a savage breast" obviously never had one. As any woman with painful breasts knows, it takes more than a little Beethoven or Beatles to make the pain go away.

Breasts can become swollen, tender, and lumpy. They can pull at your neck and back and hurt at the slightest bump. They can make running, jumping, and even rolling over in bed pure agony. "Some women demand breast reduction surgery because they have such pain," says Bernard Ginsberg, M.D., a doctor in private practice in Santa Monica, California.

MONTHLY

Breast discomfort usually occurs just prior to menstruation, when hormones stimulate fluid retention in breast tissue, says David P. Rose, M.D., D.Sc., Ph.D., chief of the division of nutrition and endocrinology at the Naylor Dana Institute of the American Health Foundation in Valhalla, New York. Breastfeeding can also cause pain.

Women sometimes hesitate to seek treatment for breast discomfort because they fear the worst. Yet doctors say that premenstrual breast changes such as swelling and lumpiness are pretty much normal. Moreover, having lumpy breasts does not in itself put you at greater risk for breast cancer, says Dr. Ginsberg.

So if you're bothered by breast pain, you should know that you can do something about it. Here's what experts recommend.

Prescriptions
TO END THE ACHE

When your breasts hurt, you want to make them as comfortable as possible, as quickly as possible. The following remedies provide prompt, effective relief.

❐ Soak in a bathtub filled with comfortably hot water for at least 20 minutes. "Settle back into the tub so that your chest is submerged," suggests Rosalind Benedet, R.N., a breast health nurse specialist with the California Pacific Medical Center in San Francisco. The water soothes your breasts and relaxes your entire body.

TIME IT RIGHT

❐ As an alternative to heat, apply a cold pack to sore breasts for up to 20 minutes whenever you need relief. Use either crushed ice or a bag of frozen peas, since either will conform to the shape of your breasts, says Benedet. And remember to wrap the ice or bag of peas in a towel so that the extreme cold doesn't injure your skin.

❐ Wear a larger-size bra while your breasts hurt. Select one that keeps your breasts secure without being uncomfortably constricting, suggests Benedet. "A sports bra with a wide elastic band may be your best bet," she says. "But every woman is different, so shop around to find the bra that's just right for you."

You may even want to plan to shop when your breasts are most swollen. When you try on the bra, move around to make sure it gives you comfortable support while you are moving.

Prescriptions
TO BANISH BREAST PAIN

NUTRITION

Whether or not you experience breast discomfort depends to some degree on your eating habits. Some foods can prevent breast symptoms, while others can make those symptoms worse. To shape a more breast-friendly diet, give the following tips a try.

❐ Take a vitamin E supplement every day. Doctors have yet to determine why, but vitamin E seems to help some women with breast pain, according to Michael DiPalma, N.D., a naturopathic doctor in private practice in Newtown, Pennsylvania. He starts his patients with 400 international units (IU) of vitamin E a day, then increases the dosage by 100 IU monthly until the women report that their breasts feel better. Dr. DiPalma sometimes prescribes up to 1,600 IU a day, but no more than that. Women who require such a high dosage may find that after a few months they can cut back without experiencing a flare-up in their symptoms.

Note: If you plan to take more than 600 IU of vitamin E a day, you should talk to your doctor first.

❒ Consume at least 30 grams of fiber a day. Both kinds of fiber—soluble and insoluble—help escort excess estrogen from your body. This prevents the hormone from stimulating breast tissue and causing discomfort, explains Dr. Rose. Unfortunately, most women get less than half the amount of fiber that Dr. Rose recommends. To boost your intake, fill your meals with whole grains, beans, fruits, and vegetables. For example, one-half cup cooked barley contains almost three grams of fiber. One-half cup boiled lima beans provides more than six grams. And one-quarter cup dried figs supplies more than four grams.

MONTHLY

❒ Drink at least eight eight-ounce glasses of water a day. Paradoxically, the more water you drink, the less likely your breasts are to swell before your period. Water flushes salt out of your body, so you retain less fluid, says Benedet.

❒ Limit your intake of dietary fat to 15 percent of calories. In one study, women who adhered to this guideline reported significant reductions in breast tenderness, swelling, and lumpiness. Incidentally, most women consume more than twice this much fat, with an average daily intake of 34 percent of calories.

MONTHLY

❒ Restrict your salt consumption. Salt makes your entire body retain fluid—including your breasts, which can swell up like water balloons. "Lots of women crave salty foods such as potato chips and pickles right before their periods," notes Benedet. "But these foods just make matters worse."

If you feel that you can't resist them, Dr. DiPalma advises, don't even bring them into your home.

MONTHLY

❒ Give up caffeine-containing foods and beverages for two menstrual cycles. Caffeine—which is found in coffee, black tea, cola, and chocolate—seems to increase the sensitivity of breast tissue to estrogen.

Although this remains controversial, some people do find that their pain decreases if they eliminate caffeine sources from their diets for a month or two. One study, conducted at Michigan State University College of Human Medicine in East Lansing, found that women who consume more than 500 milligrams of caffeine a day (the amount in about four cups of coffee) have more than double the risk of lumpy, painful breasts compared with those who abstain. Women who eliminate caffeine from their diets experience a 60 to 65 percent reduction in their symptoms.

Take notice if your breast pain improves during the month you abstain from caffeine. "Some women can then go back to drinking one cup a day without problems," says Dr. DiPalma. "Others may need to give up caffeine only during the second half of their menstrual cycles."

"If you are a big coffee-drinker, restricting or eliminating caffeine may be all you need to do to end your breast pain," adds Benedet.

Prescriptions
for Long-Term Breast Health

Rx

To reduce breast pain or even get rid of it for good, some women may need to look beyond good nutrition to other aspects of their lifestyle. "You may have to make some changes, but once you get through them, your whole body feels better, not just your breasts," Benedet says. Consider the following tactics for maintaining healthy, pain-free breasts.

Lifetime

❒ Maintain a healthy weight. If you carry too much body fat, you may have more estrogen circulating in your system than is good for you. "In women, body fat acts like an extra gland," explains Dr. Rose. "It produces and stores estrogen, which stimulates breast tissue." Also, research has established a link between weight gain after menopause and an increased risk of breast cancer.

While there are a number of complex formulas for figuring out your ideal weight, one simple formula used by some experts can tell you if you are close: If you are five feet tall, you should weigh 100 pounds. If you are taller, add 5 pounds for each additional inch of height. Then to that number, add 10 percent if you have a large frame, or subtract 10 percent if you have a small frame.

❐ Exercise for at least 30 minutes every day. Women who regularly engage in aerobic workouts (the kind that elevate your heart and breathing rates) are less likely to have premenstrual symptoms, including breast pain, according to Dr. Rose.

If exercise seems to worsen premenstrual breast pain, switch to a low-impact activity until you feel better. Running, in particular, may aggravate your symptoms, says Benedet. Try swimming, walking, or bicycling instead.

Medical Alert

If you try dietary and lifestyle changes for three months and your breasts still hurt, or if your breasts become tender and swollen over the course of a day or two, see your doctor, advises Dr. Rose. You may have a hormonal problem that requires medical treatment. Also see your doctor if your breasts become painful after you start taking oral contraceptives or hormone-replacement therapy. Your dosage may need adjustment, or you may need to switch to a different type of drug. And, of course, consult your doctor if you notice anything unusual during your monthly breast self-examination.

Coffee Nerves

Are you shaking so bad that the cup in your hand seems to have taken on a life of its own? Could be that you have OD'd on caffeine.

Caffeine is a drug. A legal drug—but a mind- and body-altering one nonetheless. That's why you may react strongly to too much of it, says Roland Griffiths, Ph.D., professor in the departments of psychiatry and neuroscience at the Johns Hopkins School of Medicine in Baltimore.

Most people drink coffee in the morning when they need a jump start, in the afternoon when their energy starts to flag, or anytime when they feel a snooze coming on and they aren't in bed. All for good reason: Caffeine, the compound that gives coffee, tea, cola, and chocolate their buzz, jolts you awake, says Manfred Kroger, Ph.D., professor of food science at Pennsylvania State University in University Park. "Your eyelids open, your fatigue evaporates, you're more alert, and your reflexes improve."

Caffeine cranks up your brain by stimulating the central nervous system. It also stimulates your sympathetic nervous system, raising your blood pressure and making your pulse and heartbeat accelerate. And caffeine acts very rapidly. A cup of coffee starts to affect you in about 10 minutes, reaches its peak in an hour, and lingers in your system for three hours or longer, says Dr. Griffiths.

Coffee, tea, cola, and chocolate vary in how big a jolt they impart, depending on their caffeine content. A six-ounce cup of coffee has about 100 milligrams. A same-size cup of tea has about 40 milligrams, as does 12 ounces of cola.

What's more, the degree of kick you get from caffeine depends on what you're used to. If you hardly ever drink the stuff, a cup of coffee will have a more pronounced effect on you than on someone who drinks several cups a day. Same with tea or cola drinks.

Your susceptibility to that sweaty, shaky, jittery feeling known as coffee nerves is also influenced by what else is going on in your life, says Stanley Segall, Ph.D., director of nutrition and food services at Drexel University in Philadelphia. "If your nerves are racked to begin with, drinking two cups of coffee can put you over the edge. Next week, when your problem—whatever it was—is resolved, drinking the same amount of coffee may not leave you as jangled."

Prescriptions
FOR JINXING THE JITTERS

Rx

As with a hangover, curing a case of coffee nerves takes time. While you wait it out, here's what to do to soothe your hyper-caffeinated nerves and avoid future fits.

❐ Steer clear of all additional sources of caffeine, including over-the-counter medicines such as Midol, No-Doz, and Excedrin. If your heart is already racing and you know you are tense, the last thing you want to do is take another stimulant, says Dr. Segall.

❐ If you react strongly to caffeine, consume it only when you really need to, as a morning wake-up boost, for example, says Dr. Segall.

MORNING

❐ To slow down absorption and lessen the jitters, drink coffee with food, not on an empty stomach, says Dr. Kroger.

❐ Cut back. "Everyone ought to be her own body's keeper, observer, archivist," says Dr. Kroger. "If you start to shake after the third cup, stop."

And cut back to one to two cups, which is considered a normal, harmless daily intake.

Medical **Alert**

Some medicines—such as antidepressants and some birth control pills—cause your body to metabolize caffeine more slowly, making you more susceptible to coffee nerves. So when you get a prescription filled, read the list of potential side effects in the package insert. If nervous tremors and irritability are listed as possible side effects, skip the caffeine. Or ask your pharmacist whether drinking caffeinated beverages while taking your medication will give you the shakes, says Dr. Segall.

Colds and Flu

Considering the hundreds of different cold and flu viruses out there and everywhere, it's amazing that we aren't all constantly hacking and heaving. Luckily, a healthy immune system stops most of these microscopic invaders before they can reproduce by the billions in our noses, throats, and lungs. Doing your best to strengthen immunity and avoid germs are the top two ways to prevent a cold, with its stuffy nose, sneezing, sore throat, and slight fever. These tactics will also reduce your chances of getting the flu, with its higher fever, muscle aches and pains, and tail-dragging fatigue.

WINTERTIME

Colds and flu really do have a season, and it's winter, says Keiji Fukuda, M.D., chief of the epidemiology section, influenza branch, at the Centers for Disease Control and Prevention in Atlanta. "During the cold-weather months, people are confined to tight quarters, so an ill child in day care or a sneezing adult at work has the opportunity to infect many others," he explains.

In fact, you don't even need to be in the direct line of a sneeze or cough to contract a cold or the flu, notes Michael Fleming, M.D., a family doctor in private practice in Shreveport, Louisiana. You don't even need to be in the vicinity at the same time. "All you need to do is to touch something—a doorknob, a telephone, a hand—that someone sick touched or coughed or sneezed on, even up to 24 hours later, then touch your face, nose, or mouth," he explains. Most cold and flu viruses are spread that way.

Antibiotics can't help when you have a mild cold or the flu. They work only against bacteria, not viruses. "That's why a strong immune system is so important," says Anne Davis, M.D., associate professor of clinical medicine at New York University and attending physician of chest service at Bellevue Hospital Center in New York City. "If you're healthy, you might harbor a cold or flu virus without coming down with symptoms, but when your resistance is low, you are more likely to get sick."

Here's how to minimize the discomfort of a cold or the flu and to make yourself less inviting to viral invaders.

Prescriptions
FOR BEATING COLDS AND FLU

Rx

You are sneezing and feel achy and wish that you could crawl into bed. In fact, the sooner you follow that inclination, the faster you are going to feel better, doctors say. So try some of the following tactics.

❏ If you're tired, go to bed. "Flu viruses often have a whole-body effect. Maintaining normal activities, including intense exercising, when you have the flu can make your symptoms worse, set the stage for secondary bacterial infections such as pneumonia, and lead to fatigue that lingers for weeks," says David C. Nieman, D.P.H., professor of health and exercise at Appalachian State University in Boone, North Carolina.

TIME IT RIGHT

"Two full days in bed is not excessive for a full-blown case of flu," says Dr. Fleming. If that's impossible, at least get eight hours of sleep at night and put off whatever can wait. Give yourself up to two weeks to ease back into your normal routine. You will bounce back faster.

You may not feel the need to rest if you simply have a head cold, Dr. Nieman says. In fact, mild exercise may help resolve head cold symptoms by boosting the number of virus-fighting white blood cells circulating throughout your body.

❏ Drink tea, chicken soup, hot lemonade, or other hot fluids. "Whether you're fighting a cold or flu virus, fluids help to keep mucus thin enough to cough up or blow out. Trapped thick mucus promotes secondary bacterial infections such as pneumonia," says Dr. Davis. And feverish sweating can dry you out, which can lead to dehydration and may drive your fever up, she adds. So the advice is to drown a cold *and* a fever. And hot liquids relieve congestion better than cold drinks.

❑ If you are feeling nauseated and achy, drink a cup of ginger tea up to four times a day. Ginger is well-known and widely used for its stomach-soothing and ache-relieving properties, so it's just the ticket for colds and flu accompanied by nausea, says Nan Kathryn Fuchs, Ph.D., a nutritionist in private practice in Sebastopol, California, and a columnist for the *Women's Health Newsletter*. To make the tea, simmer one teaspoon grated fresh ginger and one cup water in a covered pot for 10 minutes. Then strain the tea and drink it.

TIME IT RIGHT

❑ Swallow astragalus or echinacea. Astragalus, a popular Chinese herb, and echinacea, or purple coneflower, have proven antiviral, immune-boosting properties, says Dr. Fuchs. At the first sign of illness, take a dose of astragalus or echinacea tincture. Repeat every hour or two for the first day, then three times a day for about three days longer than it takes for your symptoms to resolve, she says. You can buy both of these herbs in health food stores. For dosages, follow label instructions.

❑ Take frequent, comfortably hot showers or baths. Humidity fights congestion, says Dr. Fleming. Or keep a humidifier running at 60 percent humidity or more in your bedroom for the duration of your illness. "You'll feel more comfortable and breathe easier," he says.

NIGHTTIME

❑ Prop up your head when you sleep. Sneezing, coughing, and congestion are often worse at night, Dr. Davis says. Particularly if you have postnasal drip, sleep sitting up or prop your head up with extra pillows to make it easier to breathe.

❑ Double up on your vitamin C as soon as symptoms appear. In one study, people taking 1,000 milligrams of vitamin C twice a day had less nasal discharge and sneezing and shorter colds than people not taking extra vitamin C.

If you are taking 500 to 1,000 milligrams of vitamin C a day, try increasing that amount to no more than 2,000 milligrams at the first sign of illness. Continue with your larger dose for a few days after you feel better, Dr. Fuchs recommends.

Note: If you experience diarrhea with large doses of vitamin C (as some people do), cut back to 1,200 milligrams or less a day.

❐ Zap it with zinc. Researchers at the Cleveland Clinic Foundation in Cleveland found that people who started taking zinc gluconate lozenges within 24 hours of noticing cold symptoms had colds lasting only 4.4 days, about 3 days shorter than usual. They also had less coughing, headaches, hoarseness, nasal congestion, and drainage than usual.

"Scientists think that zinc helps prevent viral replication or that it may keep viruses from entering cells," says Michael Macknin, M.D., the study's main researcher. The lozenges studied contained zinc gluconate. Theoretically, other forms of zinc can bind with sweeteners in lozenges and become inactive.

You'll find zinc gluconate lozenges in health food stores and some drugstores. Follow the dosage recommendations on the label.

Prescriptions
FOR FENDING OFF VIRAL INVADERS

Rx

To cut down on the number of cold and flu episodes you experience, you need to avoid germs, when possible, and fight them off when you are exposed.

❐ Wash your hands frequently throughout the day, especially if you are around kids who are sick, directs Dr. Davis. It's just too easy to transfer cold or flu viruses from your hands to your face, eyes, mouth, or nose.

❐ Disinfect high-traffic spots during epidemic periods to prevent the spread of infection. Spray doorknobs, phones, and faucets with a disinfectant such as Lysol, making sure that you leave it on as long as the directions call for, Dr. Davis says.

❐ Cover your mouth and nose when you sneeze. It's not just polite; a high-intensity sneeze can propel viruses a distance of up to 10 feet— clear across the room.

❐ Don't smoke, and stay away from smoke-filled cars, restaurants, and the like. Cigarette smoke impairs many of your body's respiratory defenses against cold and flu viruses, says Dr. Davis.

Medical **Alert**

See your doctor if your cold or flu hasn't gotten better after a week or so, especially if it is accompanied by yellow, green, or bloody nasal discharge; a persistent severe headache; or a fever of 101°F or higher. The same goes for if your breathing becomes difficult or painful or you experience sharp pains when you cough, pain around your eyes or cheekbones, or an earache.

Cold Sores and Canker Sores

Often confused for each other, cold sores and canker sores share similar symptoms but have very different causes.

Cold sores are tiny, red, inflamed blisters that start out by tingling. Eventually, they can break open, ooze, and become painful. They often spring up where you least want them—within easy eyesight, at the spot at which your lip meets the skin, or even on your nose. Sometimes, though, cold sores spring up inside your mouth, most commonly on the roof of your mouth or where your gums meet your teeth, says Eric Shapira, D.D.S., spokesperson for the Academy of General Dentistry and a dentist in Half Moon Bay, California.

Cold sores are caused by the herpes simplex virus. Ninety percent of us catch the virus during childhood; it remains dormant in our bodies until our resistance flags and some stimulant activates the virus. Premenstrual syndrome, getting a cold, staying out in the sun too long, smoking, drinking, and not eating or sleeping well can all contribute to an outbreak, says Katherine Sherif, M.D., assistant professor of medicine at the Institute for Women's Health at Allegheny University of the Health Sciences in Philadelphia. Cold sores are sometimes known as fever blisters, but that's somewhat of a misnomer since you don't necessarily have a fever when a cold sore strikes. After a few days, the blisters burst, dry out, crust over, heal, and eventually disappear.

Canker sores, however, are recurrent, painful, open sores—yellow at the base and red at the edges. They occur almost anywhere inside the mouth—on your tongue, inside your lips, or on the mucous lining of your cheek. No one knows what causes canker sores or why you get them, although stress, injuring your mouth (like accidentally biting your cheek or tongue), and even possibly an allergic reaction can prompt trouble.

Untreated, cold sores and canker sores generally last about two weeks. Though harmless, they are painful and unsightly. Here's what you can try.

Prescriptions
for Calming Cold Sores

Rx

Once you have a full-blown cold sore, you are usually stuck with it for one to two weeks. If you feel a cold sore coming on, however, you may be able to stop the blister in its tracks just before it erupts. If you have ever had a cold sore before, you are probably familiar with what doctors call the prodrome, a sort of introductory itching around the area where a sore is about to erupt.

At the first hint of itching or burning, taking two capsules of the prescription drug acyclovir (Zovirax) is the fastest, most effective preemptive strike for stopping the herpes virus in its tracks and heading off cold sores, says Dr. Sherif. But if you don't happen to have any acyclovir on hand and can't drop everything to get to a doctor on short notice, the following nondrug strategies may speed healing and minimize pain and discomfort.

❒ The minute you feel a cold sore coming on, wrap an ice cube in a handkerchief and hold it directly on the sore for about five minutes, every two to three hours, says Jerome Litt, M.D., a dermatologist and assistant clinical professor of dermatology at Case Western Reserve University School of Medicine in Cleveland. Viruses can't thrive in a cold environment.
Time it right

❒ Make a paste by mixing meat tenderizer with a few drops of water. For the first day, apply the paste to the cold sore every two to three hours and hold it on with a washcloth for 5 to 10 minutes. After the first
Time it right

day, reduce the treatment to three times daily. Repeat the treatment until the sore clears, advises Dr. Litt.

❏ Take 30 milligrams of zinc a day, with food or water. An essential trace mineral, zinc helps get rid of cold sores more quickly, says Nan Kathryn Fuchs, Ph.D., a nutritionist in Sebastopol, California, and a columnist for the *Women's Health Letter*. Getting this much zinc from foods alone is difficult, so you will likely need a supplement to do the job. Once the cold sore heals, cut back to 15 milligrams of zinc a day.

Note: Consult your doctor before taking more than the Daily Value of 15 milligrams because large doses of the mineral can cause side effects.

TIME IT RIGHT

❏ Stop the stress. "Cold sores are often stress-related," says Dr. Fuchs. "When you have a cold sore, sleep an extra half-hour, meditate 10 minutes a day, dress more warmly—whatever eases the stress." According to Dr. Fuchs, relaxation may help you get rid of your cold sores days earlier.

❏ Don't share towels or kiss while you have active cold sore lesions. Cold sores are contagious and can be spread easily, explains Jeffrey Jahre, M.D., chief of the infectious disease section at St. Luke's–Muhlenberg Hospitals in Bethlehem, Pennsylvania.

Rx ——— *Prescriptions*
FOR FENDING OFF FUTURE OUTBREAKS

Once you have had a cold sore, you are likely to get another. Though no one has completely figured out why cold sores occur, the link between cold sores and not taking care of yourself—physically and emotionally—seems pretty well established. To shore up your defenses and keep cold sores at bay, experts offer these preventive strategies.

❏ Eat a diet high in fruits, vegetables, and grains and low in sweets and caffeine, says Dr. Fuchs.

❏ Avoid alcohol—it seems to evoke cold sores, says Dr. Sherif.

❏ Get plenty of sleep—it strengthens your immune system, says Dr. Sherif.

❐ Slow down and temper the stress, says Dr. Sherif. "Tell yourself, 'I come first. I'm not going to be supermom or superdaughter.' You'll sleep better, and you'll be less likely to overmedicate with alcohol or eat too many sweets or become run-down."

❐ Take 500 milligrams of lysine three times a day, says Dr. Litt. Many people who get cold sores say that the essential amino acid lysine, used as a preventive measure, helps keep cold sores away. You can buy lysine supplements in health food stores.

❐ Use a lip balm with a sun protection factor (SPF) of 15 when you head outdoors. This may help prevent a sunburn-induced cold sore, especially if you have a history of recurring cold sores on your lips, explains Dr. Jahre.

Prescriptions
FOR LESS-CANTANKEROUS CANKERS

Although canker sores usually occur inside your mouth, out of sight, you'll know that they are there. And they tend to be worse at certain times rather than others. In women, canker sores occur most frequently at menstruation and times of stress, says Neil Sadick, M.D., clinical associate professor of dermatology at Cornell University Medical College in New York City.

Without treatment, canker sores last up to 14 days. To minimize pain and suffering, follow these tips.

❐ Immerse a regular tea bag in warm water for a few minutes. When the tea bag is thoroughly soaked, squeeze out the excess water and hold the tea bag directly on the canker sore for about five minutes. This treatment works best if it's used immediately after a sore appears, says Dr. Litt. You may repeat the applications two or three times a day.

The tannin in tea helps to reduce the pain associated with canker sores, although no one knows exactly how the compound works, adds Dr. Litt.

❐ Stay away from acidic and spicy foods. Canker sores often don't hurt until you drink something acidic such as orange juice, and then the inside of your mouth will be "sting city," says Dr. Sadick. Since any sharp taste will greatly irritate canker sores, bland foods are better choices.

❏ Try imagery to further reduce the ache of canker sores. Some people may find it helpful to imagine something attacking the canker sore, says Dr. Jahre.

❏ Take time out for yourself—a half-hour bubble bath, an hour of listening to restful music, or even just a five-minute break to close your eyes and relax, says Dr. Sherif. You're more prone to an outbreak during the holiday season or other stressful times, such as when you're planning to ask for a raise or you learn that your child just came home with three Ds and an F on his report card. So regular, concerted efforts to soothe stress can minimize canker sores.

Rx ——— *Prescriptions*
FOR PERMANENT RELIEF

Plagued by frequent canker sore attacks? Consider these preventive tactics.

❏ Change your toothbrush once a month. If you keep getting canker sores, bacteria living in your toothbrush may be responsible, says Peter L. Jacobsen, D.D.S., Ph.D., director of oral diagnosis and treatment planning at the University of Pacific Dental School in San Francisco.

❏ Brush your teeth gently. If canker sores always appear in the same spot inside your cheek or below your teeth, the way you are brushing your teeth may be responsible, says Dr. Jacobsen. In your zeal to scrub away every last vestige of dental debris, you may be jabbing your toothbrush too vigorously. Lighten up on your toothbrush, and your sores may vanish forever, he says.

❏ Change your brand of toothpaste. Dr. Jacobsen recommends toothpastes that contain fluoride but not sodium lauryl sulfate, an ingredient that some people associate with canker sores. He suggests Biotene or Rembrandt Natural, available in most drugstores.

❏ If you're not sure what causes your canker sores, keep a diary of what happened in your life the day or so before your canker sores broke out, says Dr. Jacobsen. Go back over what you might have done differently in the last day or so—perhaps you ate a new kind of spicy food, inadvertently bit your cheek, or experienced a lot of stress.

And watch for other factors, too. Many people also get canker sores as an allergic response to certain foods, especially walnuts; to common medications such as aspirin and ibuprofen; or to chewing gum, mouthwashes, menthol cigarettes, or lozenges, says Dr. Litt. If something that you are putting in your mouth seems to provoke trouble, avoidance is the key.

Medical **Alert**

Watch out for bumps or ulcers that look like cold sores or canker sores but don't hurt and never heal, especially if you smoke. Mouth sores that don't heal within two weeks should be evaluated by a doctor or dentist to rule out oral cancer.

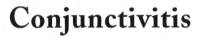

Conjunctivitis

Feel as though a mosquito is permanently lodged underneath your eyelid? Are the whites of your eyes so irritated that they're pink—or bloodshot red? Odds are that you have conjunctivitis, often referred to as pinkeye.

Conjunctivitis can be triggered by bacteria, allergies (to pollens, pets, or chemicals), or viruses (like the common cold). While anybody can get conjunctivitis at any time, the problem may sometimes be linked to the drop in estrogen levels that occurs when women reach menopause, says John Hibbs, N.D., a naturopathic physician and professor of clinical medicine at Bastyr University in Seattle.

No one knows why, but some women develop new allergies when they hit menopause, sometimes triggering conjunctivitis, says Eleanor Faye, M.D., an ophthalmic surgeon at the Manhattan Eye, Ear, and Throat Hospital in New York.

Bacterial conjunctivitis is distinguished by a puslike discharge. To prevent serious infection and loss of vision, your doctor will prescribe antibiotic eyedrops or ointment, says Dr. Faye.

If your eyes burn and are red, itchy, and swollen, but with no discharge, you probably have allergic or viral conjunctivitis, says Andrew

Farber, M.D., an ophthalmologist in Terre Haute, Indiana, and a spokesman for the American Academy of Ophthalmology.

Though the symptoms of allergic conjunctivitis will last as long as you are exposed to the allergen, viral conjunctivitis will almost always get better without treatment within 3 to 10 days. You can spur resolution with several nonprescription remedies, says Anne Sumers, M.D., an ophthalmologist in Ridgewood, New Jersey, and a spokesman for the American Academy of Ophthalmology.

Rx

Prescriptions
for Fast Relief

Time or antibiotics will clear up conjunctivitis, but in the meantime, it is bothersome and uncomfortable. What's more, infectious conjunctivitis—that is, bacterial or viral conjunctivitis—is as contagious as the common cold. If you so much as touch your finger to the affected eye, you can spread infection to the other eye. Same goes if you touch your eyes, then touch clothing, the telephone, or furniture, and then touch your eyes again. Soon, those contagious conjunctivitis germs are everywhere. So you can continue to spread conjunctivitis germs for two weeks after you are over it, and even reinfect yourself, Dr. Farber says. Just as with a cold, you want to relieve the immediate symptoms and prevent the spread of germs. Here is exactly what to do.

❒ At the first sign of redness and irritation, take out your contact lenses, if you wear them, and wear glasses instead. Not only will contacts irritate your eyes further, they keep the germs in your eye, says Dr. Farber. You can begin wearing your contacts again when your eyes are no longer red and irritated, or when your doctor gives you the go-ahead.

TIME IT RIGHT ❒ Place a cool, clean washcloth over your eyes a few times a day for 10 minutes at a time, Dr. Sumers says. Repeat the applications for as long as your eyes are irritated to reduce itching and swelling. To avoid reinfection, launder the washcloth in hot water and detergent before reuse.

❒ For allergic or viral conjunctivitis, rinse your eyes with a saline solution that's preservative-free. Sold for contact lenses in drugstores and supermarkets, saline works best when it's cold. So keep a bottle in the refrigerator and use an eyedropper to dunk several drops in your eye to reduce itching and burning, Dr. Faye says.

❏ Wash your hands with hot water and soap as soon as you touch anything, especially your eyes, says Dr. Farber. Antibacterial soap is best, as long as you aren't allergic to it.

❏ Try to keep your hands away from your eyes. Rubbing your eyes, no matter how much they itch, will irritate them and exacerbate conjunctivitis, says Dr. Farber.

❏ Change your towels after each use and be sure to launder them in hot water and detergent to get rid of germs, says Dr. Farber. Do the same with pillows.

❏ Don't share towels or eye makeup with others. If you do, you'll spread infection, says Dr. Sumers.

❏ Replace your mascara. Bacteria live in mascara wands. So if you continue to use mascara that has become contaminated, your conjunctivitis will return, says Dr. Sumers.

❏ Wait until conjunctivitis clears before wearing eye makeup. Otherwise, your eyes may remain irritated, says Dr. Farber.

❏ Remove all your makeup before you go to bed at night. Try a dab of corn oil or mineral oil on a cotton swab—it will keep your lids clean and prevent dryness and reinfection, says Dr. Faye.

NIGHTTIME

❏ Steer clear of pets and pollen. If you have allergic conjunctivitis, try to protect yourself against the source. If your eyes itch when you are caressing your cat, keep her out of the bedroom. If pollen is making you want to scratch your eyes out, close the windows, turn on the air conditioner, and stay inside as much as you can, says Dr. Farber.

❏ Try an elimination diet. If you suspect that your conjunctivitis is triggered by a food allergy (most commonly, wheat, dairy, egg, or soy) try eliminating that food from your diet for two weeks, says Dr. Hibbs. Then reintroduce the food to see if you get a reaction. If so, stop eating the offending food.

Prescriptions
FOR CONJUNCTIVITIS

HERBAL
Rx

Various herbs, applied as eyewashes, have soothing, anti-inflammatory effects and can help speed recovery from conjunctivitis, says Dr. Hibbs.

A Homeopathic Prescription for Conjunctivitis

For conjunctivitis with lots of swelling, stinging, and burning, try Apis, a homeopathic remedy made from honeybee extract. Take a 30C dose once or twice a day until you feel better, says Judyth Reichenberg-Ullman, N.D., a naturopathic doctor with the Northwest Center for Homeopathic Medicine in Edmonds, Washington, and co-author of *Homeopathic Self-Care*. For added relief, you may wish to hold a cold washcloth on your eyelids for 10 minutes. (The notation 30C is a standard measurement in homeopathy and refers to a remedy's potency, which is listed on the label.)

You can buy Apis and other homeopathic remedies in capsule form in health food stores and some drugstores.

To prepare an eye bath, place one teaspoon of the appropriate herb in one cup freshly boiled water and steep the brew for 10 minutes. Strain the mixture, then let it cool. Use a dropper to apply two drops of the solution to the affected eye. Or make a compress by soaking a soft cloth in the herbal mix, then wringing out the cloth and folding it over your closed eyelid. Leave the compress on for about 10 minutes, allowing the liquid to soak into your eye.

Select the herbal bath appropriate for your particular type of conjunctivitis, suggests Dr. Hibbs. You should be able to find these herbs in health food stores. If not, ask the store to special order the one you want. Repeat the eye bath anytime your eyes hurt, but be sure to stop using an herbal remedy if you experience any type of allergic reaction.

❒ For bacterial conjunctivitis, use an eye bath of goldenseal tea, in addition to antibiotic eyedrops from your doctor, to help soothe your eyes and fight bacteria, says Dr. Hibbs.

❒ For allergic conjunctivitis, apply a chamomile eye compress. The remedy is most effective when it's cold. So keep a solution of the tea (one teaspoon chamomile, or one tea bag, to one cup water) handy in your refrigerator to use whenever your eyes burn and feel dry from allergic conjunctivitis, says Dr. Faye.

❒ If your lids are crusty when you wake up in the morning, try using fennel eyedrops or a fennel compress. The herb fennel works as an anti-inflammatory to soothe irritated, itchy, crusty eyes, says Dr. Hibbs.

MORNING

❒ For any type of conjunctival irritation, make a super-soother from goldenseal and eyebright. Steep a pinch of goldenseal mixed with one-half teaspoon eyebright in one-quarter cup hot water for five minutes, says Dr. Hibbs. Strain, let cool, then use as an eyewash.

Medical **Alert**

If your eyes are painful and red or you experience any vision loss associated with conjunctivitis, see a doctor immediately. If your eyes don't improve at all in two days despite your efforts, see a doctor to rule out a more serious condition such as iritis, an inflammation of the iris, the colored portion of the eye, says Dr. Farber.

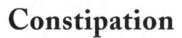

Constipation

With so many laxatives on the market today—and with each one promising to work faster, gentler, and better than the rest—which product do doctors recommend?

Truth be told, none. Relying on laxatives to get things moving, so to speak, can eventually lead to what doctors call a lazy bowel. In effect, you lose your ability to void naturally. Only in rare instances—for relief during travel, to treat side effects from medications you may be taking temporarily, or for any other short-term circumstance—do doctors advise using laxatives to relieve constipation, says Anne Simons, M.D., clinical physician and assistant clinical professor of family and community medicine at the University of California, San Francisco, Medical Center.

In fact, if you move your bowels at least once every three days, you don't even have constipation, according to Dr. Simons. Only if you void less than that, or if you suddenly go from one bowel movement a day to one a week, do you have a problem.

Constipation usually results from poor nutrition—eating too many processed foods such as potato chips, cookies, and other snacks and too few fiber-rich foods such as grains, fruits, and vegetables. Lack of exercise plays a role, too, as does rushing your toilet time so that you can't void completely.

LIFETIME

Women sometimes become constipated during their periods, whether because of hormonal fluctuations (the change in estrogen and progesterone balance decreases bowel motility) or because of cravings for fatty, sugary foods, says Dr. Simons. Constipation is also a frequent visitor during the first trimester of pregnancy, when the uterus expands and puts pressure on the abdomen and pelvis.

NUTRITION
Rx

Prescriptions
TO CONQUER CONSTIPATION

If constipation has your gut in its grip, you can restore regularity naturally with any of the following remedies.

TIME IT RIGHT

❐ Eat at least one serving of fruit and one serving of vegetables at every meal. Produce has plenty of fiber, and fiber increases the bulk and water content of your stool, says Dr. Simons. That makes the stool easier to pass. Good fruit sources of fiber include raspberries (eight grams of fiber per half-cup) and prunes (six grams per half-cup). Among vegetables, choose sweet potatoes (three grams per potato) and brussels sprouts (two grams per half-cup).

❐ Avoid apples and bananas while you are constipated. These two fruits actually bind your stool, so moving your bowels becomes even more difficult, Dr. Simons explains.

TIME IT RIGHT

❐ Take a teaspoon of whole flaxseed, mixed in an eight-ounce glass of water or juice, with each meal for two to three days, or until your symptoms improve. Though flaxseed won't dissolve completely, it does wash down easy. And it's rich in fiber, so it helps increase the bulk and water content of your stools. You will find whole flaxseed in health food

An Herbal Prescription to Soothe a Balky Bowel

Certain herbal teas can help gently coax your bowel back into action. One such tea, called Smooth Move, contains a blend of herbs (senna leaf, licorice root, ginger, cinnamon, and fennel) that gets your stool moving without side effects, explains Mitchell Fleisher, M.D., assistant clinical professor of family medicine at the University of Virginia Health Science Center in Charlottesville and a family-practice and homeopathic physician in Nellysford, Virginia. He suggests sipping one to two cups of the tea each day for three to four days. You can buy Smooth Move in health food stores and some drugstores.

stores, says Mitchell Fleisher, M.D., assistant clinical professor of family medicine at the University of Virginia Health Science Center in Charlottesville and a family-practice and homeopathic physician in Nellysford, Virginia.

❒ Take a rounded teaspoon of powdered psyllium seed, mixed in an eight-ounce glass of water or juice, with each meal until your symptoms subside. Follow this with a second glass of water or juice, says Joel Mason, M.D., associate professor in the divisions of gastroenterology and clinical nutrition at Tufts University School of Medicine in Boston.

TIME IT RIGHT

❒ Take a natural fiber supplement made with psyllium seed, such as Metamucil or Konsyl at breakfast and dinner. Simply stir a rounded teaspoon of the supplement into a glass of water, then drink up, says Dr. Mason. Take this dosage one to three times daily, depending on your needs, for up to three days. You will find Metamucil and similar products in drugstores and supermarkets.

TIME IT RIGHT

Rx

Prescriptions
to Stay Regular

The good news about constipation is that it is easy to avoid. These strategies can help.

❒ Get at least 25 grams of fiber a day (the Daily Value) by eating at least five servings of fruits and vegetables and two servings of whole grains. In addition to the foods mentioned earlier, try a half-cup serving of kiwi (3 grams of fiber), barley (2.9 grams), or broccoli (2.3 grams).

❒ Drink at least ½ ounce of water for each pound of body weight every day. For a 140-pound woman, that works out to 70 ounces—a little less than nine 8-ounce glasses. Water keeps your stool soft so that it's easier to pass, explains Dr. Fleisher.

TIME IT RIGHT

❒ Walk for 15 to 20 minutes every day. Pace yourself so that you find talking difficult but not impossible. Scientists can't explain why, but walking stimulates bowel function, so you stay regular, explains Dr. Simons.

TIME IT RIGHT

❒ Sit on the toilet for about 10 minutes after each meal. Planning your potty breaks in this way trains your body to void at the same time every day. And after you have eaten, your digestive system is on standby, ready to process food and empty waste. Stick with this schedule, says Dr. Simons, and within a few weeks, the urge to void after a meal will come naturally. But if you can't go within 10 minutes, don't force it, as straining creates problems of its own.

Medical **Alert**

See your doctor if you suddenly develop constant pain or cramping that does not resolve when the constipation is relieved, says Dr. Simons.

Also see your doctor if you experience any persistent and substantial change in your bowel movements, such as a drastic decrease in frequency—for example, from two a day to one every four days. This is especially important after age 40, when your risk for colon cancer increases, says Dr. Mason.

Cough, Sore Throat, and Laryngitis

A nagging cough. A scratchy throat. A raspy, barely there voice. Together they add up to the classic symptoms of the common cold.

But don't reach for the cold medicine just yet. While a virus may be responsible for your misery, other culprits can irritate your throat as well. Such things as pollen, dust, dry air, tobacco smoke, and even backed-up stomach acid can cause throat tissues to become painfully inflamed.

Most of the time, the inflammation goes away on its own within a matter of days even without medical intervention. But that doesn't mean that you have to suffer in the meantime. You can take steps to boost your body's natural defenses so that your throat heals faster—and stays "in the pink."

Prescriptions
TO QUIET THE COUGH

Coughing is actually a good thing—your body's way of trying to clear mucus or a foreign material from your airways. Of course, this may not be much consolation when you are wide-awake at three o'clock in the morning, hacking uncontrollably. Try the following remedies for speedy relief.

❑ Drink thyme tea three times a day for up to three days. "*Thymus vulgaris* is a traditional remedy for whooping cough and is still prescribed by naturopathic doctors for adult bronchitis," says Lisa Meserole, R.D., N.D., a naturopathic doctor and past chairman of the department of botanical medicine at Bastyr University in Seattle. "It relaxes airway muscles and acts as an antimicrobial and expectorant." To make the tea, pour six ounces freshly boiled water over 1⅔ teaspoons fresh thyme leaves or ½ to ⅔ teaspoon dried thyme. (If you are using the dried form, it is best to obtain a medicinal-quality thyme at your local health food store and

TIME IT RIGHT

reserve the thyme in your spice cabinet for culinary uses.) Cover and steep for 10 minutes, then strain. Allow the tea to cool before drinking it. If your sore throat doesn't improve within three days, stop using this remedy until you see your doctor, she advises.

❐ Add a few drops of vegetable oil to a glass of fresh carrot juice and sip frequently throughout the day. "Carrot juice is full of vitamin A, which strengthens your respiratory system and can silence your cough," notes Nan Kathryn Fuchs, Ph.D., a nutritionist in Sebastopol, California, and a columnist for the *Women's Health Letter*. "The vegetable oil coats and soothes your throat."

❐ For a dry, hacking cough, take 5,000 international units of vitamin A every day for a week. "Vitamin A supports the microbe-catching membranes of your respiratory system," explains Dr. Fuchs. The membranes can do a better job of nabbing the irritants that caused your cough in the first place.

NIGHTTIME

❐ For a cough caused by postnasal drip, sleep with your head propped on pillows. Postnasal drip gets worse when you lie down because mucus can then clog your chest and throat, says Barbara Phillips, M.D., associate professor of medicine at the University of Kentucky A. B. Chandler Medical Center in Lexington. The congestion makes you cough.

Rx ———

Prescriptions
to Soothe a Sore Throat

Coughing and sore throats often go hand in hand. You get a sore throat when some irritant—very likely the same stuff that is making you cough—dries out the mucous membrane lining your airways. A bacterial or viral infection can cause a sore throat as well. To feel better fast, take this advice from the experts.

TIME IT RIGHT

❐ Begin sucking on zinc gluconate lozenges at the first sign of a sore throat and continue until the scratchiness subsides. "Using the lozenges in this way bathes the tissue lining the throat in a zinc solution," explains Michael Macknin, M.D., a researcher in the department of pediatrics at the Cleveland Clinic in Cleveland. "This direct contact may stop a viral infection by preventing the virus from entering cells and reproducing."

Theoretically, forms of zinc other than zinc gluconate can bind with sweeteners and even vitamin C in lozenges and become inactive.

You can buy zinc gluconate lozenges in health food stores and some drugstores. Follow the directions on the label for proper dosage.

❏ Gargle with warm salt water four or five times a day. "The salt water temporarily soothes your throat by cleaning it and drawing fluids out of swollen tissues," says Dr. Phillips. You can make the solution by mixing one-half teaspoon salt in one cup warm water.

To gargle, begin by taking in a deep breath. Sip a small amount of salt water and tilt your head back. Breathe out through your mouth to create bubbles. If you are making noise, you are doing it right. Spit out the salt water when you are done gargling.

❏ Sip marsh mallow root tea as needed throughout the day. "The herb marsh mallow has a soothing, moistening quality that makes it ideal for treating a dry, irritated throat," says Dr. Meserole. To make the tea, put one-quarter cup dried, chopped herb (available in health food stores) in a glass or ceramic jar. Then pour a pint of room-temperature water over top. Cover the jar and allow the herb to steep overnight. In the morning, strain the herb and add four teaspoons honey. Sip one-quarter to one-half cup of the tea at a time throughout the day.

Prescriptions
TO OUTLAST LARYNGITIS

Rx

Much like a sore throat, laryngitis involves the drying-out of the mucous membrane. Only in this case, the membrane surrounds the larynx, or voice box. Because the membrane can't moisten and filter air properly, your speaking voice—created by air passing over your vocal cords—becomes distorted. You may even lose your voice altogether.

Fortunately, you don't have to remain speechless for long. The following tips can help treat laryngitis.

❏ Squeeze the juice from one to two fresh lemons, then mix it with a tablespoon honey and a pinch of ground red pepper. Take a small sip of the mixture every few hours throughout the day, says Dr. Meserole. Avoid this remedy if you have a very sensitive stomach or mouth.

TIME IT RIGHT

TIME IT RIGHT

❐ Inhale steam three times a day. Begin by pouring three cups water into a pot and bringing it to a simmer. Remove the pot from the stove and add one-quarter teaspoon eucalyptus essential oil or peppermint essential oil (available in health food stores) to the water. Set the pot where you can sit in front of it—perhaps on the kitchen or dining room table. Position your face over the pot (not too close, though, or you risk burning yourself) and drape a towel over the back of your head to create a mini-sauna. Breathe in the steam, coming up for fresh air after five minutes, says David Alessi, M.D., an otolaryngologist specializing in voice disorders at Cedars-Sinai Medical Center in Los Angeles.

❐ Rest your voice as much as possible—and if you must talk, use a soft, low-pitched voice rather than a whisper. "Whispering stresses your vocal cords even more," says Dr. Alessi.

❐ If your throat feels congested, sip water to soothe it. "You may think you have phlegm, but in the case of laryngitis, it's actually swollen tissue," explains Dr. Alessi. Trying to clear your throat with frequent *ahems* only aggravates your discomfort.

❐ Refrain from gargling while you have laryngitis. It only irritates your vocal cords.

Rx

Prescriptions
TO REDUCE YOUR RISK

While coughs, sore throats, and laryngitis are quite common, they are by no means inevitable. You can fortify your resistance to these ailments with the following strategies.

❐ Take 1,000 milligrams of vitamin C every day. Vitamin C may reduce your susceptibility to colds, according to Dr. Phillips. That means you are less likely to experience the coughs and sore throats that colds can bring.

❐ Give up smoking. People who smoke report that they actually cough *less* when they are puffing away. In the long run, however, they are only making matters worse. "The chemicals in cigarette smoke temporarily paralyze the cells lining the respiratory tract," explains Dr. Phillips. "These cells normally help remove virus- or bacteria-laden mucus. Since they can't do their job effectively, infection has a better chance of setting in."

If you stop smoking, you may initially cough more. That's a good sign. "It means your lungs are clearing out," says Dr. Phillips.

❒ Avoid secondhand smoke. Even if you are not the one with a cigarette in your mouth, the smoke can have a similar detrimental effect on your respiratory tract, advises Dr. Phillips.

❒ Eat your last meal no less than four hours before bedtime. Otherwise, lying down allows stomach acid to slosh back into your esophagus. The acid makes your throat burn and causes you to cough, says Dr. Phillips.

NIGHTTIME

❒ Keep tabs on your weight. Like eating too close to bedtime, carrying extra pounds prompts stomach acid to back up into your esophagus. While there are a number of complex formulas for calculating your ideal weight, one simple formula used by some experts can let you know if you are close: If you are five feet tall, you should weigh 100 pounds. If you are taller, add 5 pounds for each additional inch of height. Then to that number, add 10 percent if you have a large frame, or subtract 10 percent if you have a small frame.

Medical **Alert**

You should see your doctor if your cough lasts for more than three weeks, if your cough is accompanied by a fever, or if you are bringing up green or yellow mucus or blood. You want to rule out more serious respiratory conditions such as strep throat, a sinus infection, bronchitis, and pneumonia, says Dr. Phillips.

Cuts, Scrapes, Bruises, and Abrasions

Close encounters with paring knives, cheese graters, and sardine tins can leave your fingers nicked or slashed. Mishaps with tools, missteps on a sidewalk, and mishandling of envelopes can also break your skin. Not exactly life-threatening accidents, but they are painful and distracting nonetheless. To help cuts and scrapes heal quickly, here's what to do.

Rx ——— *Prescriptions*
TO CARE FOR CUTS AND SCRAPES

The first order of business is to keep the wound infection-free, says Barbara Yawn, M.D., director of research at the Olmstead Medical Center in Rochester, Minnesota.

❐ Wash the wound thoroughly with warm water and perfume-free soap.

❐ To get rid of grit, pour a small amount of hydrogen peroxide on a clean cloth and dab directly on the wound. Hydrogen peroxide is a safe, simple way to bubble out loose dirt or gravel caught beneath the skin, Dr. Yawn says.

TIME IT RIGHT ❐ If the cut really hurts, soak the wound in warm water for up to 10 minutes. Any longer, and the skin will pucker and you'll lose some of the essential oils that protect against the invasion of bacteria, according to Dr. Yawn.

❐ To promote healing and help clean up residual debris caught beneath the skin, first apply a tincture of Calendula officinalis, a homeopathic remedy, suggests John Collins, N.D., a naturopathic physician who is board-certified in homeopathy, associate professor of homeopathy at the National College of Naturopathic Medicine, and co-owner of Rockwood Natural Medicine Clinic, both in Portland, Oregon. Mix 25 drops of Calendula in four ounces of sterile water (available in most drugstores) and apply directly on the wound as often as needed. (If your health food store does not carry Calendula, ask them to special order it for you.)

❐ Then apply Calendula ointment directly to the wound or on a bandage. An antiseptic, Calendula has been used for more than a hundred years, says Paul Mittman, N.D., chairman of the homeopathy department at Southwest College of Naturopathic Medicine in Tempe, Arizona. Calendula ointment is available in health food stores.

❒ For puncture wounds, try Ledum palustre. A homeopathic remedy derived from wild rosemary, Ledum is particularly good for puncture wounds (for example, if you step on a nail) or for insect bites or stings, according to Dr. Collins. Take a 6X or 30C dose in tablet form or try Ledum ointment as often as needed. Both remedies are available in health food stores. (The notations 6X and 30C are standard measurements in homeopathy and refer to a remedy's potency, which is listed on the label.)

❒ To speed healing, cover the wound with an adhesive bandage, says Dr. Yawn. Change the bandage once or twice a day so that it remains clean and dry.

❒ Consider a high-tech dressing such as Nu Skin, available in drugstores. These wet gel-like dressings prevent dehydration and contamination of the wound, help immune cells do their job, and promote the growth of new blood vessels, Dr. Collins says.

Prescriptions
FOR BRUISE CONTROL

HOMEOPATHIC
Rx

Unlike cuts, which bleed on the surface, bruises occur when blood vessels break below the surface, leaking blood under your skin and causing swelling, discoloration, and soreness. So bruises call for slightly different first-aid strategies.

❒ For fast relief, apply ice directly to the bruise immediately and elevate the bruised area for 20 minutes, says Dr. Yawn. If pain persists, elevate the injured area for another 20 minutes.

TIME IT RIGHT

❒ Take Arnica. A homeopathic medicine available in tablet, ointment, spray, or drops at health food stores, Arnica has long been used for bruises and soreness. But like aspirin, no one knows why Arnica works, says Jacquelyn Wilson, M.D., a health-care consultant in homeopathy in Escondido, California. She recommends Arnica in potencies ranging from 6X to 30X or 30C. A "C" potency means that the medicine has been shaken and diluted 100 times and an "X" dose, 10 times. You can either suck on one tablet, rub ointment or spray onto the injured area, or place 5 to 10 drops under your tongue once a day or more as needed, she says. You should see your doctor if the pain has not decreased after three days, recommends Dr. Wilson.

❏ To soothe your nerves, try Hypericum perforatum. Hypericum, an herb used to make this homeopathic medicine, is particularly useful for soothing injuries to areas with lots of nerve endings, such as your fingertips, lips, or backbone. If you hit your thumb with a hammer or a chair gives out under you, Hypericum will ease the pain and shock, says Dr. Wilson. Take a 6X to 30X or 30C potency in tablet, drop, or ointment form as described for Arnica above. You can buy Hypericum at health food stores.

Medical **Alert**

If a cut is deep and more than an inch or two long or doesn't stop bleeding after you have applied firm pressure for five minutes, you may need stitches. If in doubt, call ahead and ask your doctor whether you really do need them, says Dr. Yawn. Don't delay, though. "Stitches should always be placed within a few hours," she says. In the event that your cut shows signs of infection, see a doctor, especially if you have diabetes or an autoimmune disease such as AIDS. If you get a puncture wound and haven't had a tetanus shot in 10 years, see your doctor, says Dr. Yawn.

Dandruff and Scalp Problems

Everybody sheds a little dandruff. Those little white flakes on the scalp are perfectly normal. You just don't notice it until it reaches critical mass.

"The skin is always turning over and recreating itself," explains Jerome Shupack, M.D., professor of clinical dermatology at New York University Medical Center in New York City. "Skin cells migrate to the surface and flake off. It's usually imperceptible, with the flakes coming off when you shampoo. But because of the presence of oil in hair, sometimes scale gets trapped. Don't wash your hair for long enough—say, a month— and anyone would end up with dandruff."

Other, more severe scalp problems can resemble a serious case of dandruff. Seborrheic dermatitis looks a lot like dandruff but may include itching and a visibly pink or red scalp, says Dr. Shupack.

And with "seb derm," you are likely to shed flakes from your eyebrows and nose as well as your scalp, says Jeffrey Herten, M.D., assistant clinical professor of dermatology at the University of California, Irvine, College of Medicine.

More serious are psoriasis and eczema, which are treated with prescription medications. Signs of psoriasis and eczema also include itching and a red, inflamed scalp, but the patches are more distinct, and the scale won't come off just by shampooing. You are likely to know you have psoriasis or eczema because you will have white scaly patches on your elbows, knees, and other areas of skin as well as your hair, says Dr. Shupack.

Dandruff often starts at puberty and disappears at menopause, says Diana Bihova, M.D., a dermatologist in New York City and author of *Beauty from the Inside Out*. No one knows why, but scalp problems also tend to accompany hormonal changes that occur during menstruation or pregnancy. Dandruff and seborrheic dermatitis often worsen at times of stress.

LIFETIME

Prescriptions
TO END DANDRUFF

NATURAL
Rx

If you have psoriasis or eczema, see your dermatologist, says Dr. Bihova. For dandruff or seborrheic dermatitis, a change in shampoos and a few other simple strategies should shield your shoulders from snow.

❏ Wash your hair daily. Seems simple and obvious, but if you don't shampoo, dandruff flakes have nowhere to go, says Dr. Bihova.

❏ Try a dandruff shampoo every day for two weeks. That's the easiest way to see if you have dandruff or something more serious, says Dr. Bihova. The best dandruff shampoos contain tar or selenium or zinc pyrithione (check the ingredients list on the label). They relieve the itch as well as remove scale from the scalp. With that proviso, all work equally well; experiment until you find the type of shampoo you like best. If you do have dandruff, you should see results in two weeks.

TIME IT RIGHT

❐ For dandruff shampoo to work best, leave it on for three to four minutes. This gives the shampoo enough contact with your scalp, says Dr. Bihova. "Use dandruff shampoo when you are not in a hurry, which for most people is in the evenings. When you shampoo in the morning, you are rushing to work, and every minute counts, so you won't leave it in. Three to four minutes doesn't sound like a lot, but it can make a big difference." By shampooing in the evening, you can make it a nice, pleasant, soothing experience to relieve stress.

❐ Once you have determined that you do have dandruff, use a gentle, nonmedicated shampoo every other day, says Dr. Herten. In other words, alternate a regular, nonmedicated shampoo with a stronger dandruff formula.

WINTERTIME

❐ Apply a conditioner after every shampoo, especially in the winter, to make sure that your scalp doesn't dry out, says Howard J. Donsky, M.D., a staff dermatologist at the University of Rochester in New York.

TIME IT RIGHT

❐ Oil your scalp once a week. If your scalp stays moisturized, you are likely to have less dandruff, Dr. Herten says. To prepare the oil treatment, heat an ounce (about one-eighth cup) of olive oil in a Pyrex measuring cup in the microwave or in a double boiler until it's comfortably warm but not hot or scalding. Then rub the oil into your scalp. Pull on a shower cap and let set for 30 minutes. Then lather with a gentle shampoo.

❐ To keep your scalp moist from the inside out, stay hydrated. That means drinking at least eight eight-ounce glasses of water and eating at least five servings of fruits and vegetables every day, says Dr. Donsky.

NIGHTTIME

❐ Use a vaporizer in your bedroom to keep the air moist.

❐ Wear a hat. Sun and cold dry out your scalp. If you wear a hat, your head is less likely to dry out and produce an excess of scaly flakes that cause dandruff, says Dr. Donsky.

TIME IT RIGHT

❐ Head off stress with five-minute relaxation breaks. Dandruff and other scalp problems are often brought on by stress, says Dr. Bihova. So if something is coming up that's likely to stress you out, take time to calm down—take a walk, listen to soothing music, or just stare out the window for five minutes. If you are already stressed, take a relaxation break. If you soothe yourself, you just might control your dandruff more quickly.

Medical **Alert**

If you use a dandruff shampoo every day for two weeks and your scalp is still shedding flakes, you may have psoriasis or eczema, stubborn conditions that call for medical treatment, says Dr. Bihova. Same goes if your scalp has distinct patches of white and big chunks of scale or if you are always itching. If so, you have more than simple dandruff, and you should see a doctor.

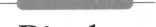

Diarrhea

Nothing can spoil a good vacation like a bad case of traveler's diarrhea. Yet a chance encounter with unfriendly bacteria has left many a tourist doing her sightseeing from the hotel bathroom.

In countries with less-stringent public-health standards than our own, food and water commonly harbor bacteria that cause diarrhea, says Randall Reves, M.D., associate professor of medicine in the division of infectious diseases in the department of medicine at the University of Colorado Health Sciences Center in Denver. Those loose, watery stools occur when the offending bugs attach themselves to the cells of your intestinal lining, where they produce a toxin that causes fluid release.

Of course, you don't even have to leave home to experience the runs. You are vulnerable to the bacteria anytime you consume improperly handled food or drink. A few disease-causing bacteria will rapidly multiply in food that is not refrigerated or kept hot.

Infectious diarrhea is common in small children. It can be passed on to other family members during diapering or by other contact.

Prescriptions
TO DERAIL DIARRHEA

Rx

A bout of diarrhea usually clears up on its own within 48 hours. In the meantime, you may find yourself making 8 to 10 trips to the toilet each day. If you would prefer more speedy relief, try an over-the-counter antidiarrheal such as Pepto-Bismol or Imodium A-D, suggests Dr. Reves.

These products relieve the runs by binding with toxins produced by the bacteria attached to the lining of the bowel. The following natural remedies can help, too.

TIME IT RIGHT

❐ Take a 6C, 12C, or 30C dose of the homeopathic remedy Arsenicum at the onset of diarrhea. (The notation 6C, 12C, or 30C is a standard measurement in homeopathy and refers to a remedy's potency, which is listed on the label.) Repeat the dose every two hours for intense symptoms and every four hours for mild symptoms, continuing until your bowel movements become firmer and less frequent, says Dana Ullman, a homeopathic practitioner in Berkeley, California, and author of *The Consumer's Guide to Homeopathy*. Arsenicum works especially well for treating diarrhea brought on by eating tainted food, he notes. But if your diarrhea doesn't improve within 24 hours, you should stop taking the remedy. You can buy Arsenicum capsules and other homeopathic remedies in health food stores and some drugstores.

❐ Drink a cup of raspberry leaf tea, advises James A. Duke, Ph.D., author of *The Green Pharmacy*. To make the tea, pour boiling water over two teaspoons raspberry leaf and let it steep for two to three minutes. Strain it before drinking. You can flavor it with peppermint leaves or lemon, if you like. Raspberry leaf contains tannins, compounds that help reduce intestinal inflammation. You can buy the herb in health food stores.

❐ Eat a slippery elm ball. "Take a few spoonfuls of slippery elm bark powder, found at health food stores, and blend it with honey until you can roll the mixture into small balls. Dust the balls with additional slippery elm powder, store in a closed container, and use as needed," says Susun S. Weed, director of the Wise Woman Center in Woodstock, New York, and author of the *Wise Woman Herbal* series. Slippery elm works because it contains a nutritive mucilage, which soothes intestinal irritation, she says. At the first sign of diarrhea, let a ball dissolve slowly in your mouth and repeat as necessary.

NUTRITION Rx

Prescriptions
TO ARREST THE RUNS

When diarrhea strikes, how long your symptoms linger depends a great deal on what you eat. A few adjustments in your diet can help temper a testy digestive tract and return your bowel movements to normal. Doctors recommend the following strategies.

❒ Consume only clear liquids for the first 24 hours after diarrhea TIME IT RIGHT
sets in. Clear liquids such as chicken bouillon, herbal tea, and soft drinks help keep you hydrated. And that's important, says Dr. Reves, because diarrhea drains a lot of water from your system. Adding sugar to your tea or drinking soft drinks without artificial sweeteners can help, too, because sugar enables your body to absorb salt and water. (If you choose an herbal tea or soft drink, check the label to be sure that it does not contain caffeine.)

❒ Avoid or minimize caffeine-containing beverages such as coffee, tea, and cola at least until your diarrhea subsides—and preferably one day longer. Caffeine may irritate your bowels, and it makes your stools even looser, according to Dr. Reves. It gives you the urge to void more frequently, too.

❒ After the first 24 hours, switch to small meals of bland foods such TIME IT RIGHT
as bananas, rice, and crackers. Continue eating this way for the duration of your diarrhea and for 24 hours after your diarrhea subsides. Eating light gives your digestive tract a chance to rest and recuperate, explains Ralph Giannella, M.D., professor of medicine and director of the division of digestive diseases at the University of Cincinnati College of Medicine.

❒ Stay away from all dairy products while you have diarrhea. Diarrhea temporarily disrupts your ability to digest lactose, the sugar found in milk and milk-containing foods, according to Dr. Reves. And that can aggravate an already-irritated digestive tract.

Prescriptions — Rx
FOR COPING WITH CHRONIC DIARRHEA

Recurrent bouts of diarrhea may signal an underlying health problem such as irritable bowel syndrome (IBS). If you frequently get diarrhea (more than two or three times a month) that is accompanied by abdominal pain—both classic symptoms of IBS—you should see your doctor. In the meantime, the following remedies can help rein in chronic runs. (And for more information on IBS, see page 215.)

❐ Avoid packaged, processed foods made with sorbitol or mannitol. These artificial sweeteners, which are often used in dietetic gums and candies, have a laxative effect on many people, says Dr. Giannella. Just five or six sticks of gum can supply enough sorbitol or mannitol to cause diarrhea, he notes.

❐ Write down what you eat and drink as well as when you experience bouts of diarrhea. After two weeks, review your notes to determine whether certain foods or beverages seem to trigger your diarrhea. Common culprits include milk, cheese, chocolate, coffee, and tea. Keep in mind that your body doesn't react for five to six hours after you have consumed something, says Dr. Giannella.

Once you have identified the potential offenders, eliminate them from your diet. You should notice a decline in the frequency and severity of your diarrhea. If your symptoms don't improve, see your doctor.

Medical **Alert**

See your doctor when your diarrhea lasts for more than 48 hours or is accompanied by blood in your stool or fever, recommends Dr. Giannella.

You should also see your doctor if you feel light-headed, have difficulty keeping liquids down, or notice a decline in your usual urine output, adds Dr. Reves.

Dry Eyes

If you're a woman of a certain age, you may suffer from dry eyes. In fact, 90 percent of those who experience dry eyes are female. Yet few women realize that along with hot flashes and night sweats, dry eyes are most common during or after menopause, when levels of the hormones estrogen and prolactin drop, says William Frey II, Ph.D., research director at the Dry Eye and Tear Research Center at the Regions Medical Center in St. Paul, Minnesota.

Not all dry eyes are related to hormonal changes. If you live in a dry and windy climate or work in a building that isn't well-ventilated, you are likely to suffer from dry eyes, says Eleanor Faye, M.D., an ophthalmic surgeon at the Manhattan Eye, Ear, and Throat Hospital in New York. Allergies and many medications, such as diuretics, antihistamines, decongestants, and blood pressure medications, can also dry out your eyes.

Eyes tend to be driest early in the morning when you wake up, particularly if you sleep in a dry bedroom, or at 5:00 or 6:00 P.M., after you have worked in front of a computer screen all day. Spending time in a dry environment like an air-conditioned car or airplane can also exacerbate dry-eye symptoms, says Anne Sumers, M.D., an ophthalmologist in Ridgewood, New Jersey, and a spokesman for the American Academy of Ophthalmology.

If you have dry eyes, you'll know it. Dry eyes itch and burn and can feel gravelly and irritated. Crying makes the problem worse. Emotional tears actually wash away the oils in the tear film. (The tear film is a thin layer of mucus, water, and oils produced in glands under the eyelids to help stabilize the eyes.) Without these oils, your eyes can rub against your eyelids, causing aggravation and dryness, says Eric Donnenfeld, M.D., program director of the cornea department and associate professor of ophthalmology at North Shore University/Cornell and co-chairman of the external diseases and cornea department at the Manhattan Eye, Ear, and Throat Hospital in New York.

MORNING

Prescriptions
for Instant Moisture

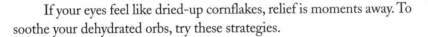

Rx

If your eyes feel like dried-up cornflakes, relief is moments away. To soothe your dehydrated orbs, try these strategies.

❏ Apply preservative-free artificial tears, which can be purchased in drugstores and supermarkets. A few drops should solve the problem right away, says Dr. Sumers. (Preservatives tend to irritate sensitive eyes, says Andrew Farber, M.D., an ophthalmologist in Terre Haute, Indiana, and a spokesman for the American Academy of Ophthalmology.)

It is especially helpful for contact lens wearers to use artificial tears for dry eyes. Contact lenses act like sponges, absorbing all the available tear film, says Dr. Donnenfeld.

An Herbal Prescription for Dry Eyes

Chamomile tea soothes the eyes, says Eleanor Faye, M.D., an ophthalmic surgeon at the Manhattan Eye, Ear, and Throat Hospital in New York. To make the tea, steep one teaspoon of the dried herb or one tea bag in one cup freshly boiled water, then strain it to remove the herbs. Keep the tea refrigerated until you need to use it.

When your eyes are dry and burning, soak cotton squares in the cold tea. Apply the compresses to your closed eyes for 10 minutes at a time, as often as needed.

TIME IT RIGHT

❐ As an alternative, wet a towel or a washcloth with warm water and place the warm cloth against your eyes for a few moments. Make sure that the water isn't hot enough to burn you. Leave the compress on just long enough to heat up the oil glands in your eyelids so that they moisten your eyes effectively, says Dr. Donnenfeld. Repeat twice a day.

Rx ——— *Prescriptions*
FOR CONTINUED COMFORT

You can permanently put an end to desert-dry eyes. These tips will tell you how.

NIGHTTIME

❐ Using a cotton swab, apply a pinhead-size drop of petroleum jelly to your lids along the edge of your lashes every night before bed. Tear production decreases at night, and petroleum jelly helps keep the tears that you do produce from evaporating quickly, Dr. Faye says. Try not to get the jelly into your eyes, or you may have a brief bout of blurry vision. (If you do get some in your eyes, rinse a soft washcloth in warm water and swipe it over your closed eye to wipe it clean.)

❐ For a severe case of dry eyes, use an eyedropper to place a drop Nighttime of corn oil in each eye before you go to sleep, says Dr. Faye. If you are going to use this remedy, be sure to keep a separate container of corn oil in your medicine cabinet. Corn oil from the pantry is likely to be contaminated, she cautions.

❐ Drizzle some olive oil on your salads. Dry eyes often stem from a deficiency in essential fatty acids, an increasing problem in this era of low-fat diets, says Dr. Faye. Olive oil is a good way of preventing a deficiency without loading up on saturated forms of fat.

❐ Take 500 milligrams of evening primrose oil in capsule form three Time it right times a day until your eyes feel less irritated, says Deirdre O'Connor, N.D., a naturopathic physician in private practice in Mystic, Connecticut. Like olive oil, evening primrose can help raise your level of essential fatty acids. Evening primrose oil may be purchased in health food stores.

❐ Be sure that you are getting 5,000 international units of vitamin A and 15 milligrams of zinc each day. Deficiencies of vitamin A and zinc can cause dry eyes, says Dr. Faye.

❐ Take one capsule of cod-liver oil daily. The essential fatty acids in cod-liver oil keep the oil glands in your eyelids from clogging up and drying out your eyes, says Dr. Donnenfeld. Cod-liver oil does contain hefty amounts of vitamin A, however. So cod-liver oil capsules are replacements for, not additions to, the vitamin A supplements recommended by Dr. Faye.

Prescriptions
to Prevent Dryness

Aside from keeping your eyes and lids well-oiled, don't forget these tried-and-true prescriptions for keeping your eyes from getting dry.

❐ If you wear contact lenses, change to glasses when you get Lifetime home from work, says Dr. Farber. If you're pregnant or going through menopause and have relentlessly dry eyes, you may want to switch to glasses entirely, he says.

❐ When you go outside on a dry, windy day, wear wraparound sunglasses to prevent the wind from blowing against your eyes and drying out your tear film, says Dr. Donnenfeld. You may want to consider wearing ski goggles, even if you don't ski.

❐ When riding in your car, turn the air vents toward your feet, not your face.

❐ At home, don't sit under or in the direct line of heating or air conditioning vents, says Dr. Donnenfeld.

WINTERTIME

❐ In the cold of winter, run a humidifier in any room where you spend a lot of time (usually your bedroom). A humidifier keeps the air moist, so it doesn't dry out your eyes, Dr. Donnenfeld says.

❐ If you smoke, stop. Smoking aggravates dry-eye symptoms of burning and tearing. It also increases your risk of macular degeneration, a condition in which the cells in the macula (the central portion of the retina) break down. Left unchecked, macular degeneration can eventually lead to blindness, says Dr. Sumers.

Medical Alert

If you find that you develop dry eyes after starting a new medication, report the symptom to your doctor. She may be able to recommend another medicine that doesn't produce dry eyes as a side effect, advises Dr. Donnenfeld.

You should also see your doctor if your eyes are red and you experience pus or discharge for more than two days, says Dr. Sumers. If you have pain in the eye or suffer any loss of vision, get medical attention immediately.

Dry Mouth

Ever suck on a cheekful of cotton wads at the dentist's office? Then you know what it feels like to have a dry mouth.

A dry mouth makes it hard to chew and swallow. Wake up from a night of sleep with a dry mouth, and your lips feel plastered shut. Worse, the absence of saliva in your mouth can lead to cavities, especially around the gum line, since saliva fights bacteria and helps restore minerals such as calcium in teeth. And a dry mouth can promote the growth of other unwanted organisms in your mouth, most notably, *Candida*, or yeast, which can cause a burning sensation and cracks around the corners of your mouth. Not fun.

A saliva shortage is most common in older people taking medications. "But it can happen to anyone, at any age, and can be caused by prescription or over-the-counter drugs, stress, or nasal congestion that makes you breathe through your mouth instead of your nose," says Phillip Fox, D.D.S., clinical director of the National Institute of Dental Research in Bethesda, Maryland. And occasionally, a dry mouth, usually along with dry eyes, is one of the first signs of Sjögren's syndrome, an autoimmune disease that strikes women much more frequently than men.

A dry mouth can trigger burning sensations from acidic foods or alcohol-based mouthwashes. But some people—especially women past menopause—have the sensation of burning in their mouths without dryness. (For more information, see burning mouth syndrome on page 246.)

Prescriptions
TO WET YOUR WHISTLE

Rx

The trick is to stimulate your salivary glands to pump out as much juice as they can and replace the deficit with other fluids as necessary. Here's how.

❒ Exercise your mouth by chewing. Chewing sends a message to your salivary glands: "Crank it up, guys. We need spit!" Sugarless gum gives your mouth a good workout, as do carrots and bagels. "I tell people to spend some time really chewing food, to get their juices flowing," explains Leo Sreebny, D.D.S., Ph.D., professor of oral medicine at the State University of New York at Stony Brook. "Chewing is the mouth's exercise. It helps keep it healthy."

❐ Suck on sugarless lemon drops. These get the biggest nod since their sour taste can jump-start sluggish salivary glands. You can also add a squeeze of lemon juice to water. But avoid putting your teeth in direct contact with straight citrus when your mouth is dry. Its strong acidity can eat away tooth enamel over time.

TIME IT RIGHT

❐ Sip water every 10 minutes or so. "As simple as it sounds, this can really provide a great deal of relief," says Dr. Fox. Fortunately, it is now socially acceptable to carry around a water bottle. Just don't wait until you are desert-dry to wet your whistle.

❐ Use a stimulating spray. A number of acidic solutions on the market can help get saliva flowing. Two to look for are ProFlow and Optimoist, suggests Dr. Sreebny. If your drugstore doesn't stock these products, ask your pharmacist to place a special order for you. The big advantage to using a spray (instead of sucking on candy) is that you minimize any potential damage to your teeth.

❐ If none of these measures stimulates your salivary glands enough to keep you comfortable, try an artificial saliva product such as ORALbalance. These products offer some relief by coating your mouth, explains Dr. Sreebny. You can find artificial saliva in most drugstores. If your drugstore doesn't carry it, ask your pharmacist to place a special order for you.

❐ Dab your lips with petroleum jelly. If your mouth is dry on the inside, chances are good that your lips are equally dry on the outside, since saliva helps keep them moist. Petroleum jelly can prevent dry lips from cracking, Dr. Sreebny says.

Rx

Prescriptions
FOR PERMANENT RELIEF

Lasting relief is likely only if you can find a treatable cause for your dry mouth. Here are some possible solutions.

❐ Find out whether any medicine that you are taking can cause dry mouth. You can ask your doctor or pharmacist, or you can check the *Physician's Desk Reference*, which you will find in the reference section of your local library. "Probably more than 400 drugs have dry mouth as a possible side effect," says Dr. Fox. The most common culprits include antihistamines, antidepressants, sedatives, blood pressure and heart drugs, diuretics, and anesthetics. "Your doctor may be able to suggest an alternative drug that is less likely to cause dry mouth, or she may be able to reduce your drug's dosage."

❒ Take 50 milligrams of B-complex vitamins three times a day, cutting back to once a day as your symptoms start to improve (usually within three to four weeks). Deficiencies of the B vitamins can lead to dry mouth, explains Craig Zunka, D.D.S., a dentist in Front Royal, Virginia, and president of the Holistic Dental Association. Make sure that you know how much vitamin B_6 you are getting in your B-complex supplement. High doses of B_6 (that is, 50 milligrams to 2 grams a day) over a prolonged period of time can cause numb feet and an unstable gait.

❒ Also take 500 milligrams of omega-3 fatty acids and 500 milligrams of evening primrose oil twice a day. As with the B-complex vitamins, shortages of these essential fatty acids can contribute to dry mouth, according to Dr. Zunka. You can buy omega-3 and evening primrose supplements in capsule form in drugstores and health food stores.

❒ Monitor your intake of vitamin A. Too little or too much of the nutrient can cause your mouth and eyes to become dry. The Daily Value for vitamin A is 5,000 international units.

❒ Avoid foods and dental-care products with ingredients that can make your mouth sting or burn, advises Michael A. Siegel, D.D.S., associate professor at the University of Maryland School of Dentistry in Baltimore. Among the more common culprits are citrus fruits, spicy foods, cinnamon and cinnamon flavoring, pyrophosphates (found in tartar-control toothpastes and mouthwashes), and alcohol (found in some mouthwashes).

Medical **Alert**

See your doctor if you suspect that a certain prescription drug may be causing your dry mouth. See your doctor, too, if dry mouth persists despite self-help efforts or if it is accompanied by dry eyes,

fatigue, or aching joints, says Dr. Siegel. You may have an autoimmune disorder, a condition in which disease-fighting antibodies attack your own cells. Your family doctor can refer you to a specialist, a doctor oral medicine, or, in the case of an autoimmune disorder, a rheumatologist.

Energy Slump

Second only to more time and more money, most people say that they could use more energy. Or at least a reliable supply that enables them to do everything they need to or want to accomplish day and night. All too often, though, energy levels slump just when we still have plenty of items remaining on our "to do" list. Blame your natural rhythms.

"An afternoon slump is natural even for well-rested people; it's reminiscent of ancestral behavior," says Scott Campbell, Ph.D., associate professor of psychiatry and director of the sleep laboratory in the chronobiology laboratory in the department of psychiatry at New York Hospital/Cornell Medical Center in White Plains. "Studies have shown that cognitive performance—how well we think and problem-solve—improves after a nap. The post-lunch dip is a biological tendency."

TIME IT RIGHT

That's because our bodies ordinarily have one long and one short sleep period within each 24-hour cycle. The shorter period occurs 12 hours after the middle of the longer one. So if you slept from 11:00 P.M. to 8:00 A.M., your body might be inclined to take a short nap at about 3:00 in the afternoon, writes Kathryn A. Cox, M.D., medical editor of *The Good Housekeeping Illustrated Guide to Women's Health*.

That said, few women can squeeze in an afternoon snooze. As we work, do errands, and take care of our families without a break, we end up feeling enervated when we should be energetic.

What, how, and when we eat also affects our energy levels. "A soda and doughnut for breakfast provides no nutritional value," says Allan Magaziner, D.O., president of Magaziner Medical Center in Cherry

Hill, New Jersey. In fact, he says, junk food depletes the body of the B vitamins, which are essential to help our digestive system convert food to energy.

Prescriptions
FOR NATURAL ENERGY

Feel sluggish in the morning? Or, feel okay when you wake up but miserably tired by lunchtime? Can't stay awake after dinner? These simple prescriptions may help.

❐ Eat early. The sooner you eat the better, but if you just can't face food first thing in the morning, make sure that you sit down to a nutritious meal within three hours, says Judith J. Wurtman, Ph.D., a nutrition research scientist at the Massachusetts Institute of Technology in Cambridge and author of *Managing Your Mind and Mood through Food.* Eating helps your body rev up after a nighttime of sleeping, when your body is at rest and you're not putting forth any energy. Eating a good breakfast will also prevent you from eating too big a lunch, which can make you sluggish in the afternoon.

MORNING

❐ Start your day with foods rich in vitamins and minerals and other essentials. For breakfast, skip the ham and cheese on a croissant. Instead, focus on fresh fruit and low-fat or nonfat plain yogurt with a bran muffin, or fruit juice and a slice or two of whole-wheat toast topped with an ounce of low-fat cheese, such as skim-milk mozzarella, says Dr. Wurtman. An ounce of skim-milk mozzarella would be equal to one to two slices.

MORNING

❐ At midday, focus on protein. The amino acid tyrosine, supplied by high-protein food, synthesizes more of the brain's alertness chemicals and keeps the brain from manufacturing the neurotransmitter serotonin, which slows you down, Dr. Wurtman says. But don't overeat. And stick with low-fat, low-calorie meats and cheeses. For example, have between three and four ounces (about a hand's-width) of meat, poultry, seafood, tofu, or fish, or one cup nonfat yogurt or nonfat cottage cheese. Avoid creamy soups, fast-food fried hamburgers, fried vegetables, and cheesy potatoes.

DAYTIME

DAYTIME

❏ For afternoon slumps, try a carbohydrate/caffeine combination. A few ounces of a carbohydrate (for example, four small fig bars or three gingersnaps) eaten with a cup of coffee, hot chocolate, or diet cola between 3:30 and 4:30 P.M. will boost your mental energy for about six hours, Dr. Wurtman says. The reason that caffeine and carbohydrates work together so well is that while caffeine boosts your mental energy, the soothing effect of serotonin in carbohydrates allows you to settle down and refocus on your tasks for the rest of the day.

NIGHTTIME

❏ Nix caffeine after 4:30 P.M. Since caffeine keeps you alert for up to six hours, it can prevent you from getting to sleep at a regular time if you consume it in the evening, says Dr. Campbell. That's all caffeine—including chocolate, cola, and tea.

MONTHLY

❏ When you are menstruating, take special care of your nutrition. Make sure that you include good sources of iron, such as lean meat, poultry without skin, fortified cereals, and legumes. "These foods keep your energy up and prevent iron-deficiency anemia, which can tire you out," says Wahida Karmally, R.D., director of nutrition at the Irving Center for Clinical Research at Columbia-Presbyterian Medical Center in New York City.

❏ Supplement your diet. Most people don't get enough nutrition from food, Dr. Magaziner says. To store up your energy supply, he recommends a daily multivitamin/mineral supplement that includes 400 milligrams of magnesium, 15 milligrams of zinc, 400 micrograms of folic acid, 400 international units of vitamin E, 200 micrograms of chromium, and 50 milligrams of B-complex vitamins such as thiamin, riboflavin, niacin, B_6, and B_{12}.

Note: If you have heart or kidney problems, be sure to check with your doctor before you begin taking supplemental magnesium. Supplemental magnesium may cause diarrhea in some people.

TIME IT RIGHT

❏ Drink one glass of water every hour for eight hours. Dehydration can cause your performance to flag measurably. Drinking enough water—eight eight-ounce glasses a day—allows you to keep up your energy levels, says Wayne Askew, Ph.D., professor of nutrition and director of the division of foods and nutrition at the University of Utah in Salt Lake City.

Keeping a ready supply of water nearby throughout the day will encourage you to drink as much as you need, when you need it. Try leaving a quart bottle on your desk or taking a bike bottle with you in the car.

❏ Take a 20-minute walk after breakfast or by lunchtime. Repeat three to five times a week. Exercise will buoy up your energy as much as eight hours afterward, says Dr. Campbell. But don't exercise within several hours of bedtime, he cautions. You may be too energized to fall asleep.

TIME IT RIGHT

"Give exercise the same priority that you would any prescription medicine," says Barb Tobias, M.D., assistant professor of family medicine in the department of family medicine at the University of Cincinnati.

❏ In winter, get outdoors for 30 minutes a day. Seasonal affective disorder (SAD) is a condition marked by a loss of energy in the cold, dark winter months, says Brenda Byrne, Ph.D., director of the seasonal affective disorder program affiliated with the light research program at Jefferson Medical College in Philadelphia. SAD is often accompanied by depression, mood and appetite changes, and a tendency to withdraw and sleep a lot. But even people without SAD are often affected by the seasons and will respond to light, she says.

WINTERTIME

If you think that you are affected by the shortening of the days in the winter months, start by increasing your exposure to daylight at that time of the year, Dr. Byrne says. "Take a 30-minute walk first thing in the morning even if it's cold. Do it for a week and see if you feel more energetic. If you do, keep up your walking to maintain a higher energy level."

❏ Treat yourself. Sometimes, energy levels slump not so much because of how much you do but because you are expending so much for everyone but yourself. "So, give yourself a prescription to do something for yourself today—take a half-day off, get child care, and do something just for you," says Dr. Tobias.

A "Common-Scents" Prescription to Recharge Your Batteries

Is your energy spent by midday or early evening with no oomph to spare? Sit for 20 to 30 minutes in a warm or comfortably hot bath scented with one of the following essential oils: lavender, rosemary, pine, eucalyptus, or juniper. The overall effect will be one of relaxation and renewed energy, says Kathleen Maier, an herbalist and co-director of the Dreamtime Center for Herbal Studies in Flint Hill, Virginia.

"A relaxed system actually functions with greater energy and stamina," explains Maier. "These oils are stimulating in that they bring us back to our senses and help us to feel a general wellness."

If you are a newcomer to the benefits of essential oils, try lavender essential oil first. "Lavender is the safest, most universal bath, no matter what someone is needing. It helps reduce stress by quieting the mind and bringing mental clarity," says Maier. "Close the door to your bathroom so that you receive the full benefit of the aromatherapy from the steam in your bath. And be sure to remember that a few drops of essential oil go a long way."

Medical Alert

Occasional energy slumps are normal. Unrelenting fatigue is not. If four weeks have passed without improvement and nothing seems to restore your energy levels to your satisfaction, consult your doctor, says Peter Manu, M.D., director of medical services at the Hillside Hospital division of the Long Island Jewish Center in Hyde Park, New York.

Gas

Flatulence is funny—as long as it befalls someone else. Unfortunately, it tends to be an equal-opportunity deployer. Which means that every one of us has, on occasion, fallen victim to an odorous ill wind.

Most of the gas you pass is formed when undigested food makes its way into your colon and gets broken down by bacteria that live there, explains Michael Levitt, M.D., professor of medicine at the University of Minnesota School of Medicine and associate chief of staff for research at the Veterans Affairs Medical Center in Minneapolis. The process produces a bad-smelling brew that includes carbon dioxide, hydrogen, methane, and sulfur, with its distinctive rotten-egg aroma.

For many of us, flatulence is nothing more than an embarrassing annoyance. For others, it can actually cause discomfort and pain. The sheer volume of gas in their intestines leaves them feeling bloated.

Women pass gas an average of 12 times a day—the same as men. "But while women have slightly higher concentrations of odorous gases, men produce more gas per emission," says Dr. Levitt. In terms of volume, men release roughly four ounces per day, compared with women's three ounces.

Gender doesn't influence flatulence much, but eating style may. Carnivores tend to eat more protein than vegetarians, and protein is a major source of sulfur, one of the compounds in gas.

Prescriptions
TO DEFUSE FLATULENCE

Rx

While gas may be a normal state of affairs, you don't have to just grin and bear it. Try these tactics for prompt relief.

❏ Take two to four capsules of activated charcoal. Activated charcoal is considered a universal antidote because it absorbs whatever is in your intestines, including gas and food particles that might later form gas in your colon, says Michael DiPalma, N.D., a naturopathic doctor in private practice in Newtown, Pennsylvania. Ideally, you should take activated charcoal while you are eating a food that you know will give you problems later, but you can take it at the first sign of symptoms. You can buy activated charcoal in drugstores and health food stores.

❐ Chew one-half teaspoon fennel seeds. Fennel is a carminative, meaning that it helps dissipate or expel gas. "It helps to correct digestive disturbances such as gas by relaxing muscle spasms," explains Dr. DiPalma.

❐ Drink tea made from peppermint, ginger, or chamomile. Like fennel, these herbs are carminatives, according to Dr. DiPalma. To make the tea, steep one teaspoon dried herb in one cup freshly boiled water for approximately five minutes. Strain the tea and allow it to cool before drinking it.

❐ Engage in 5 to 15 minutes of physical activity such as yoga or walking immediately after eating. "Any physical activity assists the digestive process," says Dr. DiPalma.

TIME IT RIGHT   ❐ Lie down with your knees bent, then raise each knee in turn toward your chest until you feel relief. This exercise eases the pressure in your lower abdomen, according to Dr. DiPalma.

Rx ——— *Prescriptions*
TO CONTROL EMISSIONS

With a few adjustments in your eating habits, you can limit the frequency and severity of flatulence. Experts say that the following strategies yield the greatest gas-reducing benefits.

❐ Whenever you eat, chew each bite of food until it's liquefied. "The saliva in the mouth contains digestive enzymes that break down many foods," says Dr. DiPalma. "Even liquids should be 'chewed' before swallowing to start the digestive process." For people who eat fast, thoroughly chewing food takes some getting used to. But it really improves digestion. Eating in a relaxed atmosphere rather than in the car or at your desk can help.

❐ Season your meals with turmeric, cumin, and cardamom. All three spices aid digestion and help prevent gas, according to Dr. DiPalma. They are also ingredients in curry powder, a spice blend that's a trademark of Indian cuisine.

❐ Increase your fiber intake slowly. Eating more fiber is a good thing. In fact, you should be getting at least 25 grams a day—enough to meet the Daily Value. But if your intake has been on the low side and you start consuming large amounts of fiber, you could end up with big-time gas. Instead, take your time, advises Malcolm Robinson, M.D., director of the Oklahoma Foundation for Digestive Research at the University of Oklahoma Health Sciences Center in Oklahoma City. Start with less than 10 grams and add about 10 grams a week. That way, your intestines have a chance to adjust to your new, high-fiber diet. And you'll have less gas as a result.

❐ Monitor your reaction to dairy products. If you seem to develop gas whenever you drink milk or eat ice cream, you may be lactose intolerant, according to Dr. Robinson. That means your small intestine produces little or no lactase, an enzyme that's necessary to digest lactose, a sugar found in milk and milk products. Not all "moo foods" cause problems, however. Processed cheeses may tie your gut in knots because they are made with whey. (Whey has the highest concentration of lactose.) But aged cheeses such as Cheddar, blue, Roquefort, and Stilton may pass through without incident because the lactose has already been broken down or removed.

Since dairy products are such an important source of bone-building calcium, think twice about giving them up completely. Instead, you can make them more digestible with the help of a lactase supplement such as Lactaid or Dairy Ease. Or look for lactose-reduced milk, which is widely available in supermarkets. Yogurt has its own lactase if it contains active yogurt cultures.

❐ Identify other gas-producing foods in your diet. Ironically, many of the healthiest foods are also the gassiest: broccoli, brussels sprouts, cabbage, cauliflower, corn, eggplant, garlic, onions, and radishes. If fruit causes you problems, try eating it by itself rather than with other foods, suggests Dr. DiPalma. For some people, combining protein, which is digested in

De-Breezing Beans

Beans are far too healthy to exclude from your diet, says Michael DiPalma, N.D., a naturopathic doctor in private practice in Newtown, Pennsylvania. But their reputation as the musical food may make you a little leery of them. You can take some of the wind out of beans' sails with these tips.

❏ Choose thin-skinned beans that contain less of the indigestible carbohydrates that cause gas, such as anasazi beans and black beans. Bypass kidney beans and other pink beans.

❏ Choose canned beans rather than dried. The canned variety has already been thoroughly cooked. Undercooked beans are more likely to produce gas. Just be sure to rinse canned beans well since the liquid that they are packed in contains a lot of salt.

❏ If you do use dried beans, soak them overnight, then cook them until they are practically melting in their liquid.

❏ Add a few drops of Beano to your beans before eating them. Beano contains enzymes that break down the carbohydrates and proteins in beans. You can buy Beano in drugstores and health food stores.

the intestines, with vegetables or complex carbohydrates, which start digesting in the mouth, can create havoc.

Other potential intestinal offenders include the artificial sweeteners sorbitol, mannitol, and even aspartame (NutraSweet). Any of these can cause gas pain in some people, says Dr. Robinson.

❏ If you take vitamin C supplements, be aware of your bowel tolerance. Some people develop gas and diarrhea when they take too-large doses of vitamin C. If this happens to you, simply reduce your dose until your symptoms subside, recommends Andrew Weil, M.D., director of the integrative medicine program at the University of Arizona College of Medicine in Tucson and best-selling health book author. You may find that you can take the same amount of vitamin C daily, as long as you divide it into smaller doses—say, 400 milligrams twice a day instead of 800 milligrams all at once.

❐ Look for a product that can restore beneficial bacteria to your intestines, such as Megadopholus. These products are available in the refrigerated section of health food stores, usually in powder or capsule form. Once in your intestines, they supply good bacteria, which then multiply to crowd out bad bacteria, says Dr. DiPalma. The good bacteria improve the digestive process, so gas is less likely to form. Follow the suggested dosage on the label.

Medical **Alert**

From a medical perspective, gas is usually nothing to worry about. Still, you should see your doctor if gas hangs around for more than three days and is accompanied by severe stomach or abdominal pain or unexplained weight loss, says Dr. Robinson.

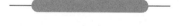

Gum Disease

It turns the pearliest of pearly whites a dingy shade of yellow. But plaque saves its dirtiest work for your gums. In fact, it's the number one cause of gum disease, which is responsible for at least 80 percent of dental problems in adults.

Plaque is actually a thin, sticky film of bacteria that forms on and between your teeth and under your gum line. If you don't brush and floss this film away, it hardens into a substance called tartar (also known as calculus). Tartar can irritate your gums, causing them to swell and bleed. This soreness is usually the first sign of gingivitis, an early stage of gum disease.

(continued on page 80)

A Prescription for Mouth Maintenance

Experts agree that your best weapon against gum disease is good oral hygiene. That means brushing and flossing regularly, using the following strategies.

BRUSHING BASICS

❏ Choose the best brush. Many dentists think that electric brushes do a better job because of their quick, short, vibrating strokes. Whether you opt for electric or manual, be sure it has soft bristles, says Flora Parsa Stay, D.D.S., a dentist in Oxnard, California, and author of *The Complete Book of Dental Remedies*. Also be sure the handle allows you to maneuver the brush easily.

❏ Brush after every meal. The sooner you clean up those food particles lingering in your mouth, the less opportunity bacteria have to grow and thrive there, explains Dr. Stay.

❏ Take your time. A good toothbrushing lasts about three minutes, Dr. Stay says.

❏ Choose a brushing technique that you are comfortable with. Any of the following is acceptable, Dr. Stay says.

PROPER BRUSHING TECHNIQUE

Place the brush at a 45-degree angle to the length of the tooth. Then gently vibrate the brush at the gum line and on the surface of the tooth.

Place the brush at the gum line and roll or sweep it toward the top of the tooth.

Rotate the brush in a circular motion on the gum line and tooth surface.

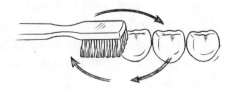

❏ First brush the outside surfaces of your upper and lower teeth, starting with your back teeth on one side and working your way around to the other side. Then brush the inside surfaces of your upper and lower teeth. Finish by brushing the chewing surfaces. Always follow the same sequence, Dr. Stay advises.

❏ Brush gently but thoroughly, no matter which technique you choose. Too-rough brushing could actually damage your teeth and gums, Dr. Stay says. It wears away the enamel, exposes the dentin (the inside of the tooth), and traumatizes the gums, causing them to recede.

❏ Store your brush in a solution of either hydrogen peroxide or rubbing alcohol to keep it sterile and bacteria-free, Dr. Stay suggests. Rinse your brush before using it, and replace the solution when it gets cloudy.

❏ Replace a manual brush every month—or sooner if the bristles begin to bend or fray, Dr. Stay says.

❏ Invest in a new brush when you have had a cold or another respiratory infection. The bristles may still harbor the virus that made you sick in the first place, Dr. Stay explains.

FIRST-RATE FLOSSING
❏ If you floss only once a day, do it at bedtime. This helps prevent plaque from building up overnight, when your saliva flow slows down and your mouth becomes especially vulnerable to bacteria, says Heidi Hausauer, D.D.S., assistant clinical professor in the department of operative dentistry at the University of the Pacific in San Francisco and spokesperson for the Academy of General Dentistry.

❏ Pick the right floss for you, advises Dr. Stay. If you have rough fillings or if your teeth are very close together, waxed

(continued)

A Prescription for Mouth Maintenance—Continued

floss works best. Unwaxed floss is thinner than waxed, but it also frays more readily. If your teeth are widely spaced or if you have a hard time flossing, dental tape is a good choice.

❐ Floss correctly. If you are unsure about proper technique, follow these steps recommended by Dr. Stay.

1. Tear off a strand of floss about 18 inches long. Wrap the ends around the middle fingers of both hands until just 6 to 8 inches of floss is exposed.

2. Pinch the floss between the thumb and index finger of one hand. With the index finger of your other hand, guide about one inch of floss between your teeth.

3. Using a back-and-forth motion, slowly and gently move the floss up and down between your teeth.

4. Curve the floss around the base of one tooth. Gently move the floss back and forth under the gum line.

5. To remove the floss, use the same back-and-forth motion to bring it up and away from your teeth. Never snap or force the floss, or you might bruise delicate gum tissue.

❐ If you have difficulty holding and maneuvering the floss with your fingers, try a floss holder, suggests Dr. Stay. You will find them in supermarkets and drugstores.

LIFETIME

A woman's chances of developing gingivitis increase during pregnancy, says Heidi Hausauer, D.D.S., assistant clinical professor in the -department of operative dentistry and spokesman for the Academy of General Dentistry at the University of the Pacific in San Francisco.

The teeth and gums are most vulnerable to problems during the first trimester, which is why you should see your dentist as soon as you know you are pregnant, adds Dominick DePaola, D.D.S., Ph.D., president and dean of Baylor College of Dentistry in Dallas.

What's behind the rise in risk? Experts believe it has something to do with the female hormone estrogen. While changes in estrogen levels can affect your dental health while you are menstruating and if you take birth control pills, they seem to wreak the most havoc when you are pregnant. The hormones that prepare the uterine tissue for pregnancy can also have a great impact on gum tissue by making it more susceptible to irritation by bacterial plaque, explains Dr. Hausauer.

During pregnancy, gums can become sore and sensitive or bleed easily. When that happens, women ease up on brushing and flossing. And that's not helpful, says Peg Terp, dental hygienist supervisor for the Seattle–King County Department of Public Health. Bacteria can multiply, increasing problems. What started as minor gum irritation can evolve into full-scale gingivitis.

Left untreated, gingivitis can lead to periodontitis, a condition characterized by severely receding gums and destruction of the jawbone, which anchors your teeth in place, says Flora Parsa Stay, D.D.S., a dentist in Oxnard, California, and author of *The Complete Book of Dental Remedies*. But gum disease doesn't have to get nearly that far. You can keep your teeth and gums in the pink, mainly by brushing and flossing thoroughly and frequently and by seeing your dentist every six months for a professional cleaning and an exam.

Prescriptions
TO SOOTHE SORE GUMS

Rx

If, despite your best efforts at mouth maintenance, your gums bleed each time you brush, pick up the phone and call your dentist's office for an appointment. Until she can squeeze you in for an appointment, try these tips for temporary relief.

❐ Rinse your mouth with a 3 percent hydrogen peroxide solution. Hydrogen peroxide (available in drugstores or supermarkets) helps destroy bacteria and clean gum tissue, according to Dr. Stay. Don't use the solution for more than three days in a row, however. It may damage delicate gum tissue.

❐ Avoid spicy foods such as chili and Buffalo wings. They will only irritate your already inflamed gums.

❐ Steer clear of candy, baked goods, and other sweets. Bacteria—including the kind that form plaque—thrive on sugar, explains Dr. Stay.

❐ Switch to a toothpaste that contains aloe vera and baking soda. (One brand, Grace, is available in many health food stores.) It is gentler on your gum tissue than many commercial toothpastes, which contain harsh chemicals, says Dr. Stay.

❐ Prepare your own toothpaste by mixing one tablespoon of the herb goldenseal with enough water to form a paste. Then brush your teeth as you normally would. Goldenseal (which is available in health food stores) can help heal inflamed, diseased gums, Dr. Stay explains.

❐ Use an alcohol-free mouthwash. A product that contains alcohol can irritate and dry your gum tissue. So before you buy, check the label to see whether alcohol is an ingredient, advises Dr. Stay.

❐ Take 60 milligrams of coenzyme Q_{10} every day for as long as your gums are inflamed and bleeding. A natural compound, coenzyme Q_{10} is chemically similar to vitamin E and shares E's antioxidant properties. It helps treat gum disease by increasing the flow of oxygen to cells. You will find coenzyme Q_{10} supplements in health food stores.

HERBAL
Rx ———

Prescriptions
for Healing

Certain herbs have medicinal properties that are effective in easing aching gums. Dr. Stay recommends the following herbal preparations to her patients.

❐ Sip a soothing tea made from a mixture of anise and sage. To prepare the tea, Dr. Stay says, add two tablespoons of each dried herb (available in health food stores) to one cup freshly boiled water. Steep for 10 minutes, then strain the tea and drink up. You can use the tea as needed for relief.

❐ Consume garlic, which Dr. Stay calls nature's antibiotic. It helps fight plaque-forming bacteria, which means that they are less likely to set up shop in your mouth. You can increase your intake of fresh garlic simply by adding it to most of your meals. Worried about garlic breath? Then take supplements instead—250 milligrams a day, suggests Dr. Stay.

Prescriptions
to Keep Gums Healthy

Along with regular, thorough brushing and flossing, proper nutrition is essential to good dental health, says Dr. Stay. A balanced diet does its part to keep your teeth and gums in A1 condition. A number of nutritional supplements can help, too.

❐ Boost your intake of vitamin C to 500 milligrams a day. This nutrient not only keeps your gums healthy but also helps them heal properly after tooth extraction or surgery, Dr. Stay explains. In fact, a vitamin C deficiency can lead to bleeding gums and gingivitis, which may cause teeth to become loose and even fall out. Fresh fruits and vegetables, including citrus fruits such as oranges, are good sources of vitamin C. If you opt for a supplement, avoid the chewable vitamin C tablets. They can promote tooth decay by leaving acid residue on your teeth, says Dr. Stay.

❐ If you are between ages 19 and 50, make sure that you are getting 1,000 milligrams of calcium a day. Women need this mineral to help prevent osteoporosis, which can cause bones—including the jawbone—to become brittle, according to Dr. Hausauer.

❐ Aim for at least 750 milligrams of magnesium a day. Magnesium helps your body use calcium properly and so plays an important role in maintaining healthy bones, including the jawbone, according to Dr. Stay. If you prefer to get your magnesium from foods rather than supplements, spinach, brown rice, and baked potatoes are all good sources of the mineral.

Note: If you have heart or kidney problems, be sure to check with your doctor before you begin taking supplemental magnesium. Also, if you experience diarrhea when taking these supplements, cut back your dosage until your symptoms subside.

❐ Make sure that you are getting the Daily Value of zinc, which is 15 milligrams. According to Dr. Stay, zinc fights gum disease in two ways: It helps build new immune cells, and it supports the production of collagen, the connective tissue needed to heal "wounded" gums.

❐ Limit your intake of vitamin A. While A is essential for good oral health—it helps maintain the mucous membranes inside your mouth—

too much can cause gingivitis as well as mouth ulcers and cracked lips, Dr. Stay says. If you take vitamin A supplements for any reason, keep your daily dose below 15,000 international units (IU), or 10,000 IU if you're pregnant. Higher amounts should be taken only with medical supervision. Beta-carotene, which your body converts to vitamin A, doesn't appear to have these side effects even in high doses.

Medical **Alert**

See your dentist immediately if you notice any redness or soreness in your gums, if your gums bleed when you brush and floss your teeth, or if you have unrelenting tooth pain, Dr. Hausauer says. And if you find out that you're pregnant, make an appointment with your dentist as soon as possible.

In fact, if you're considering becoming pregnant, Dr. Hausauer suggests seeing your dentist first. A cleaning can help prevent gingivitis during pregnancy. And taking care of dental problems can eliminate the need for involved dental procedures during the first trimester.

Heartburn

Stomach acid is about as caustic as the acid used in car batteries. As long as it stays in your stomach, though, it does no harm. Your stomach's lining is specially designed to withstand the potent gastric juices essential to the digestion of food.

But once in a while some factor prompts stomach acid to make a trip north, into your esophagus. You feel it as an uncomfortable burning sensation that begins behind your breastbone and seems to move upward, toward your throat. That's heartburn, or, in medical terms, acid reflux.

LIFETIME

Heartburn often results from what you ate or, just as likely, from how much you ate. Smoking and drinking can increase risk, as can being severely overweight. Pregnancy plays a role as well. In fact, about 25 percent of all moms-to-be experience heartburn, as hormonal changes cause the gastroesophageal sphincter muscle—the gatekeeping muscle situated at the end of the esophagus—to relax. This allows stomach acid to splash into the esophagus.

New medicines, such as Zantac and Pepcid, promise to prevent heartburn by inhibiting the production of excess stomach acid. They are available in both over-the-counter and prescription strengths. Antacids still reign as the over-the-counter treatment of choice. Still, you don't have to rely on drugs for relief.

Prescriptions
to Douse the Flames Fast

Rx

When you feel as though a bonfire is blazing in your belly, let natural remedies put out the fire for you. The following have been found to be especially effective in treating heartburn.

❒ Chew gum. This tactic relieves heartburn in two ways. "For starters, when you chew gum, you produce saliva. Since saliva is alkaline, it counteracts the acidity in your esophagus," says Swarnjit Singh, M.D., a gastroenterologist in private practice in Scottsdale, Arizona. "Plus, swallowing saliva triggers a downward muscular wave that pushes acid back into your stomach." Any kind of gum will do the trick, he adds.

❒ Loosen or remove tight clothing such as bras, girdles, and control-top panty hose. These garments put the squeeze on your innards and make acid reflux more likely, says Dr. Singh.

❒ Walk rather than lie down. "Lying down is the worst thing that you can do for heartburn," explains Dr. Singh. "You want to get gravity on your side in order to clear any acid from your esophagus. To do that, you should be on your feet and moving around." Staying mobile is especially helpful after a big meal, he adds.

Prescriptions
to Spurn the Burn

Rx

Once you have had a bout of heartburn, no doubt you'll want to avoid a recurrence. The following mealtime evasive maneuvers can help.

❒ Eat slowly. When you gulp down food, you swallow a lot of air. The air distends your stomach and leads to belching and acid backwash, according to Douglas Drossman, M.D., professor of medicine and psy-

Time It Right

chiatry in the division of digestive diseases at the University of North Carolina at Chapel Hill. He instructs people to become aware of how fast they eat. To help you do that, you may want to try counting the number of times you chew each bite or putting down your fork between bites. "The main thing is to remain focused on the process of eating," he says.

TIME IT RIGHT

❏ Stop eating when you start to feel full, not when you have no room for another bite. This may seem obvious, yet people often continue stuffing their faces long after their stomachs have had enough—especially in social situations. Overeat in this way, and you're just begging for heartburn, says Malcolm Robinson, M.D., director of the Oklahoma Foundation for Digestive Research at the University of Oklahoma Health Sciences Center in Oklahoma City.

NIGHTTIME

❏ Eat your last meal of the day no less than two hours before bedtime. Otherwise, the food hits your stomach at just about the time you lie down, which means stomach acid is likely to slosh back into your esophagus. "Damage to the esophagus most often occurs overnight, while you sleep," notes Dr. Singh.

❏ Limit your daily intake of dietary fat to 25 percent of calories. "The more fat a meal contains, the slower the meal leaves your stomach," explains Dr. Robinson. "This increases the likelihood that all gastric contents, including stomach acid, will find their way into your esophagus."

MEALTIME

❏ Drink no more than one cup of fluid with a meal. While fluid can be beneficial by diluting the acidic contents of your stomach, it can also cause them to liquefy so that they easily splash into your esophagus. Limiting your intake of fluids at mealtimes prevents your stomach from becoming overfilled, according to Michael DiPalma, N.D., a naturopathic doctor in private practice in Newtown, Pennsylvania. Unfortunately, some people have problems no matter how little they drink.

❏ Skip the coffee. Caffeine stimulates the production of stomach acid, whether or not you drink it with a meal, explains Dr. Robinson. It may also relax the gastroesophageal sphincter muscle, the muscle that helps keep stomach acid in its place.

And if you think that drinking decaf will solve the problem, keep in

Herbal Prescriptions to Banish the Burn

Prone to heartburn? You can reduce the frequency and severity of flare-ups with the following herbal remedies, recommended by Michael DiPalma, N.D., a naturopathic doctor in private practice in Newtown, Pennsylvania. You'll find these herbs in health food stores.

❒ Take marsh mallow root, plantain, or slippery elm immediately after each meal. All are available in tablet or tea form. "These herbs are demulcents, which means that they coat mucous membranes. This lessens the corrosive effects of stomach acid and promotes healing," explains Dr. DiPalma.

❒ Take two tablets or capsules of deglycyrrhizinated licorice root 15 minutes before each meal. Deglycyrrhizinated licorice root stimulates the cells that line the stomach to produce mucus. The mucus then protects your stomach against its own acidic juices and reduces the acidity if you have a reflux reaction.

mind that some people report heartburn even when they switch. Decaffeinated coffee still contains tannic acid, which irritates the lining of the esophagus.

❒ Bypass the after-dinner mints and chocolates, too. Like caffeine, mint and chocolate relax the gastroesophageal sphincter muscle, allowing stomach acid to escape into the esophagus, says Dr. Robinson.

Prescriptions
to Stay Heartburn-Free

Beyond your eating habits, other lifestyle factors can influence your susceptibility to heartburn. Experts recommend the following to reduce your risk.

❏ Give up smoking and drinking—or at the very least, curtail your indulgences. As with caffeine, chocolate, and mint, nicotine and alcohol may relax the gastroesophageal sphincter muscle, the muscle that confines acid to your stomach. "Plus, the deep inhalations associated with smoking act as a siphon, drawing stomach acid up into your esophagus," says Dr. Robinson.

NIGHTTIME

❏ Raise the head of your bed four to six inches. This tactic positions your body in such a way that you're less likely to experience nighttime acid reflux, even though you are lying down, explains Dr. Singh. To do this safely, cut a four- by four-inch piece of wood so that it matches the width of your bed. Nail jar caps onto the wood, positioning them far enough apart that the legs or casters of your headboard fit in them. The caps hold the legs or casters in place, so your bed won't slide off the wood during the night.

NIGHTTIME

❏ As an alternative to raising the head of your bed, use a wedge-shaped support to elevate just the upper half of your body while you sleep. Don't use extra pillows that raise only your head because that will not help prevent reflux, says Dr. Singh.

Medical **Alert**

See your doctor if you experience heartburn more than twice a week, advises Dr. Singh. Chronic heartburn is one of the symptoms of gastroesophageal reflux. Left untreated, gastroesophageal reflux can cause asthmalike symptoms, bleeding in the esophagus, and possibly cancer of the esophagus.

Also see your doctor if your heartburn is accompanied by difficulty swallowing or the feeling that food is getting stuck at the end of your throat. You may have scar tissue on your gastroesophageal sphincter muscle, says Dr. Singh.

Hemorrhoids

According to the folks who count such things, more than 75 percent of us develop hemorrhoids at some point during our lives. These painful protuberances occur when veins stretch and weaken, causing them to bulge outward. Often hemorrhoids show up in and around the anus, where you can see and feel them. But they can also affect the rectum, where they are tucked out of sight.

Anything that produces pressure inside your abdomen can, over time, lead to hemorrhoids. Constipation—with its accompanying straining and pushing—is among the most common causes, according to David E. Beck, M.D., chairman of the department of colon and rectal surgery at the Ochsner Clinic in New Orleans. Overweight is also a contributing factor, as are heavy lifting and just plain sitting around too much.

Pregnancy can also increase a woman's odds of developing hemorrhoids. The intense pushing during delivery can make anal veins pop out, explains Dr. Beck.

LIFETIME

Hemorrhoids tend to announce their presence with a painless streak of blood on toilet paper or drops of blood in the toilet, usually after a bowel movement. Other symptoms to watch for include itching and burning.

Rectal bleeding can also be a sign of other common anal problems, such as fissures, abscesses, polyps, and even cancer. That's why you shouldn't just assume that you have hemorrhoids, says Debra Ford, M.D., chief of the division of general surgery and head of the section for colon and rectal surgery at Howard University Hospital in Washington, D.C. You should always have rectal bleeding checked out by your doctor, she advises.

Prescriptions
FOR IMMEDIATE RELIEF

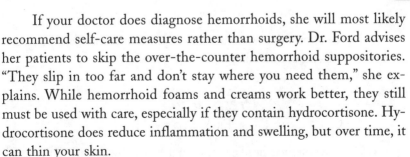

Rx

If your doctor does diagnose hemorrhoids, she will most likely recommend self-care measures rather than surgery. Dr. Ford advises her patients to skip the over-the-counter hemorrhoid suppositories. "They slip in too far and don't stay where you need them," she explains. While hemorrhoid foams and creams work better, they still must be used with care, especially if they contain hydrocortisone. Hydrocortisone does reduce inflammation and swelling, but over time, it can thin your skin.

So what options do you have? If you are looking to stop the pain and itching, experts recommend the following tactics.

TIME IT RIGHT ❏ Lie facedown with a pillow under your stomach for 15 minutes two or three times a day to elevate your hemorrhoids higher than your heart. "This helps reduce blood flow to the anal area, which decreases swelling," explains Dr. Beck.

❏ Avoid lying on your back or sitting for long periods of time. Both positions can aggravate hemorrhoids, according to Dr. Beck. When you lie on your back, your hemorrhoids are below the level of your heart. Consequently, blood flows to that area, which increases swelling.

TIME IT RIGHT ❏ Put a wet washcloth in the freezer until it freezes, then apply it to the anal area for 10 minutes. Repeat as often as necessary over the next 24 hours to relieve pain, suggests Dr. Beck. Cold treatments seem to work especially well if you have a thrombosed hemorrhoid—that is, a hemorrhoid marked by an exquisitely tender lump at the edge of your anus.

TIME IT RIGHT ❏ Sit in a bathtub of comfortably hot water for 10 to 15 minutes, three times a day. Draw your knees toward your chest so that the water can reach the anal area. Heat works better than cold for chronic hemorrhoids characterized by swelling and dull pain, says Dr. Beck.

❏ Some experts recommend shallow baths, or sitz baths, for the treatment of hemorrhoids. But Dr. Beck believes that the depth of the water doesn't matter, as long as your anal area is submerged. Do skip bath additives such as Epsom salts, though. They just irritate your hemorrhoids, according to Dr. Ford.

❏ Use a cotton ball to dab cornstarch onto protruding hemorrhoids two to three times a day. The cornstarch absorbs moisture and keeps the anal area dry, which prevents irritation, explains Dr. Beck.

❏ As an alternative to cornstarch, try a zinc oxide–based powder such as Gold Bond or any other antifungal powder.

Rx ——— *Prescriptions*
FOR PAIN-FREE POTTY TIME

If you have hemorrhoids, you may dread nature's call. Of course, you can't ignore it either. The following tips can help you make peace with the potty until your hemorrhoids heal. (And if you don't have hemorrhoids, these strategies may help stop them from forming in the first place.)

❏ Sit on the toilet only when you feel the urge to move your bowels. Never force yourself to go, which puts tremendous pressure on hemorrhoids. "Besides, if you're getting enough fiber and fluids in your diet, you won't have to sit and push," notes Dr. Ford.

❏ Refrain from using your bathroom as your library. "Spending too much time on the toilet is hard on your hemorrhoids," says Dr. Ford. "Yet so many people do it that I tell my patients to keep reading material out of the bathroom altogether." If your bathroom truly is the only place in your house where you can enjoy peace and quiet, at least put the lid down on the toilet before you sit on it.

❏ When you do move your bowels, gently wipe the anal area using unscented white toilet paper moistened with water. Then pat the area dry. You can aggravate hemorrhoids by wiping too vigorously, especially if you use a cloth-based product such as a wet wipe, says Dr. Beck.

❏ Instead of wiping with toilet paper, squirt the anal area with water from a squeeze or pump bottle, then pat dry. This technique is less likely to irritate sensitive anal tissues, according to Dr. Beck.

Prescriptions
to Avoid Hemorrhoids

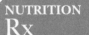
NUTRITION
Rx

While hemorrhoids are quite common, they are also quite preventable. You can give them the slip simply by increasing your fiber intake. Fiber makes stools easy to pass, which in turn makes hemorrhoids a thing of the past. "Ideally, your bowel movements should have the texture and consistency of cottage cheese," says Dr. Beck. The following dietary strategies can get you there.

❏ Eat enough fiber-rich foods every day to meet the Daily Value of 25 grams. That means plenty of whole-grain breads and cereals as well as beans, fruits, and vegetables. "I always give my patients a list of good fiber sources," says Dr. Ford. "Otherwise, they think they can eat nothing but lettuce and still get the fiber they need." In fact, one cup shredded iceberg lettuce contains less than one gram of fiber. By comparison, a half-cup cooked great Northern beans supplies more than six grams of fiber. As for the whole grains, choose breads and cereals that provide three to five grams of fiber per serving, recommends Dr. Ford.

❑ Take one or two doses of a fiber supplement containing psyllium (as in Metamucil and Konsyl) or methylcellulose (as in Citrucel or Cologel) every day. You will want to base the quantity and timing of your doses on the frequency and consistency of your stool. A total of 10 to 15 grams of supplemental fiber a day is usually adequate.

Both psyllium and methylcellulose are forms of fiber that absorb water. "The fiber in stool forms a gelatinous mass that keeps it soft, bulky, and easy to pass," says Dr. Beck. "Stools move through the intestines more easily, which means less straining."

You may have to try different doses and types of fiber until you find one that's right for you. "The amount you take doesn't really matter, as long as you're having bowel movements that don't irritate your hemorrhoids," says Dr. Beck.

❑ Drink at least eight eight-ounce glasses of water a day. "If you become dehydrated, your body draws water out of the feces in your intestines," explains Dr. Beck. "This makes the feces rock-hard and painfully difficult to pass."

And since soluble fiber requires fluid to do its job, you can become quite stopped up if you are taking a fiber supplement but not drinking enough water, adds Dr. Ford.

Medical **Alert**

If you notice any rectal bleeding, don't assume that you have hemorrhoids, cautions Dr. Ford. You should make an appointment with your doctor so that she can rule out other causes of bleeding. And you should go back to your doctor if self-help measures don't improve your symptoms within four to six weeks or if your symptoms worsen. Your doctor may need to remove the hemorrhoid with a simple in-office procedure.

Sometimes hemorrhoids become thrombosed, or clotted, which makes them very painful. If this happens to you, your doctor can likely remove the clot—or the entire hemorrhoid. Removing the external hemorrhoid is the treatment of choice, since removing only the clot can lead to a recurrence.

Post-Workout Soreness

You'd think a body would learn: You venture outside to dig out your garden in April, and the next day, you feel stiff and sore. You finally get to the gym after procrastinating for months. And now you are hobbling. Your legs and arms feel as if they are going to fall off—or you wish they would.

Relax. "Some soreness is perfectly normal," says Barbara Yawn, M.D., director of research at the Olmsted Medical Center in Rochester, Minnesota. "As long as it's not screaming pain, a little tenderness is okay, not a sign to back off."

In fact, you can even time it. "The 'boot-camp period' seems to last about two weeks," says Lynn Van Ost, a physical therapist and sports medicine specialist at the Jefferson Sports Medicine Center in Philadelphia. "If you have never exercised before or are just getting back into it, figure that for two weeks, you'll ache all over."

Though men and women both experience post-workout soreness, women often ache more if they use machines to try to strengthen their upper body muscles, says Karen Rucker, M.D., chairman of the department of physical medicine and rehabilitation at Virginia Commonwealth University in Richmond. That's because workout machines are designed for men, who often have as much as 85 percent more muscle fiber than women.

Some women experience muscle soreness when they menstruate, Dr. Rucker says. Though no one is entirely sure why that is, experts believe that monthly hormonal changes can make your joints less flexible.

Monthly

LIFETIME

Our muscles are also more likely to be prone to soreness as we age, because our body tissues become progressively less flexible, says Dr. Rucker. By age 35, you may find that you need to do more warmup and cooldown activities to prevent soreness than when you were sweet 16.

Rx ——— *Prescriptions*
TO SOOTHE SELF-INFLICTED BATTERY

You felt so proud of yourself for working out or raking the leaves—at the time. And you didn't feel sore at all. Often, post-workout soreness is a delayed reaction. It may not be till the next morning or even the day after that you'll feel as if you went through a 10-round boxing match. If you are uncomfortably sore, try the following prescriptions.

❏ Taper off. If you have been hard at work, it's tempting to collapse into a chair afterward. To stay limber, continue the exercise in moderation—that is, not so intensely that you break into a sweat or feel sharp pain. For example, if your legs are sore, slowly walk around the block, increasing your pace as the soreness or stiffness decreases, advises Dr. Yawn.

❏ Stretch each muscle group slowly and methodically. Focus on the calves, quadriceps, hamstrings, groin, hips, chest, arms, neck, and shoulders. Stretching after exercise reduces soreness by breaking the cycle of muscle contraction and decreased blood flow that leads to a painful buildup of lactic acid in your muscles. When you stretch, you send more blood flowing through your muscles, which helps to spread the lactic acid more evenly through your body, explains Dr. Yawn.

❏ To help prevent cramping, gently massage the painful area yourself or get someone else to do so, Dr. Yawn says.

TIME IT RIGHT

❏ Put a bag of ice right on whatever part of you feels sore. And do it as soon as possible, advises Van Ost. If you know that you are going to be working out at a gym where they might not have ice, think ahead. Take along a small cooler filled with ice and resealable plastic bags. Then, you have an ice bag at your fingertips whenever you need it. Wrap the bag of ice in a damp cloth and apply it for no more than 10 minutes at a time.

❐ Use ice when you eat. If you work out in the afternoon, ice your sore limbs then, again at dinnertime, with your bedtime snack, and when you eat breakfast the next morning, says Van Ost.

Prescriptions
FOR SORENESS

HOMEOPATHIC Rx

According to practitioners, homeopathy works a little like a vaccine: A nontoxic dose of a natural substance—usually a plant or mineral—that causes symptoms like those that ail you may actually cure you. Large doses of the daisylike plant arnica, for example, may make you feel as though you have a sprain or injury if you take it when you're not bruised and sore, says Jacquelyn Wilson, M.D., a health-care consultant in homeopathy in Escondido, California. But if you feel as though you just ran a marathon or if you haven't worked your muscles in a long time, an extremely dilute amount of Arnica will help your bruises and soreness heal faster.

❐ Put three pellets of Arnica under your tongue as soon as you can after exertion and let them dissolve. Repeat every few hours until your soreness subsides, says John Collins, N.D., a naturopathic physician who is board-certified in homeopathy, associate professor of homeopathy at the National College of Naturopathic Medicine, and co-owner of Rockwood Natural Medicine Clinic, both in Portland, Oregon. Arnica is available in pellet form in 6C to 30C potencies at health food stores and drugstores. (These potencies are standard measurements in homeopathy and should be listed on the label.)

❐ Try a homeopathic preparation called Sportenine. Available in health food stores, Sportenine contains arnica, zinc, and lactic acid in lozenge form. Dr. Collins recommends taking one lozenge before and one lozenge after your workout. If you are having an intense workout, you may even benefit from taking one during a rest period, he says.

❐ Rub an over-the-counter homeopathic ointment containing arnica on your sore muscles. Dr. Collins suggests Traumeel, a product available in health food stores and some drugstores. Massage the ointment into

(continued on page 102)

Warmup and Cooldown Stretches

Preparing your muscles for exertion—and coddling them afterward—will prevent soreness. To warm up, jog in place for 5 minutes and then stretch for 5 to 20 minutes, depending on the length and intensity of your workout and your age, says Karen Rucker, M.D., chairman of the department of physical medicine and rehabilitation at Virginia Commonwealth University in Richmond. Some people may need to warm up longer and stop to stretch during a workout as well as before cooling off completely.

Stretch the muscles that you are actually going to use while you exercise. "If you're going to go out for a jog, stretch your calves, quadriceps, hamstrings, and groin muscles, not your arms," advises Dr. Rucker. And pay special attention to any muscles that you have previously injured, she adds.

The following stretches can help prepare the major muscle groups for activity. At the very least, spend 30 to 60 seconds on each stretch and repeat each one twice, says Dr. Rucker. Then repeat the entire stretching sequence after your workout.

QUADRICEPS STRETCH

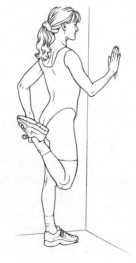

Stand on your left foot, touching a chair or wall with your right hand for support. Bend your right knee and grab your right foot with your left hand. Gently pull your right foot up behind you so that your heel presses against your buttocks. Keep your upper body upright to maximize the stretch. Hold, then repeat with your left leg.

CALF STRETCH

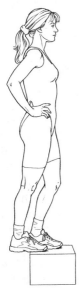
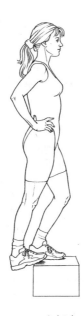

Stand on a step with your left leg slightly bent and your hands on your hips. Look straight ahead and slide your right foot behind you until you feel your heel protruding over the edge of the step.

Drop your right heel below the level of the step until you feel a stretch. Hold, then repeat with your left heel.

You can also stretch a higher part of the Achilles tendon if you do this stretch with your right knee slightly bent.

(continued)

Warmup and Cooldown Stretches—Continued

HAMSTRING STRETCH

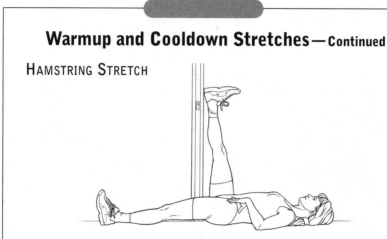

To stretch the muscles at the back of your upper leg, lie on the floor in a doorway so that you can keep your left leg straight on the floor. Bend your right leg and raise it above you, leaving 3 to 5 inches between the back of your thigh and the wall. Rest your foot on the wall and then straighten your leg by moving your foot up the wall until just your heel is touching it. Make sure to arch your lower back and rest your hands on your hipbones so that your hips are even with the rest of your body. (If one hip is higher than the other, your hamstring muscles won't get as good a stretch as they should.) Hold. Repeat on the other side of the doorway with your left leg. Stop if you notice your feet starting to fall asleep. And get up very slowly after completing this stretch, or you might feel lightheaded.

GROIN STRETCH

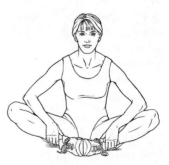

To stretch your groin, sit on the floor with your legs bent butterfly-style, the soles of your feet pressed together. Gently press your knees toward the floor with your hands or elbows and feel the stretch along your inner thigh muscles. Hold.

Hip Stretch

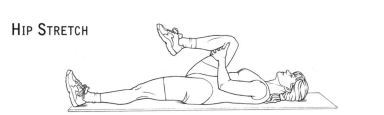

Lie on your back with your legs straight. Clasp your hands together behind your upper right thigh and pull your right knee toward your chest while keeping your back flat. Hold, then return to the starting position before repeating with your left leg.

Lower Back Stretch

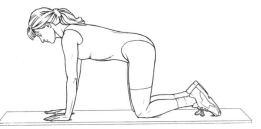

Get on all fours, with your hands directly under your shoulders and your knees below your hips.

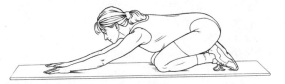

Without repositioning your hands, sit back onto your heels so that your arms are outstretched and you feel a stretch along your back. Hold.

(continued)

Warmup and Cooldown Stretches—Continued

NECK STRETCH

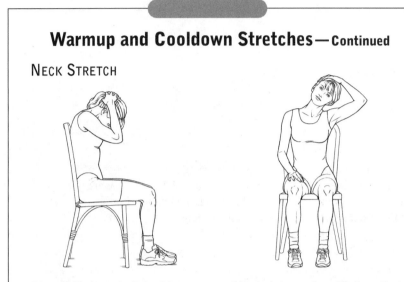

Sit upright in a chair and interlock your fingers behind your head. Gently press your head so that your chin moves toward your chest. Keep your arms relaxed and stop when you feel a tug along your neck. Release your fingers and lower your arms to your sides before repeating the stretch.

Slowly let your head fall so that your ear moves toward your left shoulder. Use your left hand to pull your head downward—but not too far. Relax the opposite shoulder as you hold this pose. Don't shrug, and remember to breathe throughout the exercise. Repeat on the other side.

SHOULDER STRETCH

Extend your right arm straight out, even with your chest. Use your left hand to grasp your right arm just above your elbow and pull it gently toward your left shoulder. Repeat on the other side.

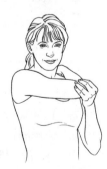

UPPER ARM STRETCH

Raise both arms in the air, letting your right
arm bend at the elbow behind your head. Hold your
right elbow with your left hand and gently extend the
stretch by slowly pulling the elbow further down and
back. Repeat with the other arm.

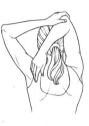

ARM STRETCH

Look straight ahead and relax your shoulders. Bring
your arms behind your back, clasping your right wrist
with your left hand. Keeping your right arm straight,
let your left arm pull the right one toward your left
hip, as shown. Gently complete the stretch by slowly
leaning your left ear toward your shoulder. Relax, then
repeat on the other side.

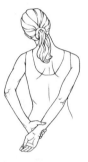

UPPER BACK STRETCH

Interlace your fingers in front of you and
turn your palms outward as you raise
your hands to shoulder level. Extend
your arms forward to feel the stretch
in your shoulders, upper back, arms,
hands, fingers, and wrists.

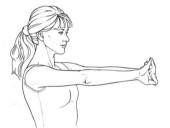

CHEST STRETCH

Hold on to both sides of a doorway
with your hands behind you at about
shoulder level. Slowly lean forward
until your arms straighten. Keep your
chest up and your chin slightly in
toward your chest as you hold this
position.

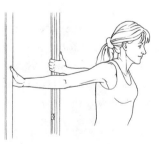

sore areas four times a day until you get relief. Then repeat only when soreness returns. Athletes who have used this remedy report more endurance and less cramping, he says.

Rx —— *Prescriptions*
FOR PAIN-PROOF EXERTION

Weekend warriors—or backyard horticulturists—can save themselves a lot of agony by preparing their bodies for exertion. That goes for shoveling snow, gardening, yard work, and other household tasks as well as walking, running, cycling, hiking, or lifting weights. Here's the foolproof plan.

❒ Start slowly. If you have a huge garden to plant and you have been hibernating in front of the television screen all winter, divide the work over two or three days instead of trying to prepare the soil, pull out dead plants, get rid of rocks, haul mulch, and plant everything in one day, advises Dr. Yawn.

Similarly, if you are finally going to honor that vow to work out at the gym, don't try to make up for lost years of workouts in one day, or you'll suffer in soreness. "It's not helpful to the body to start working at a level way beyond anything you have ever done," says Dr. Rucker.

❒ Stretch the muscles that you'll be using ahead of time. Pay special attention to your hamstrings, quadriceps, and arm muscles, says Dr. Rucker.

❒ If you feel pain or fatigue, stop. Many women find themselves doing more than they are prepared for because they want to keep up with their friends at aerobic workouts or in lifting weights, says Dr. Rucker. When you overdo your workout, though, you'll end up with achy, sore muscles, so it's important to pace yourself. Don't do more than you feel comfortable with.

TIME IT RIGHT ❒ Drink water before, during, and after activity. "I cannot stress this enough," Dr. Yawn says. "Even a little dehydration will make you feel much more fatigued." It can also decrease circulation and slow down recovery, adds Dr. Collins.

❑ Drink orange-banana fruit juice every day. Or eat a banana and drink some orange juice. When you are dehydrated, your blood concentrations of potassium and other key minerals—called electrolytes—change, leading to soreness and cramps. Consuming high-potassium foods like orange juice and bananas keeps your electrolytes in balance, says Dr. Yawn.

Medical **Alert**

If you exercise regularly, muscle soreness associated with overexertion should subside in a day or two. If you experience sharp, intense pain, can't move your muscles, or can't bend or move one of your limbs, see a doctor, says Dr. Yawn. You may have strained or torn a muscle or ligament.

Queasy Stomach

Forget butterflies. The churning and cramping of a queasy stomach can feel more like the entire insect population taking up residence in your belly.

Any number of factors can cause stomach upset. At the top of the list is stress. "Stress not only tightens your abdominal muscles but also increases your stomach's acid production," explains Barbara Majeroni, M.D., assistant professor of family medicine at the State University of New York at Buffalo. "That's why you feel nauseated in stressful situations."

Of course, you can also get a queasy stomach from something that you have eaten. Food that is improperly stored, cleaned, or prepared invariably picks up bacteria, says Dr. Majeroni. In fact, just about any food, if mishandled, can attract troublesome bacteria. But red meat, eggs, and poultry are particularly susceptible. And when those bacteria get into your system, they can leave you with a mild case of food poisoning.

MEALTIME

Even certain medications—particularly antidepressants—have stomach upset as a side effect. If you start a new prescription, you may be nauseated for a week or two until your body adjusts to the drug, says Dr. Majeroni.

Rx

Prescriptions
TO SOOTHE AN UNSETTLED STOMACH

No matter what its cause, stomach upset usually goes away on its own within 24 hours. Chewable antacids such as Tums and Extra Strength Rolaids and liquid antacids such as Mylanta and Extra Strength Maalox can speed relief along, says Dr. Majeroni. The following remedies can help as well.

TIME IT RIGHT

❐ Drink tea made from chamomile or peppermint three or four times a day until you feel better. Both herbs work gently to relieve digestive distress. You can buy the herbs in tea bag form in health food stores and some supermarkets, says Dr. Majeroni.

Note: Women who are pregnant should watch their intake of peppermint tea. Some herbalists have noted that large amounts of peppermint tea may lead to miscarriage.

TIME IT RIGHT

❐ Take a 6C, 12C, or 30C dose of the homeopathic remedy Ipecacuahna (or Ipecac) every 2 to 8 hours until you feel better. (The notation 6C, 12C, or 30C is a standard measurement in homeopathy and refers to the remedy's potency, which is listed on the label.) Which dosage you choose depends on the severity of your symptoms, according to Dana Ullman, a homeopathic practitioner in Berkeley, California, and author of *The Consumer's Guide to Homeopathy*. If your symptoms don't improve within 24 hours, stop taking the remedy and talk to your doctor. You will find Ipecacuahna in drugstores.

❐ Sip warm ginger ale. Ginger ale stimulates the production of saliva, which in turn neutralizes stomach acid, says Dr. Majeroni. Taking frequent small sips can help prevent dehydration.

TIME IT RIGHT

❐ Chew a stick of gum for 30 minutes at the onset of stomach upset. Like ginger ale, chewing gum gets saliva flowing, says Bob Marks, M.D., a gastroenterologist in private practice in Alabaster, Alabama. Avoid chewing gum that contains artificial sweeteners such as sorbitol or mannitol. These sweeteners have been known to have a laxative effect on some people.

Prescriptions
TO EASE QUEASINESS

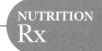

When your stomach is doing more somersaults than the U.S. gymnastics team, it takes a toll on your appetite. But you still need to eat—and the fact is that some foods may help you feel better. To stop your stomach from churning, Dr. Majeroni suggests these dietary strategies.

❐ Eat small but frequent meals every three to four hours for the duration of your digestive distress. Your stomach can better tolerate and process mini-meals compared with the standard three squares, explains Dr. Majeroni. Small meals are easier on your abdominal muscles, too, which helps keep your food down.

❐ Stick with bland foods such as bananas, cereal, rice, and chicken soup until your symptoms subside. These foods move smoothly through your digestive tract and help soothe a tumultuous tummy.

❐ Snack on crackers or a slice of unbuttered bread. These foods absorb excess stomach acid and relieve queasiness.

❐ Avoid coffee, black tea, diet soda, and fried foods until you feel better. These all cause your stomach to produce more acid, which worsens your discomfort, explains Dr. Majeroni.

Prescriptions
FOR A TRANQUIL TUMMY

Once your stomach has settled down, you can take steps to stave off a recurrence of queasiness. For starters, give these tips a try.

❐ Breathe deeply for five minutes whenever you feel stressed. Sit in a straight-back chair and inhale slowly, feeling your lungs fill with air. Focus on your abdomen as it expands. Then exhale slowly, feeling your diaphragm (the muscle at the base of your rib cage) relax. This exercise calms you down, which helps keep your stomach from churning, says Dr. Majeroni. It also gives you time to compose yourself so that

TIME IT RIGHT

you can deal with the stressful situation in a constructive, non-gut-wrenching way.

❑ Wear clothing with comfortable waistbands. Tight-fitting garments that cinch your waist put pressure on your stomach. When you eat, this pressure forces food to back up into your esophagus, leaving you nauseated, says Dr. Marks.

TIME IT RIGHT

❑ After a meal, wait at least two hours to lie down. This gives your stomach time to digest what you have eaten, explains Dr. Majeroni. Otherwise, stomach acid can easily slosh into your esophagus when you are in a horizontal position. You will end up feeling queasy.

❑ When you do lie down, lie on your left side rather than your right. Because the stomach rests in the left side of the abdominal cavity, this position minimizes the chances of stomach acid backtracking into your esophagus, says Dr. Majeroni.

Medical **Alert**

If you have stomach upset that lasts for more than two weeks after starting a new medication, notify your doctor, says Dr. Majeroni. She may want to examine you to make sure that you don't have another, underlying health problem. And she may be able to prescribe medication to relieve the nausea.

Sinusitis

The average person breathes 23,000 times a day. Every one of those breaths invites airborne particles and disease-causing viruses into the nose and sinuses. So is it really any wonder that the average person gets at least an occasional case of sinusitis?

Sinusitis simply means inflammation of the sinuses, the hollow cavities located behind and around your nose and eyes. It usually occurs when many airborne particles (such as smoke, dust, and pollen) or a virus finds its way into your nasal passages and irritates the delicate mucous membrane lining there. The membrane swells, blocking off your sinus cavities so that they can't drain, explains Robert Ivker, D.O., clinical instructor of family medicine and otolaryngology at the University of Colorado School of Medicine in Denver, president of the American Holistic Medical Association, and author of *Sinus Survival*. The result is pressure and pain across your forehead and around your eyes and nose, along with a stuffed-up, can't-breathe feeling.

While cold and flu bugs account for their fair share of sinus problems, Dr. Ivker says that more of us are getting sinusitis these days because we are breathing more polluted air. "Your nose and sinuses act as your body's primary air filter," he explains. "When they have to filter polluted air, it's as though they are getting rubbed with very fine sandpaper—23,000 times a day. The very act of breathing has become an irritant to the mucous membranes in the nasal passages and sinuses."

Prescriptions
to Clear the Airways

Rx

Of course, you must breathe, which automatically makes you a candidate for sinusitis. If you find yourself coping with a clogged schnozz, the following remedies can provide prompt relief.

❒ Use a natural, nondrug nasal spray. Dr. Ivker recommends a product that he helped to develop called Sinus Survival Spray, which contains salt water, aloe vera, goldenseal, and grapefruit seed extract. This combination soothes inflamed mucous membranes by irrigating them and keeping them moist. The ingredients help the mucous membranes heal, while eliminating bacteria and viruses—unlike traditional decongestant sprays, which shrink swollen mucous membranes only temporarily. Look for Sinus Survival Spray in some health food stores or order it direct from Klabin Marketing by writing them at 2067 Broadway, Suite 700, New York, NY 10023. You may also want to check out other brands of nondrug nasal spray in health food stores and drugstores. Whichever product you choose, use it according to the directions on the label.

❒ Sip a cup of ginger tea as needed for relief. Due largely to its high zinc content, ginger reduces inflammation and helps open clogged nasal passages, explains David Nickel, O.M.D., a doctor of Oriental medicine in Santa Monica, California, and author of *Acupressure for Athletes*. To make the tea, finely chop a quarter-inch slice of fresh ginger, add it to one cup water, and gently boil in a covered non-aluminum pot for 10 to 15 minutes. Strain the tea and allow it to cool before drinking it.

Another alternative is to add about one level teaspoon powdered ginger to one cup freshly boiled water. And if you are daring (or desperate), throw a pinch or two of ground red pepper into your ginger brew for a real sinus-clearing blast. According to Chinese medicine, "hot" substances like ginger and red pepper work best if your cold or sinusitis is accompanied by a runny nose with clear or light mucus, explains Dr. Nickel. But these substances could aggravate your sinus condition if you have yellow or green mucus, he adds.

TIME IT RIGHT

❐ To relieve congestion fast, use your index finger to press into the small depression on the outside of each nostril. You can close one nostril at a time or pinch both closed simultaneously. As you press, exhale through your mouth for about five seconds. Then stop pressing and inhale through your nose for five seconds. Repeat several times. "You can expect to breathe better within minutes," says Dr. Nickel.

❐ Massage a dab of mentholated ointment—such as Tiger Balm (available in health food stores) or Vicks VapoRub—into the depression on the outside edge of each nostril. Both of these products provide a nose-opening sensation of heat, Dr. Nickel says.

TIME IT RIGHT

❐ Apply a comfortably hot, moist towel to your face, from the middle of your forehead to your upper lip, for 5 to 15 minutes, twice a day. The moist heat improves blood and lymph circulation and helps open sinuses, explains Dr. Nickel. It also brings additional oxygen and nutrients to the area, which helps your sinuses to heal, he adds.

❐ Take a comfortably hot shower, allowing the water to run over your face and head. Inhale the steam, too. "It feels great, and it provides fast relief," says Michael Borts, M.D., co-director of the Comprehensive Sinus Clinic at St. Louis University School of Medicine.

A Yoga Prescription for Stuffed-Up Sinuses

Many sinusitis sufferers have found gentle, long-lasting relief by using a yoga healing technique called neti. No, it doesn't involve twisting yourself up like a pretzel. In fact, it's nothing more than rinsing your nasal passages with salt water. Here's what you need to do, according to Andrew Weil, M.D., director of the integrative medicine program at the University of Arizona College of Medicine in Tucson and best-selling health book author.

1. Dissolve one-quarter teaspoon salt in one cup warm water.

2. Pour the solution into your cupped hand or into a small cup or glass.

3. Dip one nostril into the solution and inhale while holding the other nostril closed with your index finger. Or use a rubber nose dropper (available in drugstores) to put the solution in one nostril, then inhale while holding the other nostril shut. You want to take in enough of the solution that you can spit it out of your mouth.

4. Switch nostrils and repeat.

5. Rinse each nostril two or three times, then gently blow your nose.

6. Repeat the nasal wash up to four times a day until your sinus infection clears.

You should know that you will probably cough, sputter, and spill until you get the hang of this technique. But don't get discouraged. You will learn to inhale the salt water neatly and efficiently—and to like the way it feels, according to Dr. Weil.

❏ As an alternative to taking a shower, inhale steam from boiling water, suggests Dr. Borts. Be sure to pour the water into a bowl or cup first—never inhale steam directly from a pot of boiling water on the stove. Repeat this treatment at least twice a day, and if possible, three or four times a day, recommends Dr. Borts.

Rx ——— *Prescriptions*
to Combat Chronic Clogging

If you have had sinusitis once, you are likely to get it again, observes Andrew Weil, M.D., director of the integrative medicine program at the University of Arizona College of Medicine in Tucson and best-selling health book author. "The disease-fighting cells that the body sends in to kill bacteria can themselves damage the sinus walls," he explains. "The walls become weak and prone to further infection."

To prevent a recurrence, you need to keep your immune system strong. That means eating healthfully, exercising regularly, and reducing stress as much as you can, says Dr. Ivker. And try to avoid environments that expose you to the airborne particles that cause sinusitis—places like smoky bars, dusty attics, even smoggy cities.

The following strategies can also help you to reduce congestion and to breathe easier.

❏ Drink at least ½ ounce of water for each pound of body weight every day. For a woman who weighs 140 pounds, that's 70 ounces, or almost nine 8-ounce glasses. If she exercises regularly, she should aim even higher—to ⅔ ounce of water per pound. Staying hydrated thins the mucus so that it drains more easily, explains Dr. Ivker.

MEALTIME

❏ Eliminate milk, cheese, yogurt, and other dairy products from your diet. The protein in milk stimulates the production of mucus, which can aggravate chronic sinusitis, says Dr. Weil. "A number of my patients have reported dramatic improvements in their sinus problems after two months without dairy products," he notes.

❏ Take a multivitamin as well as 1,000 milligrams of vitamin C, 400 international units of vitamin E, and 100 micrograms of selenium daily, recommends Dr. Ivker. These antioxidants help keep your immune system strong and may prevent another bout of sinusitis, he explains.

❒ Never stifle a sneeze. Sneezing creates tremendous pressure in your respiratory tract. If you suppress a sneeze by pinching your nose shut, you force bacteria-laden mucus into your sinuses, says Dr. Borts. (You can hurt your ears this way, too.)

❒ To clean your nose, close one nostril and *gently* blow through the other into a tissue. Continue alternating nostrils until your nose is clear. "Force out air and mucus in several puffs, not one all-or-nothing blast," advises Dr. Borts.

❒ Cry if you need to. Holistic medicine attributes sinusitis, in part, to a buildup of unshed tears and repressed anger, according to Dr. Ivker. Whether or not you buy into the notion that sinusitis has an emotional component, take notice of what happens when you try to suppress crying—especially when it's driven by anger. "You may actually feel the congestion build in your face," says Dr. Ivker.

❒ Humidify the air in your home and office in winter as well as summer. People tend to run their humidifiers only when they have the heat turned on. But an air conditioner sucks almost as much moisture out of the air as a heater does, says Dr. Ivker. And those cold, dry blasts can really irritate your sinuses.

SUMMERTIME

❒ Create a clean-air zone in at least one room of your home with a negative-ion generator or high-efficiency particulate air (HEPA) filter. You can buy these products at home centers and general merchandise stores. They are somewhat expensive—between $100 and $200—but you can install them yourself.

Also, if you have a furnace, put a pleated filter on it to help keep the air in your home reasonably clean. You can find pleated filters in home centers.

Medical **Alert**

See your doctor if your sinusitis is accompanied by a fever, cough, or headache that lasts longer than 24 hours or if you notice any

swelling, especially around your eyes. Also see your doctor if your nasal discharge is persistently yellow or green. This can be a sign of a bacterial infection, which might benefit from treatment with antibiotics, says Dr. Borts. Prompt treatment is important. On rare occasions, a sinus infection may extend into the brain.

Sleep Problems

Sooner or later, everyone has a sleepless night. A conflict with a co-worker or family member preys on your mind. You have a long "to do" list for the next day. You drank more coffee than usual, and you're wired. Whatever the cause, sleep eludes you.

An occasional sleepless night might make you tired and irritable the next day, but it won't ruin your life. Habitual insomnia is another story.

Doctors define insomnia as difficulty getting to sleep or staying asleep, waking up too early, or experiencing poor-quality sleep with frequent awakenings, says Mark Rosekind, Ph.D., research scientist at NASA's Ames Research Center in Moffet Field, California.

NIGHTTIME

Based on decades of research, sleep specialists have found that, barring unusual circumstances, women naturally sleep between 8 and 8½ hours a day. Over time, losing even as little as an hour or so of sleep a night leads to irritability, difficulty performing tasks well, and memory loss, says Virgil Wooten, M.D., associate director of the Sleep Disorders Center at Eastern Virginia Medical School of the Medical College of Hampton Roads in Norfolk.

Scientists have found that we actually have an internal biological clock that operates on a circadian rhythm, or cycle, of slightly more than 24 hours. Among its other functions, our biological clock prepares us for sleep, says Timothy Monk, Ph.D., professor of psychiatry and director of the human chronobiology research program at the University of Pittsburgh School of Medicine.

To ready itself for sleep, the body suppresses your level of alertness and your need to eat or go to the bathroom. About an hour or two before bedtime, the pineal gland responds to signals from the biological clock and secretes a hormone called melatonin, which makes you sleepy (among other things). The clock also slows down your heart rate and lowers your body temperature and blood pressure. It then reactivates these vital signs a few hours before you wake up, Dr. Monk says.

Your biological clock works under the assumption that you sleep at night. Therefore, its timing is governed by the cycles of daylight and darkness. This is one reason that some people who are blind suffer from insomnia. It is also why some people lose sleep if they don't get enough light during the day or wake up too early if light streams in through their bedroom windows. Other factors—like drinking too much coffee or exercising late at night or just plain nervousness—can keep you awake, too, says Dr. Wooten.

In addition to these factors are several that are unique to women.

Strike 1: Women require more sleep than men. In a unique series of experiments, women were studied in an isolation chamber with no competing demands on their time. It turned out that they naturally slept 1 to 1½ hours more than men in identical studies. Although women very often have less time available for sleep than men do, says Dr. Monk, they actually need more sleep than their male counterparts.

Strike 2: Insomnia often accompanies premenstrual syndrome, presumably because of monthly hormonal changes, and for some women, from increased consumption of caffeine and sweets at that time, says Joyce Walsleben, Ph.D., director of the Sleep Disorder Center at the New York University Medical Center in New York City.

Strike 3: Hormonal shifts and weight gain often affect sleep when women are pregnant, Dr. Walsleben says. "Twenty extra pounds on the diaphragm (the muscle underneath your rib cage that influences breathing) disrupts sleep."

MONTHLY

LIFETIME

Of course, once you have the baby, your sleep patterns also will be disrupted by the baby's need to nurse or be fed at inconvenient hours, Dr. Walsleben says.

Women who are going through menopause often get less sleep because of hot flashes and night sweats. "The sheer force of hot flashes can be extraordinarily disruptive," Dr. Walsleben says.

Rx ——— *Prescriptions*
FOR GETTING A GOOD NIGHT'S SLEEP

If you are lying in bed and can't sleep, these tactics may help.

❐ If hot flashes or night sweats keep you awake, lower the temperature of the room, says Dr. Walsleben. Or slip into lightweight nightclothes and turn on a fan or an air conditioner.

NIGHTTIME

❐ Keep your eyes closed and try to stay in that semiconscious state between sleep and waking. You will be more likely to fall back asleep, says Sonia Ancoli-Israel, Ph.D., professor in the department of psychiatry at the University of California, San Diego, and author of *All I Want Is a Good Night's Sleep.*

TIME IT RIGHT

❐ If you can't fall back asleep within 15 to 30 minutes, get out of bed and do something relaxing for a half-hour, like reading. Then try to go back to bed. Repeat as often as you need to until you fall asleep, says Dr. Rosekind.

MORNING

❐ Even if you can't sleep at all, get out of bed at your regular time and don't worry about it. No one can stay awake forever, but worrying can make it a chronic problem, says Dr. Wooten.

Rx ——— *Prescriptions*
FOR CURING INSOMNIA FOR GOOD

If you find yourself nodding off in front of the television, at a meeting, or any time during the day or evening when you expect to be awake, you are clearly not getting enough sleep, says Dr. Wooten. You should feel alert and refreshed when you wake up and as you go through your day, says Dr. Ancoli-Israel.

"Falling asleep when you don't want to is a sign that your body is physically tired," Dr. Walsleben says. "On the other hand, if you turn off the television set, hop into bed and—voilà!—are wide-awake again, you may have a psychological problem with sleep." Either way, try these non-drug strategies for better sleep.

TIME IT RIGHT

❐ Try an herbal tincture or tea. Don't wait until bedtime to take herbs that soothe the nervous system and promote restful sleep. Passionflower, skullcap, St.-John's-wort, or kava kava root—taken in a

A Visualization Prescription for Insomnia

Can't sleep? Try this technique, recommended by Henry Lahmeyer, M.D., a physician in private practice in Northfield, Illinois.

Close your eyes and relax. Count backward slowly from 100 to 0. As you do, visualize the numbers in some beautiful way. Maybe you see them being written by a calligrapher. Or try seeing the numbers being drawn on a huge blackboard across a giant sky. Continue until sleep overtakes you.

tincture or tea morning, noon, and night—can help you relax so that you are not tense when it is time to go to bed, says Kathleen Maier, an herbalist and co-director of the Dreamtime Center for Herbal Studies in Flint Hill, Virginia. Have one-half to one teaspoon tincture (available in health food stores) three times a day. To make a tea, mix one tablespoon dried herb in one cup freshly boiled water and steep for an hour.

Valerian can be taken as a tincture or a tea at bedtime. It should not be taken during the day because it has a sedative effect. Lemon balm, oatstraw, nettles, and red clover blossoms also are relaxing teas. You can use one herb at a time or mix them into a blend. Mix one tablespoon dried herb in one cup freshly boiled water and steep for an hour.

MEALTIME

❒ Don't eat heavy meals within four hours before bedtime. Otherwise, digestion—or indigestion—may keep you awake, says Dr. Wooten.

NIGHTTIME

❒ Do have a glass of milk and half of a turkey sandwich one to two hours before you sleep. Milk and turkey contain tryptophan, an amino acid that makes you drowsy, says Dr. Walsleben.

MORNING

❒ If you have difficulty getting up in the morning, set your alarm and walk around the block before breakfast so that you can get more light, Dr. Monk says.

NIGHTTIME

❒ Cut out caffeine in any form—coffee, tea, cola, and chocolate—after dinner. Caffeine is a stimulant that can hold sleep at bay, Dr. Rosekind says.

MONTHLY

❒ Cut out caffeine and sweets during menstruation, Dr. Walsleben advises.

❒ Don't smoke. Nicotine acts as a stimulant that can keep you awake, and coughing disturbs sleep further, Dr. Wooten says.

MORNING

❒ If you tend to waken too early, walk outdoors at sunset and stay away from windows and natural light early in the morning, recommends Dr. Monk.

NIGHTTIME

❒ Exercise no later than three to four hours before bedtime. "You may think that a two-mile run will tire you out, but what it's really doing is accelerating the heart rate," Dr. Rosekind explains. Though your heart will calm down when you stop, the body still needs hours to cool down and recover from the exertion.

NIGHTTIME

❒ Drink no alcohol after dinnertime. Though it will initially put you to sleep, alcohol actually disturbs deep sleep. You are likely to be wide-awake at four in the morning and groggy the following day, says Dr. Wooten.

❒ Do nothing but sleep or have sex in bed, says Timothy Roehrs, Ph.D., director of research at the Henry Ford Hospital Sleep Disorders and Research Center in Detroit.

If you use your bed as Action Central—the hub from which you read, watch television, and call your friends—it may be hard to sleep when you turn off the light because you no longer associate the bed with sleep, says Dr. Wooten.

❒ Don't stay in bed for 10 or 11 hours to try to make up for lost sleep time. If you usually need 8 hours of sleep, you will just have an extra 2 hours to toss and turn. You won't get more sleep, says Dr. Rosekind. If you extend your sleep time too much, you may begin to wake up too early in the morning. It is more important to get the sleep you need on a regular basis.

❏ Try a 30-minute to one-hour nap in midafternoon. If you work, you may be able to nap when you get home. But don't nap closer than four hours to bedtime, or you may not be able to sleep, says Dr. Roehrs.

DAYTIME

❏ Set aside time in the early evening as "worry time" to deal with the racing thoughts that will otherwise keep you up when you should sleep. Spend a half-hour writing down all the things that you have to worry about, choose an action to take, and then put the list in a drawer till morning, Dr. Rosekind recommends.

NIGHTTIME

Many people lie awake at night because it's the first time all day that they have had to think over the day's problems. But bedtime is the wrong time to think, Dr. Ancoli-Israel says.

❏ Take a hot bath. A hot bath taken in the early evening will cause your temperature to go up and then drop more quickly when you hit the hay, so you can fall to sleep easily, says Dr. Roehrs.

NIGHTTIME

❏ Develop a regular pre-sleep routine. Have a glass of milk, comb your hair, brush your teeth, and put on your nightie (or whatever variation feels comfortable). This signals your brain that it's time to sleep, says Dr. Rosekind.

NIGHTTIME

❏ Keep your bedroom dark and quiet to make it easier to fall asleep and stay asleep, says Dr. Rosekind.

❏ Before you go to bed, turn the clock around so that you can't see the time if you wake up in the middle of the night. It doesn't matter what time it is when you wake up, you should be sleeping, Dr. Ancoli-Israel says.

NIGHTTIME

Medical **Alert**

If you take over-the-counter or prescription medications and you have trouble sleeping, read the list of potential side effects in the package insert. Some medications keep you awake, says Dr. Roehrs. If pain is keeping you awake, consult your doctor for advice. It's also a good idea to check with your doctor if nondrug strategies don't improve your sleep within two weeks.

Stiff Joints

You used to bound out of your chair and take steps two at a time to answer the phone. You could sit cross-legged on the floor—and jump right up with little effort. Lately, though, you notice that if you sit watching a movie for two hours, your knees feel stiff and weak when you walk up the aisle to leave the theater. Or you find that creaky joints, not a poor night's sleep, make getting out of bed in the morning a struggle.

Relax. Stiff joints aren't necessarily a sign of arthritis. Rather, they are simply a sign that you're getting older. Our joints lose elasticity as we age, so if we sit still for a couple of hours, we don't bounce back as quickly as we did in our youth, says Lee Tarsitano, exercise physiologist and physical therapist at the Rehabilitation Institute of Chicago. "The less active you are, the more prone you are to injury and joint stiffness as you age," she says.

Rx

Prescriptions
FOR MORNING STIFFNESS

In your thirties and forties, it is normal for your joints to feel stiff for about five minutes when you first get out of bed in the morning, says Leslie Kahl, M.D., associate professor of medicine in the division of rheumatology at Washington University in St. Louis.

TIME IT RIGHT

❏ Take a 20-minute comfortably hot shower or steam bath, or place warm towels directly on a stiff joint first thing in the morning, says Joan Merrill, M.D., assistant chief of rheumatology in the division of rheumatology and connective tissue disease at St. Luke's/Roosevelt Hospital in New York City.

TIME IT RIGHT

❏ After you have warmed up the joint a bit, stretch slowly and gently, without bouncing, for 30 to 60 seconds. Stretching for too little time or bouncing can actually tighten the joint, says Karen Rucker, M.D., chairman of the department of physical medicine and rehabilitation at Virginia Commonwealth University in Richmond. Pause after each stretch, then repeat. (If you feel pain while stretching, back off a little and then gradually increase the pressure.) Dr. Rucker recommends the following remedies.

MORNING STRETCH

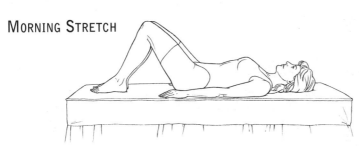

Lie on your back with one side of your body close to the edge of your bed and your knees bent.

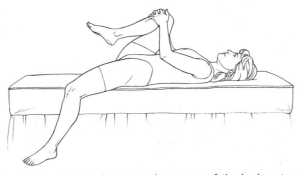

Slowly bring the leg that is closest to the center of the bed up to your chest and hold it with your hands. Slide the other leg straight out over the edge, so that it dangles off the side of the bed at midthigh. Be careful not to arch your back. Hold this position for 30 to 60 seconds, then return both legs to the bent-knee position. Repeat three times. Then change position to repeat with your other leg.

TIME IT RIGHT

❑ Stand facing a wall (a little more than an arm's-length away) with your feet firmly planted on the floor. Using the wall to support yourself and keeping your knees straight, lean toward the wall. This will bend your ankles and stretch your calf muscles, explains Dr. Rucker. Hold for 30 to 60 seconds. Repeat twice.

❑ Wash the dishes. Plunging your hands in a sink full of warm water in the morning is the perfect way to restore flexibility to fingers that are stiff and sore when you wake up, says Dr. Kahl.

NIGHTTIME ❐ If your hands tend to feel stiff in the morning, wear a pair of stretchy gloves (such as Isotoner) to bed at night, says Dr. Kahl.

NIGHTTIME ❐ Sleep on your back with a small pillow under your knees, says Dr. Rucker. If you sleep on your side, avoid the fetal position, where your neck is bent and your chin tucked. Rest your head on a pillow that doesn't tilt your head and neck. Otherwise, you'll be sleeping in an awkward position that strains your joints. You can also lessen strain by using a body pillow, available in mail-order catalogs, department stores, and medical supply stores. If you must sleep on your stomach, put a pillow under one side of your body and bend your hip and knee on that side so your head and neck aren't strained.

STRETCHING
Rx

Prescriptions
FOR A STIFF NECK

Many women who spend hours working (or playing) at a computer, doing business over the phone, or reading a lot complain of neck stiffness, says Dr. Rucker. To ease the strain, she prescribes the following stretches. Repeat them at least once an hour, or as often as needed to prevent stiffness.

❐ Look forward, relax your shoulders, then slowly turn your head to the right as far as you comfortably can. Make sure that you keep your head and chin level. Then stretch a bit farther, holding for 20 to 30 seconds and exhaling near the end. Return to the starting position and repeat, this time turning your head to the left.

❐ Facing forward, slowly tilt your head forward until your chin touches your chest. Then clasp your hands behind the lower part of your neck and slowly tilt your head up so that you are looking at the ceiling. Make sure that your hands stay on the back of your neck to help you support and extend your neck. Hold for 30 to 60 seconds.

Rx

Prescriptions
FOR DAY-TO-DAY FLEXIBILITY

A number of small changes in your daily routine and diet can go a long way toward staving off joint stiffness. Doctors prescribe the following strategies.

❐ Step into crepe-soled footwear or walking shoes. Soft-soled shoes will lessen the impact on your feet and back, says Dr. Kahl.

❐ Place arch supports in your footwear, especially if your feet pronate, or roll inward. Without adequate arch support for your body frame, you may end up with foot, knee, or ankle stiffness, says Dr. Rucker. Often, you won't notice the pain until you go to bed and your joints suddenly feel stiff and achy.

❐ Rest your joints periodically throughout the day. If your fingers ache after working at the keyboard for hours, rest your hands periodically. If embroidery taxes your fingers, put it aside and read instead, says Dr. Merrill. If baskets full of laundry are burdensome for creaky joints, make several, smaller loads. Or push the basket along the floor with your legs instead of carrying it.

DAYTIME

❐ If you work at a computer, make sure that your paperwork and computer screen are at eye level so that you don't have to crane your neck, says Dr. Rucker.

❐ If you are on the phone a lot, use a headset. Cradling the phone between your head and shoulder will put a crick in your neck, says Dr. Rucker.

❐ Take a stand. Just as overuse can tax joints, so can underuse. If you are taking a long car ride, get out every hour or so and walk around for five minutes. In an airplane, unbuckle and move around the cabin as often as possible, says Dr. Kahl.

TIME IT RIGHT

❐ Lose excess weight. Carrying as little as 10 extra pounds places added stress on your joints, especially your knees, and increases your risk of arthritis, says Dr. Kahl.

Twenty or 30 extra pounds (or more) is even more taxing, says Yvonne Sherrer, M.D., director of clinical research at Rheumatology Associates of South Florida in Pompano Beach.

❐ Walk or cycle at least twice a week for half an hour, recommends Dr. Sherrer. Work up to three to four times a week, or even every day. Regular exercise will help you lose weight and keep your joints from stiffening, she says.

TIME IT RIGHT

❐ If you have access to a warm pool, try swimming. Swimming has the double advantage of warming and limbering your limbs and avoiding strain on your joints since you're practically weightless in the water.

MEALTIME

❐ Eat salmon, mackerel, or tuna two or three times a week. Oils in these fatty cold-water fish contain essential fatty acids, which have an anti-inflammatory effect, easing joint swelling, says Dr. Sherrer.

Medical **Alert**

If your joint stiffness lasts more than 30 minutes a day and is accompanied by redness, warmth, or pain in the joint, see a doctor. You might have symptoms of rheumatoid arthritis, an inflammatory joint condition that requires medical attention, says Dr. Rucker.

Tension Headaches and Migraines

From bad-hair days to bounced checks, life sometimes seems like one headache after another. But truth be told, most of us would prefer these minor annoyances to the real McCoy—the persistent, pounding, stop-the-world-I-want-to-get-off variety of pain that grips our heads from time to time and then stubbornly refuses to let go.

Headaches occur for any number of reasons. They can be driven by emotional factors, such as depression or anxiety, or by high blood pressure, says Seymour Diamond, M.D., director of the Diamond Headache Clinic in Chicago and co-author of *The Hormone Headache*. Blocked or inflamed sinuses can trigger headache pain. Even changes in your sleeping or eating pattern can make your head hurt because they disrupt your body's internal clock, explains Joseph P. Primavera III, Ph.D., a psychologist at the Jefferson Headache Center at Thomas Jefferson University Hospital in Philadelphia.

But the most common, by far, are tension headaches. Almost everyone—about 90 percent of the population—has experienced a tension headache at some point, says Fred D. Sheftell, M.D., founder and co-director of the New England Center for Headache in Stamford, Connecticut, and co-author with Alan M. Rapoport, M.D., of *Headache Relief for Women*. The pain typically starts in the muscles at the back of your head and neck and works its way to your forehead. You may feel mild throbbing in your temples or just behind your eyes.

Tension headaches are usually a by-product of stress, but even sitting in a cramped position or straining your eyes at a computer screen can provoke pain. Fortunately, these headaches generally last no more than a few hours, and they often respond to over-the-counter pain relievers or just quiet relaxation, Dr. Sheftell says.

A migraine, on the other hand, can last from four hours to three days, says Dr. Diamond. And the pain's duration only magnifies its intensity. Typically, a migraine begins as a dull ache that progresses to an overwhelming, throbbing agony. Sometimes the pain is preceded by an aura, a visual disturbance characterized by brightly colored lines, flashes of light, dots, or spots. The pain itself usually affects only one side of the head. But you may feel ill all over with nausea, numbness, weakness, and extreme sensitivity to light and noise.

MONTHLY

Approximately 65 percent of female migraine sufferers get their headaches around the time of their periods—a fact that Dr. Diamond attributes to changing levels of the hormone estrogen throughout the menstrual cycle. Scientists can't yet explain the mechanics of it, but somehow these hormonal fluctuations make women more susceptible to the chemical chain reaction that causes blood vessels feeding the brain to rapidly constrict and then expand, producing pain. For similar reasons, some women who take hormone-replacement therapy during or after menopause also experience migraines during the interval when they are not taking estrogen. For example, if a woman takes hormone replacement for 21 days and then is off for 7 days, she may experience a headache during the 7-day, drug-free period.

Prescriptions
FOR RAPID RELIEF

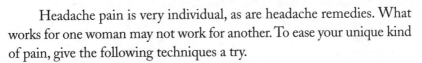
Rx

Headache pain is very individual, as are headache remedies. What works for one woman may not work for another. To ease your unique kind of pain, give the following techniques a try.

TIME IT RIGHT ❏ Run comfortably hot water over your hands for 10 minutes as soon as you feel a headache coming on. The heat draws blood away from your head, making this remedy effective against both tension headaches and migraines, according to Robert Kunkel, M.D., of the headache section for the Cleveland Clinic Foundation in Cleveland and president of the National Headache Foundation.

TIME IT RIGHT ❏ Place a warm, moist towel or a hot-water bottle wrapped in a towel across your shoulders for 20 minutes to an hour. If you have a tension headache, the heat helps relax your muscles, explains Dr. Kunkel. If you have a migraine, the heat helps relax constricted blood vessels before pain occurs.

Nutrition Prescriptions for Menstrual Migraine

Are your migraines as predictable as your periods? That's no coincidence. For many women, monthly hormonal fluctuations set the stage for migraine both before and during menstruation. You can reduce your chances of developing a migraine at "that time of the month" with the following vitamin and mineral supplements, recommended by Fred D. Sheftell, M.D., founder and co-director of the New England Center for Headache in Stamford, Connecticut, and co-author with Alan M. Rapoport, M.D., of *Headache Relief for Women*.

❏ Take 200 to 400 milligrams of riboflavin every day. Riboflavin might play a role in the way your brain's energy system works, improving its ability to short-circuit migraine pain.

❏ Take 50 milligrams of vitamin B_6 a day the week before your period. Then increase your dosage to 100 milligrams a day and continue the supplements right through your period. Vitamin B_6 stimulates production of serotonin, a brain chemical that constricts blood vessels and so staves off migraine. Don't rely on

Do watch the clock with this remedy: Applying heat for more than an hour at a time can damage your skin.

❐ Practice imagery for 3 to 10 minutes. For example, try to visualize your headache as a certain color, shape, and size, suggests Dennis Gersten, M.D., a psychiatrist in San Diego and author of *Are You Getting Enlightened and Losing Your Mind?* Perhaps it is bright red, the shape of a heart, and the size of a football, with jagged edges all over. Then "see" your pain as it turns into a liquid and runs into your shoulder, down your arm, and out through your fingertips. In your mind, allow your pain to leave the room, then your house, as if pulled out by gravity. Watch it as it flows down the street and

TIME IT RIGHT

the benefits of B₆ on a daily basis, however. Unstable gait and numb feet may occur with doses of vitamin B₆ at 50 milligrams to 2 grams daily over a prolonged time.

❐ Take 400 international units of vitamin E every day. Vitamin E helps to stabilize your body's level of the hormone estrogen. The vitamin's antioxidant properties may have some benefit as well.

❐ Take 200 to 400 milligrams of magnesium a day. Research has shown that women who get migraines during their periods tend to have low levels of this mineral in their brain cells.

Note: If you have heart or kidney problems, check with your doctor before taking magnesium supplements. Some people who take 350 milligrams or more of supplemental magnesium a day may experience diarrhea.

❐ Take a daily multivitamin in addition to the supplements above. That way, you can be sure that all your nutritional bases are covered.

into the ocean. If you practice this imagery regularly when you have mild pain, you will find that it is more effective when you have a lot of pain.

Note: Guided imagery is not appropriate for people with severe mental illness.

HERBAL Rx

Prescriptions
FOR TENSION HEADACHES

Tension headaches respond well to certain herbs. When pain sets in, turn to one of these herbal remedies for relief. (All of these herbs are available in health food stores and some drugstores.)

TIME IT RIGHT

❐ Take one dose of the herb cramp bark or feverfew every hour for up to three hours or until your headache passes, suggests Eve Campanelli, Ph.D., a practitioner of holistic medicine in Beverly Hills, California. For the proper-size dose, follow the directions on the product label. Cramp bark is a natural antispasmodic, so it helps relax tense muscles. And feverfew naturally contains salicylic acid, the active ingredient in aspirin, she explains.

❐ Make yourself a soothing herbal tea of equal parts wood betony, chamomile, vervain, and lavender. These herbs are tonics that relieve pain, gently relax your body, and help release tension. They can improve the way your body handles stress and, if used regularly, can help reduce the frequency of tension headaches, explains Elizabeth Wotton, N.D., a naturopathic physician in Plymouth, Massachusetts.

To make the tea, simply steep one heaping teaspoon of the herb blend in one quart freshly boiled water for 10 minutes, says Dr. Wotton. Strain the herbs and allow the tea to cool before sipping it. If you have a tension headache, drink one to two cups. If you are prone to tension headaches, drink up to four cups a day.

TIME IT RIGHT

❐ Soak in a lukewarm herbal bath for 20 minutes. Steep two tablespoons lavender and two tablespoons lemon balm in one cup hot water for 10 minutes, then pour the tea into your bathwater, says Dr. Wotton.

Prescriptions
TO TAME TENSION-INDUCED PAIN

Rx

Like herbs, the following remedies can ease a tension headache naturally—without drugs. Try them all to see which are most effective for your kind of pain.

❒ Get relief with peppermint or lavender essential oil. Choose peppermint if you have a headache in the front of your head, because the scent's stimulating effects help improve circulation and draw energy away from the pain. Choose lavender if you have pain in the back of your head, because the scent's relaxing properties help soothe muscle spasms.

To use either oil, moisten your fingertip with less than a drop. Then rub the oil on your temples, across your forehead, and on the back of your neck, suggests Michael Scholes, director of the Michael Scholes School of Aromatic Studies in Los Angeles. If the oil is working, you should feel a slight tingling sensation. Repeat again within the hour, if necessary. You can buy essential oils in health food stores.

TIME IT RIGHT

❒ Take 30 seconds to roll a golf ball about 50 times along the length of the palmside of one thumb. Then switch thumbs and repeat. Use this technique once an hour while you have a tension headache. (You can also use it once a day as a preventive if you are prone to tension headaches.) Practitioners of reflexology—a healing art based on the principle that applying pressure to specific areas of the hands or feet benefits other parts of the body—believe that stimulating this area of your thumb relieves muscular tension in your head, explains Kevin Kunz, a reflexology researcher in Albuquerque, New Mexico.

TIME IT RIGHT

❒ Try a two-minute self-massage at the onset of a tension headache. Begin by placing your fingertips on your scalp along the middle of your head. Press your fingers down firmly so that you move your scalp slightly from front to back with your fingertips. Continue to loosen your scalp by moving your hands down toward your ears about an inch at a time, massaging from the front of your hairline to the back of your head each time. Then use the same technique to massage your head in a different direction, moving your hands over your head from ear to ear. You should spend about 20 seconds massaging in each direction, covering your entire head in about 40 seconds.

Next, press directly on your forehead with the heels of your hands and hold for 5 to 10 seconds. Then find the tender spot between the thumb and index finger of one hand and press directly on it with the thumb of the other hand. Hold for 5 seconds, then switch hands.

Finally, use your thumb to massage along the bony ridge at the base of your skull where your head and the back of your neck meet. Bend your head forward slightly, position your right thumb in the center of the ridge, and massage gently by firmly pressing your thumb against your skin and making small circles. Move your thumb slightly to the right and repeat. You should take about 30 seconds to work your way along the right side of your skull from the center of your head to just behind your ear. Use your left thumb to repeat along the left side of your skull. If any points along the way feel too tender, decrease the amount of pressure you apply.

Remember to breathe slowly and deeply while doing this massage sequence so that you don't tense up, says Elliot Greene, massage therapist in Silver Spring, Maryland, and past president of the American Massage Therapy Association. You may repeat this routine if you find it helps.

Rx — *Prescriptions*
TO MINIMIZE MIGRAINE

Among headaches, migraine is exceptionally excruciating—and stubborn, too. But you don't have to just live with the pain. The following remedies can help rein in migraine and its symptoms.

TIME IT RIGHT

❏ Apply ice for 10 minutes to the part of your head that hurts. Some women find that cold works better than heat in relieving their migraines. Cold helps constrict expanded blood vessels and block pain messages to your brain. If you get headaches a lot, Dr. Kunkel suggests filling a paper cup with water and putting it in your freezer. Then when you need a cold compress, just tear off the top inch of the cup and rub the ice against your head. You can also buy a gel pack and keep it on the ready in your freezer.

❏ Sip a cup of coffee. The caffeine helps constrict dilated blood vessels in the brain, says Patricia Solbach, Ph.D., director of the Center for Clinical Research at the Menninger Center for Clinical Research in

Topeka, Kansas. Be careful, though: Too much coffee can make your pain even worse. Limit your daily intake to one five-ounce cup, which contains about 100 milligrams of caffeine.

❐ Take 400 to 500 milligrams of ginger two or three times a day to quell migraine-related nausea, suggests Dr. Sheftell. You can buy ginger capsules in health food stores and some drugstores.

Prescriptions
FOR STAYING HEADACHE-FREE

Rx

If you are prone to headaches, you can take steps to reduce their frequency and intensity. Get a head start on preventing pain with the following strategies.

❐ Keep a headache diary to track down what triggers your pain. MONTHLY
When you get a headache, make note of what you have eaten in the previous 24 hours, what you are doing when the pain sets in, whether you are under stress, whether your period is approaching—any factors that you think may be connected to your headache, Dr. Primavera says. Then after two weeks, see if you notice any pattern to your pain so that you can start to eliminate or regulate those triggers in your life.

❐ Bypass cured meats such as frankfurters, bologna, and salami. These foods contain nitrites, which trigger migraine in some people. Other common offenders include monosodium glutamate (found in Chinese food as well as lunchmeats and frozen dinners), aspartame (an artificial sweetener that goes by the brand name NutraSweet), and tyramine (an amino acid found in aged cheeses, pickled herring, and the pods of lima beans and snow peas). In general, if you end up with a migraine more than half the time after you eat a particular food, then you should not be eating it, advises Dr. Sheftell.

❐ Limit yourself to one drink a day. Alcoholic beverages—particu- TIME IT RIGHT
larly red wine and beer—are notorious for triggering migraine, because the
alcohol makes blood vessels dilate. In fact, if you consistently get a migraine after imbibing, you should cut out the booze entirely, advises Dr. Diamond. A drink, incidentally, is defined as one 12-ounce beer, one 5-ounce glass of wine, or a mixed drink made with 1½ ounces of liquor.

❐ Take a brisk walk for 20 minutes every other day. Walking tones your cardiovascular system, including the blood vessels that cause headache pain, and helps relieve stress, notes Dr. Wotton.

❐ Breathe deeply for five minutes, several times a day. Dr. Diamond recommends the following exercise: Sit or stand up straight, with your feet flat on the floor. Exhale completely, pulling in your abdominal muscles. Then inhale slowly and gently through your nose while simultaneously expanding your abdomen. Imagine that you are breathing in a sense of ease, quiet energy, and well-being. Take this breath down to the bottom of your lungs, allowing your chest to expand slightly. Don't raise your shoulders, though. When your lungs feel full, make a slow, smooth transition between inhaling and exhaling. Exhale slowly through your mouth while contracting your abdominal muscles. Again, don't raise your shoulders. As you exhale, imagine that you are bringing up from within you any discomfort and muscle tension. Blow your breath gently from your mouth, allowing a sense of quiet to take over your body. Repeat this exercise three times.

Medical Alert

If your headache is accompanied by any of the following symptoms, have someone take you to an emergency room right away, advises Dr. Diamond: fainting; seizures; clear fluid or blood coming from your nose or ears; vomiting; a stiff neck, along with nausea and fever; problems with speech, coordination, or vision; weakness or numbness on one side of your body; fever of 101°F or higher; or lethargy immediately after a head injury.

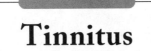

Tinnitus

The ocean surf may be nature's greatest tranquilizer. Its lilting lullaby calms and comforts—so much so, in fact, that we spend a small fortune on relaxation tapes that duplicate the sounds.

But for folks with tinnitus, it's as though the tape never stops playing. They can't turn it off or walk away from it or shut it out in any way. The surf seems to pound incessantly deep inside their ears.

Tinnitus is characterized by ringing, roaring, swooshing, buzzing, or chirping in the ears. (The word *tinnitus* literally means "tinkling like a bell.") The sounds may be high- or low-pitched, constant or intermittent. They are sometimes accompanied by hyperacusis, or extreme sensitivity to noise.

Tinnitus usually results from damage to the inner ear. The top two troublemakers are medications and excessive noise. But tinnitus can also be a symptom of an underlying health problem such as high blood pressure, poor circulation, hardening of the tiny bones in the middle ear (called otosclerosis), or a tumor of the auditory nerve. Even a buildup of wax in the external ear canal can cause problems.

That's why if you suspect you have tinnitus, you should see a hearing specialist pronto, says Maurice H. Miller, Ph.D., professor of audiology and speech language pathology in the School of Education at New York University in New York City. Your hearing specialist can make a proper diagnosis, rule out more-serious ailments, and recommend ways to manage the condition.

Prescriptions
to End the Noise Now

Rx

How you manage tinnitus depends a great deal on what caused it in the first place. While treatments for the condition abound, keep in mind that no one treatment helps everyone, says Michael Seidman, M.D., medical director of the Tinnitus Center at Henry Ford Hospital in Detroit.

That said, the following prescriptions have good track records as tinnitus therapies. Give one—or all—of them a try.

❐ If you develop tinnitus after starting a new medication, discontinue the drug and alert your physician right away. Certain prescription and over-the-counter medicines can permanently damage the nerve cells in your ears, says Dr. Seidman.

Among the worst offenders are furosemide, a common diuretic; cisplatin, a cancer chemotherapy drug; mycin-based antibiotics; and gentamicin and other aminoglycosides, often used to treat pneumonia. Even aspirin and ibuprofen can cause your ears to make their own music, although tinnitus associated with some of these drugs may be reversible, says

Dr. Miller. Still, your physician may recommend a lower dosage or switch you to a different medication.

TIME IT RIGHT

❐ Take 40 to 80 milligrams of ginkgo biloba extract (available in health food stores) three times a day. Ginkgo is widely used in Japan and Germany to improve poor blood circulation in the brain, which can cause tinnitus. Several studies have suggested that the herb may help improve the symptoms of tinnitus, according to Jennifer Brett, N.D., a naturopathic doctor in private practice in Stratford, Connecticut. "I always recommend ginkgo, even if the cause of the tinnitus cannot be determined," she says. "At the very least, the herb won't hurt. And in about half of the cases I treat, it helps."

She suggests taking ginkgo for six weeks to see if you notice any improvement in your symptoms. If you do, continue at the same dosage for up to one year. "Besides less ringing in their ears, some people report warmer hands and feet or less-severe migraines, if they're prone to them," notes Dr. Brett.

If you have a bleeding disorder or are taking blood-thinning drugs such as heparin, you should talk to your doctor to see if ginkgo would be an appropriate natural prescription for you, Dr. Brett adds. Also, be sure not to exceed 240 milligrams of ginkgo daily. In large amounts, the herb may cause diarrhea, irritability, nausea, vomiting, and restlessness.

❐ Use a masking noise to make the ringing in your ears less perceptible. As the name suggests, a masking noise works mainly by drawing your attention away from the tinnitus, says Dr. Seidman. Quiet music or a whirring fan can help. Or you may want to invest in a specially designed device that emits what sounds like radio static. Some models fit in your ears, while others sit on a tabletop or desktop. You can get these devices from an audiologist.

Rx ——— *Prescriptions*
TO KEEP THE PEACE

To silence tinnitus, you have to get to the source of the problem. The following strategies can help you minimize the factors that may be causing or contributing to your condition. (And if you don't have tinnitus, these strategies can help protect your ears from harm.)

❒ Take a multivitamin/mineral supplement that supplies the Daily Values of vitamins A, B_{12}, C, and E as well as the minerals magnesium, selenium, and zinc. Various studies have shown that all of these nutrients play roles in protecting your ears from damage caused by excessive noise or poor circulation. "I advise all my patients with tinnitus to take a good multivitamin," says Dr. Seidman. Read the label to make sure that the multi you choose fills the bill.

❒ Limit your daily fat intake to 25 percent of calories. Holding the line on dietary fat helps improve poor blood circulation, which has been implicated in some cases of tinnitus. Dr. Seidman often recommends a lower-fat diet to his patients with tinnitus. "It may help their ears, and it certainly helps their overall health," he says.

❒ Eliminate—or at least restrict—caffeine and alcohol. Both substances can increase your likelihood of developing tinnitus, according to Dr. Brett. Caffeine exacerbates the fluid and mineral imbalances experienced by those with tinnitus, while alcohol has a direct inflammatory effect on the inner ear. "Often, people who have tinnitus notice improvement in their symptoms when they cut back on caffeine and alcohol consumption," she says.

She suggests limiting yourself to no more than 100 milligrams of caffeine a day. That's the equivalent of about a 6-ounce cup of brewed coffee, a 10-ounce cup of instant coffee, or two 16-ounce cans of cola.

As for alcohol, one drink a week is one too many, advises Dr. Brett. "Alcohol alone can cause tinnitus, as it is ototoxic (has harmful effects on the ears)," she explains.

❒ Quit smoking. Like caffeine and alcohol, nicotine seems to put you at greater risk for tinnitus. That's because smoking is a risk factor for cardiovascular disease and arteriosclerosis, both of which can bring on tinnitus. And if you already have tinnitus, nicotine may make your symptoms worse, says Dr. Brett.

❒ Protect your ears from loud noises. Your best bet is to avoid high-volume situations whenever possible, advises Dr. Miller. But when you can't, at least plan to wear earplugs whenever you are exposed to potentially hazardous noise levels—for example, when using a lawn mower, vacuum cleaner, or hair dryer or when attending a rock concert or wedding reception. And when loud noise comes up unexpectedly, simply hold your ears shut with your fingers until it quiets down.

Medical **Alert**

See your doctor if the ringing in your ears (or any other tinnitus-related sound) lasts for more than 24 hours, if you have dizziness along with the ringing, or if the ringing affects only one ear, Dr. Seidman advises.

Urinary Tract Infections

AUTUMN

"Every year around the third week in September—just as predictably as the leaves turn color—teachers in the state of Maine show up in my office with urinary tract infections," says Brenda Sexton, M.D., director of Internal Medicine for Women in Yarmouth, Maine.

The cause, says Dr. Sexton, can be traced to a typical schoolteacher morning: a cup of coffee at home, a quick rest-room break before classes begin, then no opportunities to void until lunchtime. And after lunch, no toilet breaks occur again for several hours, until the children go home. To avoid the discomfort of a full bladder, schoolteachers avoid drinking water.

"Even eight ounces of water means disaster," says Dr. Sexton.

Within a few weeks of limited water intake and infrequent voiding, a teacher will wake up in the night with the urge to urinate. Yet when she goes to the bathroom, she feels burning, stinging pain, accompanied by the feeling that she hasn't completed voided—signs of a urinary tract infection, or UTI, says Dr. Sexton.

The constant need to urinate and feeling pain along with a stinging sensation when urinating are the classic characteristics of UTIs, says Paul Nyirjesy, M.D., associate professor of obstetrics and gynecology and reproductive sciences and director of the Vaginitis Referral Center at Temple University School of Medicine in Philadelphia.

Schoolteachers aren't the only ones who get them. One out of five women will get a UTI at some time in her life—eight times as often as men do. And if a woman gets one infection, she has a good chance of getting more. UTIs account for nearly seven million doctors' visits a year, more than for any other cause besides colds and flu. And treatment costs are estimated at $1 billion a year, according to the American Medical Women's Association.

Dr. Sexton's experience—treating women for UTIs at the same time every year—demonstrates just one of the many classic conditions that foster this infection.

Urinary tract infections occur when bacteria make their way up the urethra, the little pipe through which your urine exits, says Richard J. Macchia, M.D., professor and chairman of the department of urology at the State University of New York Health Science Center at Brooklyn. Bacteria often get pushed up the urethra during intercourse, and condoms and diaphragms also have been associated with an increase in the number of infections.

Other peak times for UTIs are right before menstruation, when hormonal changes are thought to have an effect, and at menopause, when the vaginal walls thin out and become more susceptible to bacteria, says Helene Leonetti, M.D., an obstetrician/gynecologist in private practice in Bethlehem, Pennsylvania. UTIs also often occur within the first few weeks of having a new sex partner, though no one knows exactly why (although it probably has something to do with the frequency of sex).

LIFETIME

These year-round conditions set the stage. Cut back on your water intake and voiding habits—as did the schoolteachers Dr. Sexton observed—and you eliminate one of nature's means of flushing the system of bacteria.

Prescriptions
FOR SOOTHING THE STING

Rx

If you are otherwise healthy, urinary tract infections will usually clear themselves within three to seven days, says Dr. Macchia. But most women don't want to live with the pain that long, so doctors generally prescribe a three- to five-day regimen of antibiotics. If you can't get to a doctor for some reason or you want some relief in addition to medication, try these natural prescriptions.

❑ Drink one glass of water every hour for eight hours. Drinking a lot of water increases urine flow, explains Kristene E. Whitmore, M.D., chief of urology and director of the Incontinence Center at Graduate Hospital in Philadelphia and co-author of *Overcoming Bladder Disorders*. This washes out the bacteria that are attempting to adhere to the cells lining your urethra.

❑ Take 2,000 milligrams of vitamin C every day for up to three days. Vitamin C inhibits the growth of bacteria, says Dr. Macchia.

Note: Taking more than 1,200 milligrams of vitamin C a day may cause diarrhea in some people. If this happens to you, switch to a buffered supplement.

❑ Drink three eight-ounce glasses of cranberry juice cocktail every day until you urinate normally again, says Dr. Macchia. For decades, women and their doctors have been using cranberry juice as a treatment for UTIs. This modern folk remedy was once thought to stunt bacterial growth by acidifying urine. But several studies now suggest that cranberry juice contains a substance that prevents bacteria from sticking to the walls of the urethra, thus helping to control infection.

❑ As an alternative to drinking cranberry juice, take three cranberry capsules a day, suggests Dr. Leonetti. Available in health food stores, cranberry capsules provide the healing effect of cranberry juice cocktail without filling you up with sugar.

❑ Avoid coffee, tea, colas, alcohol, and citrus fruits and juices. The acids in these foods and beverages act as stimulants, increasing the frequency and urgency of urination, says Gretchen Lentz, M.D., assistant professor of obstetrics/gynecology at the University of Washington in Seattle.

❑ Wear cotton underwear. Bacteria grow in warm, moist environments. Cool, absorbent cotton won't allow bacteria to thrive. Cotton underwear is especially helpful if you are experiencing external discomfort such as swelling, rawness, or dryness, says Betsy Foxman, Ph.D., associate professor of epidemiology at the University of Michigan School of Public Health in Ann Arbor.

Herbal Prescriptions for Urinary Tract Infections

The plant world offers a number of herbal remedies for urinary tract infections. Uva ursi, juniper berry, dandelion, and parsley root are all natural disinfectants, which you can drink as soothing teas, says Helene Leonetti, M.D., an obstetrician/gynecologist in private practice in Bethlehem, Pennsylvania. All are available in health food stores, sometimes already in tea bags. Pour one cup of hot water over a teaspoon of the dried herb or a tea bag, then let the tea steep for 5 to 10 minutes. If you use the dried herb, be sure to strain the tea before drinking it. Have one to two cups a day for up to four days, says Dr. Leonetti.

Other helpful bacteria-inhibiting herbs include buchu, Oregon grape, and pipsissewa, says Judyth Reichenberg-Ullman, N.D., a naturopathic doctor with the Northwest Center for Homeopathic Medicine in Edmonds, Washington, and co-author of *Homeopathic Self-Care.* These herbs are also found in health food stores and can be prepared as teas, following the directions above. Drink the tea every two hours for up to 10 days.

With any of these teas, if your symptoms persist beyond the recommended treatment period, stop drinking the tea and see your doctor.

Prescriptions
FOR PREVENTING FUTURE INFECTIONS

Rx

Once your urinary tract is free and clear of infection, experts offer these prescriptions for keeping it so.

❒ Continue drinking three eight-ounce glasses of cranberry juice cocktail every day, especially if you are prone to UTIs. You will know that you are sufficiently hydrated when your urine appears clear like water rather than deep yellow, says Dr. Macchia.

TIME IT RIGHT

❏ Go whenever you need to. The more you urinate, the less chance bacteria have to grow and thrive, says Dr. Lentz. Try to urinate every three to four hours daily.

❏ Void before and after sex. Urinating before intercourse means that bacteria won't have a place to breed; urinating afterward will flush out any bacteria that might have been pushed up the urethra during intercourse, says Dr. Lentz.

❏ Skip the panty hose for a month. You may be getting UTIs because you wear nylon panty hose and synthetic underwear, says Dr. Foxman. Switch to stockings and cotton underwear to discourage colonization of bacteria. If you still end up with an infection, at least you know that your undergarments aren't causing the problem.

❏ Check your birth control method. The use of the diaphragm as a birth control method, with and without spermicidal jelly, has been linked to UTIs. So if you are prone to bladder infections, consider another form of birth control, such as a cervical cap, an intrauterine device, or oral contraceptives, says Dr. Lentz.

Condoms have been associated with UTIs, too, says Dr. Foxman. By all means, don't stop using condoms when you have sex. But if you are getting UTIs, try switching to a different type of condom. For example, if you use a spermicidally treated condom, try a lubricated condom instead, says Dr. Foxman. If you have been using a lubricated condom, try a condom with a different type of lubricant.

Medical **Alert**

Before treating symptoms of what may be a UTI, make an appointment with your doctor to rule out vaginitis or a sexually transmitted disease such as chlamydia. You want to be sure that you're about to treat the right condition.

If your symptoms are accompanied by fever, upper back pain, or blood in the urine, call your doctor immediately. This could be a sign of a more serious problem. And always see a doctor if you have any symptoms of a UTI and you are pregnant, have diabetes, or have any other serious illness, says Dr. Macchia.

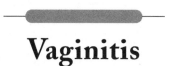

Vaginitis

Vaginitis is a catchall term for any inflammation of the vagina. Generally, the itching, burning, and discharge that typify vaginitis can be traced to one of three causes: infection, irritation, or hormones.

Yeast infections are one form of vaginitis. Another is trichomoniasis, which is an inflammation triggered by a protozoan that invades the genitourinary tracts of men and women alike. Trichomoniasis is transmitted sexually and causes itching, burning, and an abnormal, fishy-smelling discharge.

The most common form of vaginitis is bacterial vaginosis, an infection often associated with, but not caused by, sex. Like trichomoniasis, bacterial vaginosis is characterized by an abnormal, often yellowish, fishy-smelling discharge that often becomes worse after intercourse. Much less commonly, the infection can cause itching and burning pain, says Paul Nyirjesy, M.D., associate professor of obstetrics and gynecology and reproductive sciences and director of the Vaginitis Referral Center at Temple University School of Medicine in Philadelphia.

As for irritants, reactions to chemicals or other substances in douches, bubble baths, soaps, or even sperm can disturb the vagina, leaving you vulnerable to vaginitis, says Helene Leonetti, M.D., an obstetrician/gynecologist in private practice in Bethlehem, Pennsylvania.

Vaginitis can plague a woman any day of the year. But because of   changes in hormone levels, women tend to experience symptoms more often before menstruation, during pregnancy, or after menopause, when the vaginal walls become thinner and more susceptible to infection as women lose estrogen, Dr. Leonetti says.

LIFETIME

If you think you might have vaginitis, see your doctor without delay, especially if you are sexually active. Though trichomoniasis rarely leads to more serious illness, it may put women at risk for other sexually transmitted diseases. Untreated, bacterial vaginosis may lead to an upper uri-

Homeopathic Prescriptions for Vaginitis

Homeopathic remedies can effectively relieve vaginal infections, says Judyth Reichenberg-Ullman, N.D., a naturopathic doctor with the Northwest Center for Homeopathic Medicine in Edmonds, Washington, and co-author of *Homeopathic Self-Care*.

Widely available in most health food stores as tablets, pilules, or granules, homeopathic remedies are extremely dilute doses of substances that would otherwise cause the symptoms that you are experiencing. According to homeopathic practice, the correct remedy depends on your particular constellation of symptoms. Dr. Reichenberg-Ullman suggests trying these remedies.

✓ Caladium for vaginal infections when itching is the primary symptom
✓ Mercurius solubilis or Mercurius vivus for infections with an offensive discharge accompanied by rawness and soreness
✓ Apis (or honeybee) for vaginal infections accompanied primarily by swelling, but also by redness and soreness, in the genital area
✓ Kreosotum for vaginitis with extreme burning, rawness, and abrasions in the genital area

Take a 6X dose of the remedy that most closely matches your symptoms up to three times a day, says Dr. Reichenberg-Ullman. (The notation 6X is a standard measurement in homeopathy and refers to a remedy's potency, which is listed on the label.)

Start the remedy at the first sign of symptoms — vaginal discharge, pain, itching, and swelling — and stop as soon as your symptoms improve. "If they are no better after three doses, change to another remedy," advises Dr. Reichenberg-Ullman.

nary tract infection, pelvic inflammatory disease, premature labor in pregnant women, and posthysterectomy infection in other women, says Dr. Nyirjesy. For vaginitis, doctors generally prescribe antibiotics or vaginal creams, which can soothe the irritation in two to three days and prevent complications.

Prescriptions
FOR VAGINAL DISCOMFORT

NONDRUG
Rx

After you have seen a doctor and have your medical prescriptions in hand, try these natural prescriptions as well. They may help speed relief of itching and discomfort.

❐ Avoid bubble baths. Soaps often contain harsh chemicals, which can provoke an allergic reaction leading to vaginitis, says Dr. Leonetti. For similar reasons, don't use commercial douches, feminine hygiene sprays, or scented panty liners while you have vaginitis. Let your insides clean themselves, she advises.

❐ Take time for yourself. Repeated rounds of vaginitis seem to be TIME IT RIGHT related to stress, according to Dr. Leonetti. Stress seems to depress immune defenses. And it often triggers cravings for sugary, processed foods, which some experts believe may lead to bacterial imbalances that cause vaginitis.

"Check that you're sleeping enough and not eating junk food," says Dr. Leonetti. "Focus on eating lots of fruits and veggies. Stay away from colas and other caffeinated beverages, which act as stimulants. And most of all, try to relax." She suggests that you choose whatever technique works best for you—breathing deeply, listening to music, or just "taking five" for yourself.

Medical **Alert**

If you have vaginitis and your symptoms don't start to subside after two to three days of treatment, consult your health care provider, who can rule out more serious medical conditions such as pelvic inflammatory disease, says Dr. Nyirjesy.

Varicose Veins

We marvel at their pyramids and puzzle at their sphinxes. But the ancient Egyptians also left us with another, less well-known artifact: a 5,000-year-old medical text on the subject of varicose veins. Even back then, it seems, women had to contend with bulging purplish blue lines snaking down their legs.

A varicose vein occurs when a valve in a leg vein doesn't work properly, explains John Mauriello, M.D., medical director of the Vein Clinic of Charlotte in North Carolina. Normally, the valve opens to let blood flow toward the heart, then closes tightly. When the valve malfunctions, it allows blood to flow backward, causing the blood to pool in the vein. Eventually, the pressure created by the pooled blood stretches the vein wall. That's when the vein becomes visible on the surface of the skin.

Varicose veins are generally thought of as a cosmetic problem. But they can produce a variety of physical symptoms, too, including throbbing pain, burning or itchy skin, and swollen legs and feet, says Dee Anna Glaser, M.D., assistant professor of dermatology and internal medicine at St. Louis University School of Medicine.

Why do some women get varicose veins and others don't? Heredity is often to blame, according to Dr. Mauriello. If either one of your parents has varicose veins, chances are that you will, too.

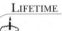
LIFETIME

Pregnancy can also contribute to the development of varicose veins, for a couple of reasons. First, the hormonal changes that occur during pregnancy allow the veins to stretch to accommodate extra blood flow, explains Dr. Mauriello. Second, the weight of the fetus can interfere with blood flow and put greater pressure on leg veins, especially during the third trimester.

Varicose veins that occur during pregnancy sometimes vanish within months of the baby's birth. The more pregnancies a woman has, however, the more likely the telltale blue bulges will stick around.

Other factors can increase your risk for developing varicose veins, says Dr. Mauriello. These include overweight, any blow or crushing injury that would rupture the valve, and even standing for six or more hours a day.

Prescriptions
TO PROBLEM-PROOF YOUR LEGS

Whether or not any of these risk factors apply to you, you can take steps now to stop varicose veins from developing. Doctors recommend the following preventive measures.

❒ Maintain a healthy weight. Carrying around extra pounds stresses your veins, causing them to stretch and even collapse, explains Dr. Glaser. While there are a number of complex formulas for calculating your ideal weight, one simple formula used by some experts can let you know if you're close: If you're five feet tall, you should weigh 100 pounds. If you're taller, add 5 pounds for each additional inch of height. Then to that number, add 10 percent if you have a large frame, or subtract 10 percent if you have a small frame.

❒ Exercise for at least 30 minutes every day. Physical activities such as walking, bicycling, and jogging strengthen your calf muscles and push pooled blood back into circulation, says Dr. Glaser.

TIME IT RIGHT

❒ Stretch your calf muscles when you sit for long periods of time. You can do this simple exercise just about anywhere: Push your foot down for one to two seconds as though you were stepping on the gas pedal in your car, then pull it up. Do this for a few minutes each hour. This movement contracts your calf muscle. "Every time you contract your calf muscle, it pushes the blood from your leg toward the central part of your body," explains Dr. Glaser.

TIME IT RIGHT

❒ On long car trips, move your legs around as much as you can. Try wiggling your toes, flexing your feet, rotating your ankles, or bending and straightening your knees. Motions like these help keep your blood circulating, says Dr. Glaser.

❒ If your family has a history of varicose veins, wear compression hose from the beginning of your pregnancy up until your ninth month or until your obstetrician instructs otherwise. Compression hose put pressure on leg veins to keep them from dilating. This keeps the veins' valves working more efficiently. Put the hose on first thing in the morning and don't take them off until you go to bed, advises J. A.

LIFETIME

Olivencia, M.D., medical director of the Iowa Vein Center in West Des Moines and president of the American Society of Phlebectomy. You can find nonprescription compression hose in drugstores and medical supply stores. Some are designed specifically for use during pregnancy.

NUTRITION
Rx —————

Prescriptions
FOR HEALTHY VEINS

You can further reduce your risk of developing varicose veins with the help of a few simple dietary strategies. Consider incorporating the following into your daily eating habits.

❐ Eat at least 25 grams (the Daily Value) of fiber every day. A fiber-rich diet, featuring whole grains, fruits, and vegetables, helps prevent constipation by making stool easier to pass. If you must strain to move your bowels, you create pressure in your abdomen that can block the flow of blood to your legs. Over time, the increased pressure may weaken the walls of the veins in your legs, says Dr. Mauriello.

One-half cup great Northern beans supplies more than 6 grams of fiber. Certain breakfast cereals can be good sources of fiber as well. For example, 100% Bran contains more than 8 grams and All-Bran contains 10 grams, each per one-ounce serving.

TIME IT RIGHT

❐ Take 500 milligrams of vitamin C twice a day. Your body uses vitamin C to build collagen and elastin, connective tissues that help strengthen vein walls, says Dr. Mauriello. And because it's an antioxidant, vitamin C also protects your veins from free radicals, unstable molecules that occur naturally in your body and that damage cells and tissues.

TIME IT RIGHT

❐ Take 500 milligrams of bioflavonoids twice a day. Bioflavonoids, which are chemical compounds found naturally in deep-colored berries such as cherries, blueberries, and blackberries, help keep veins and capillaries strong. They also enhance your body's absorption of vitamin C, so it's best to take them with your vitamin C supplement, notes Dr. Mauriello. You can buy bioflavonoid supplements in health food stores.

Herbal Prescriptions for Painful Veins

A handful of herbs have been successful in improving the condition and appearance of varicose veins. If you have varicose veins, consider giving one or more of the following remedies a try. You can buy all of the herbs in health food stores.

❒ Take 80 milligrams of bilberry in capsule form at breakfast, lunch, and dinner. This European blueberry restores the connective tissue sheath surrounding the vein, explains John Mauriello, M.D., medical director of the Vein Clinic of Charlotte in North Carolina. This prevents the vein from bulging, so blood doesn't pool in it. Bilberry also aids circulation by stimulating new capillary formation and strengthening capillary walls.

❒ Take 500 to 1,000 milligrams of bromelain in capsule form with each meal, for a total of three times a day. Varicose veins have difficulty breaking down fibrin, an insoluble protein that is essential to blood clotting. When fibrin doesn't break down, it causes the skin around the vein to get hard and lumpy. Bromelain, an enzyme extracted from unripe pineapples, helps varicose veins break down fibrin, according to Joseph E. Pizzorno Jr., N.D., a naturopathic doctor and founding president of Bastyr University in Seattle and co-author of *Encyclopedia of Natural Medicine*.

❒ Take 150 milligrams of butcher's-broom in capsule form every day. Native to Mediterranean countries, butcher's-broom contains anti-inflammatory compounds that help vein walls maintain their shape, says Dr. Mauriello.

❒ Take 40 milligrams of ginkgo biloba in capsule form three times a day, preferably at breakfast, lunch, and dinner. More than 50 studies, many from Germany and France, have shown that ginkgo improves blood circulation and reduces the discoloration of varicose veins, according to Dr. Mauriello.

Prescriptions
TO STOP THE THROBBING

If you already have varicose veins, the following remedies can help minimize symptoms and improve the veins' appearance.

TIME IT RIGHT

❏ Elevate your legs at or above the level of your heart for at least 20 minutes, three to four times a day. You can use pillows to raise your legs to the proper height. This helps drain your veins of pooled blood, explains Dr. Olivencia.

TIME IT RIGHT

❏ If your job has you on your feet all day long, elevate your legs for at least 30 minutes as soon as you get home, suggests Dr. Olivencia.

TIME IT RIGHT

❏ When you don't have your legs elevated, sit with your feet flat on the floor. Crossing your legs puts pressure on your veins and ultimately blocks the flow of blood in your legs. While 5 minutes of leg-crossing probably won't do any long-term damage, 25 minutes or more can cause problems. "You might as well put a tourniquet on your leg," observes Dr. Mauriello.

MORNING

❏ If you wear compression hose or support panty hose, put them on before you get out of bed. (For this to work, you'll need to shower at night rather than in the morning.) Once you stand up, gravity pulls blood backward through the vein valves in your legs, explains Dr. Mauriello. The blood then pools in your veins, causing them to swell.

❏ Avoid wearing knee-high nylons and socks. These garments usually have tight elastic bands that grip just below the knees and leave long-lasting indentations in the skin. "If you have varicose veins, tight-banded knee-highs are going to cause the veins to swell and stretch even more," says Dr. Mauriello.

❏ Wear sneakers or low-heeled shoes as often as possible. High heels can aggravate varicose veins. "When you step into a high-heeled shoe, you are no longer using your calf muscle," notes Dr. Mauriello. "And your calf muscle is what pushes blood up into the central part of your body."

❏ When outdoors, protect your legs with sunscreen with a sun protection factor (SPF) of 15 or higher. Some women try to conceal their varicose veins with a tan. But tanning may actually make varicose veins worse, says Dr. Olivencia. The sun's ultraviolet rays can damage the walls of very superficial veins and may cause the veins to dilate more easily.

❐ Avoid placing your legs near a heating vent to warm them in winter. Heat dilates your veins, so blood pools in your legs, especially in your feet and ankles, explains Dr. Olivencia.

❐ Limit your time in a hot tub or whirlpool to no more than 10 minutes. In fact, if you have severe varicose veins, you should avoid hot tubs and whirlpools altogether. The heat dilates your veins, and sitting compounds the problem by increasing pressure on your veins. If you must indulge, try to keep your legs at water level. This prevents blood from pooling and dilating the veins even further, according to Dr. Olivencia.

TIME IT RIGHT

❐ Keep your showers brief and lukewarm or cool in temperature. Starting your day with a hot half-hour shower will only exacerbate already dilated veins. Because your veins are below the level of your heart while showering, the blood will pool and the hot water will dilate the vein, explains Dr. Olivencia.

Medical **Alert**

If you have severe pain, redness, or hardness in a vein or the vein area of a leg or foot, you should see your doctor right away, says Dr. Olivencia. You could have a blood clot, which is a complication of varicose veins.

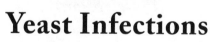

Yeast Infections

Many women are all too familiar with the intense itching, burning, and cottage-cheese-like white discharge that epitomizes a yeast infection. While yeast infections can—and do—occur anytime, many episodes fall just before menstruation, when the normal balance of "good" and "bad" organisms in the vagina is disrupted. The bacterial balance can also be upset by hormonal shifts that occur during pregnancy

LIFETIME

or menopause, use of oral contraceptives or antibiotics, or flagging immunity from fighting a cold or another viral infection. Under these circumstances, a yeast called *Candida albicans*, a type of fungus, runs rampant in the vagina.

Yeast infections also have been linked to wearing nylon underwear and wet bathing suits. Wet, or tight, sticky clothes trap heat and moisture, providing a wonderful arena for fungal growth, says Mary Lake Polan, M.D., Ph.D., professor and chairman of the department of gynecology and obstetrics at Stanford University School of Medicine.

Yeast infections are only one form of vaginitis and can also mimic urinary tract infections or sexually transmitted diseases. In fact, women misdiagnose themselves at least half the time, says Betsy Foxman, Ph.D., associate professor of epidemiology at the University of Michigan School of Public Health in Ann Arbor.

"The data suggest that most women who think that they have a yeast infection actually have something else or nothing at all," adds Paul Nyirjesy, M.D., associate professor of obstetrics and gynecology and reproductive sciences and director of the Vaginitis Referral Center at Temple University School of Medicine in Philadelphia. "Getting an accurate diagnosis is very important before beginning treatment."

So, if this is your first experience with symptoms of a yeast infection or if you are pregnant or have an underlying condition such as diabetes, head to your doctor. She can take a laboratory specimen and determine whether or not you have a yeast infection or another type of vaginal infection, says Mary Beth Hasselquist, M.D., staff physician at the Group Health Cooperative of Puget Sound in Seattle.

Rx ———

Prescriptions
FOR EASING THE ITCH

If, in fact, yeast is what's vexing you, your doctor will almost certainly prescribe an antibiotic or suggest an over-the-counter anti-yeast medication. (The best known are Gyne-Lotrimin and Monistat-7.) But over-the-counter antibiotics have been found to work only a little more than half the time, says Helene Leonetti, M.D., an obstetrician/gynecologist in private practice in Bethlehem, Pennsylvania.

If your system needs extra help fending off yeast infections, try these natural prescriptions.

❐ For external itching, apply a yogurt compress. Place one-half cup plain yogurt on a clean cloth or towel and place it on the outside of your vagina for 15 minutes. Rinse off the yogurt with warm water, then use a blow-dryer on the warm setting to make sure that you are totally dry, says Dr. Leonetti.

❐ Buy your guy some polyurethane condoms. Allergies to latex condoms may be associated with increased susceptibility to yeast infections, says Margaret Polaneczky, M.D., assistant professor of obstetrics and gynecology and medical director of women's health at New York Hospital/Cornell Medical Center in New York City. So, if you use condoms for protection and get frequent yeast infections, consider switching to a nonlatex brand.

Prescriptions
FOR PREVENTING THE RETURN OF THE ITCH

If only yeast infections were like mumps—once you have had it, you're immune. Nope. In fact, if you have had one yeast infection, chances are that you will get another, doctors say. Try these natural prescriptions, however, to fend off repeat or resistant episodes.

❐ Beat it with boric acid. Boric acid suppositories are an effective way to treat yeast infections and may be particularly effective against resistant ones, says Dr. Nyirjesy.

Buy a bag or box of boric acid and a package of No. 1 gelatin capsules at your drugstore or health food store, then fill the capsules with boric acid. Insert one suppository in the vagina in the morning and another before bedtime for two weeks, says Dr. Nyirjesy.

Caution: Boric acid is poisonous, so never take it orally or leave the capsules around where children could get at them, Dr. Nyirjesy says.

❐ Alternate boric acid suppositories with acidophilus suppositories. Some doctors believe that this combination works best to maintain the delicate bacterial balance in a woman's vagina. Alternate one boric acid suppository in the morning with one acidophilus suppository (available in

A Homeopathic Prescription for Yeast Attacks

To help relieve the discomfort of yeast infections marked by a burning sensation, lots of white, curdy discharge, and violent itching, you might consider trying Kreosotum, a homeopathic remedy, says Judyth Reichenberg-Ullman, N.D., a naturopathic doctor with the Northwest Center for Homeopathic Medicine in Edmonds, Washington, and co-author of *Homeopathic Self-Care.*

Homeopathic remedies like Kreosotum work by using very dilute doses of the same substance that causes symptoms to cure them, according to practitioners. The minuscule doses used in homeopathy can't hurt and often help, says Dr. Reichenberg-Ullman. She suggests taking a 6X dose of Kreosotum up to three times a day, stopping as soon as your symptoms subside. If you see no improvement after three doses, try another remedy.

Kreosotum is one of several remedies that homeopathic practitioners commonly prescribe for yeast infections and other types of vaginitis. For more, refer to "Homeopathic Prescriptions for Vaginitis" on page 140. Remember to choose the remedy that most closely matches your symptoms. (The notation 6X is a standard measurement in homeopathy and refers to a remedy's potency, which is listed on the label.) The remedies ae usually sold in most health food stores as tablets, pilules, or granules.

health food stores) every night for five nights, suggests Judyth Reichenberg-Ullman, N.D., a naturopathic doctor with the Northwest Center for Homeopathic Medicine in Edmonds, Washington, and co-author of *Homeopathic Self-Care.* Don't use these suppositories while you menstruate, or you may actually upset the bacterial balance rather than prevent infection.

❒ Skip the soap. Never wash inside the vagina with soap, or you may have an allergic reaction that leads to a yeast infection, says Dr. Leonetti. And don't worry that your vagina won't get clean; indeed, the vagina has a self-cleaning mechanism in no need of soaps or lotions.

❒ Wear cotton undies. Yeast thrive in the dark, moist, dank environment that nylon underwear and panty hose provide. Cotton underwear will reduce yeast's ability to thrive, says Dr. Leonetti.

❒ Wrap yourself in a sack. Not literally, of course, but you can be fashionable in looser clothes and keep out the yeast-infection-creating fungi that thrive in the environments created by tight, constricting outfits, says Dr. Leonetti.

❒ Sleep in the altogether. Sleeping nude, or at least without underwear, will "air out" your vagina and keep the yeast-infection-causing bacteria from having a place to thrive, says Dr. Leonetti.

TIME IT RIGHT

❒ Avoid sweets for one month. No one is sure if eating too much sugar really leads to yeast infections, but if you know that you get a yeast infection whenever you have gone overboard on chocolates, try avoiding sugary confections for a month and see if your yeast infections disappear, doctors say.

Medical **Alert**

If itching and soreness don't subside after two or three days of using antibiotics and these natural prescriptions, consult your doctor. And if lower abdominal pain, fever, or painful urination accompany your symptoms, see a doctor immediately, says Dr. Polaneczky.

Chapter 2

Prescriptions for Fighting Disease

According to experts, we have the potential to live 120 years. That's almost a half-century longer than the current life expectancy for the typical American woman.

What's more, say the experts, these extra years can be filled with vibrant, robust health—without many of the diseases that we so commonly associate with "growing old." We may even be able to dodge heart disease and cancer, the biggest killers among postmenopausal women.

So what's the catch, you say? Well, you need to take care of yourself starting *now*. How you treat your body in the present is going to have tremendous impact on your health down the road.

That's where this section can help. It offers dozens of simple self-care strategies for protecting yourself against the sorts of health problems that can whittle years off your life. And we do mean simple. For instance, you can reduce your risk of cancer just by eating tomatoes every day. Maintain a healthy cholesterol level by taking a daily dose of vitamin C. Cut your odds for osteoporosis simply by walking for 30 minutes at least five days a week.

You'll also find out how to successfully manage chronic conditions such as arthritis, diabetes, food allergies, and irritable bowel syndrome. If you have been diagnosed with any of these conditions, natural prescriptions—used in conjunction with any treatment program your doctor has recommended—can help minimize their impact on your health and preserve long-term quality of life.

Remember: The human body is built to last for more than a century. With proper maintenance, you can keep your body in the pink for the duration—and live to be a ripe *young* age.

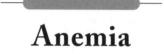

Anemia

Medical dictionaries list 90 different kinds of anemia. Various and sundry factors—such as bacterial or viral infections or nutritional deficiencies, among others—can deplete your total blood volume and reduce your red blood cell count. Red blood cells contain hemoglobin, the protein that carries oxygen through the blood. Oxygen gives you energy. So anything that disturbs the quality and quantity of your red blood cells leaves you feeling lousy. Tired all the time. Pale. Cold. Lifeless.

That's where iron (or lack of it) comes into play. Embedded in every hemoglobin molecule are iron atoms that bind with oxygen in the lungs and transport it to the heart, muscles, and body tissues. If iron stores are low, your body makes fewer and smaller red blood cells, with less hemoglobin.

In conversation, we use *anemic* as an adjective to describe someone who lacks energy or vitality. No wonder: Iron-deficiency anemia leaves you exhausted.

Iron-deficiency anemia is the most common type of anemia among reproductive-age women. When you menstruate, you lose blood and hemoglobin, and with blood, iron. If your periods are heavy, you lose a lot of iron on a regular basis. Women can also become anemic during pregnancy because blood is diverted to the fetus, and a considerable amount is lost during childbirth. Women who crash diet or chronically watch their weight often don't eat enough to have sufficient iron in their blood. Iron-

LIFETIME

deficiency anemia is rare in women past menopause. At that time, too much iron can be a problem.

Less often, anemia is caused by a deficiency of the B vitamin folic acid, vitamin B_6, or vitamin B_{12}.

DIETARY Rx

Prescriptions
FOR IRON DEFICIENCY

If blood tests show that you have iron-deficiency anemia, your doctor will probably recommend a strategy geared toward improving the quality and quantity of iron consumed.

MEALTIME

❑ Eat one three-ounce serving of beef a day, says Barry Skikne, M.D., associate professor of hematology in the department of medicine at the University of Kansas Medical Center in Kansas City.

❑ Buy lean cuts, such as ground sirloin, flank steak, or top round. (Three ounces of broiled top round supplies 2.5 milligrams of iron, for example.) Or buy cheaper cuts of beef such as strip or chuck steak and trim the fat, suggests Fergus Clydesdale, Ph.D., head of the department of food science at the University of Massachusetts at Amherst.

❑ Try meat from game animals. It provides an excellent source of heme iron, the form most readily absorbed by the body. Roasted venison provides 3.8 milligrams of iron per three-ounce serving. Quail weighs in at 4.2 milligrams per bird.

❑ Chew each morsel thoroughly. This ensures that the meat is digested properly and the iron is properly absorbed, says Eleanor Young, Ph.D., retired professor from the department of medicine, gastroenterology, and nutrition at the University of Texas Health Science Center at San Antonio.

❑ Have minestrone made with ground beef and spinach. Aside from supplying a hefty amount of highly absorbable heme iron, meat enhances the absorption of nonheme iron, found in vegetables such as spinach, says Dr. Skikne.

❑ Make shish kebabs. Combining meat with vegetables high in vitamin C, such as peppers and tomatoes, enhances iron absorption.

Foods That Pump Iron

To achieve and maintain a healthy blood level of iron, try eating more iron-rich foods. The following chart highlights some of the best dietary sources of the mineral.

FOOD	PORTION	IRON (mg.)	% DV
Pumpkin seeds, hulled, dried	⅔ cup	13.8	77
Clams, steamed	About 20	11.9	66
Oysters (eastern), steamed	About 6 medium	10.2	57
Tofu, firm, uncooked	¼ block	8.5	47
Quinoa, raw	½ cup	7.9	44
Cream of Wheat, cooked	¾ cup	7.7	29
Soybeans, boiled	½ cup	4.4	25
Quail	1 bird	4.2	23
Cassava (tapioca)	4 oz.	4.1	23
Venison, roasted	3 oz.	3.8	21
Pot roast, lean, braised	3 oz.	3.2	18
Spinach, chopped, cooked	½ cup	3.2	18
Flank steak, lean, braised	3 oz.	3.0	16
Potato, baked	1	2.8	15
Kidney beans, boiled	½ cup	2.6	14
Sirloin steak, lean, broiled	3 oz.	2.6	14
Top round steak, lean, broiled	3 oz.	2.5	14
Ground beef, extra lean, broiled	3 oz.	2.0	11
Parsley, raw, chopped	½ cup	1.9	10
Pumpkin, canned	½ cup	1.7	9
Apricots, dried	¼ cup	1.5	9
Spaghetti, enriched, cooked	½ cup	1.0	5
Raisins, seedless	¼ cup	0.85	5

❑ If you're a vegetarian, focus on legumes and soy foods. Vegetarians can get enough protein to ensure their iron count is high enough, says Allan Magaziner, D.O., president of Magaziner Medical Center in Cherry Hill, New Jersey. Three ounces of tofu, a soy food, supplies 8.5 milligrams of iron, for example. And three-quarters cup of hot and healthy Cream of Wheat cereal provides 7.7 milligrams. You may also want to try quinoa, a plant protein similar to rice. It's available in health food stores.

MEALTIME

❐ Drink orange juice with meals. Vitamin C also helps the body absorb iron, says Dr. Clydesdale. So drinking orange juice with tofu, vegetables, or iron-fortified ready-to-eat breakfast cereals helps you absorb as much iron as possible.

Rx ——— *Prescriptions*
FOR IRON SUPPLEMENTS

Women need 18 milligrams of iron a day. If you're careful, you may be able to satisfy your iron needs through a diet rich in meat, fortified cereal, and iron-rich plant foods like kidney beans and apricots, say experts. Otherwise, you may not be getting your fair share of absorbable iron, especially if you are a vegetarian, since iron from vegetable sources is harder to absorb. And if you have particularly heavy monthly menstrual flows—bleeding heavily for five days—you may lose so much blood that you still need a daily supplement with iron even if your dietary intake is adequate, says Dr. Magaziner. So for some, a daily multivitamin/mineral supplement with iron makes sense.

Taking iron tablets daily may cause diarrhea or constipation. So most experts don't recommend iron supplements unless your doctor confirms the need with a blood test. If that's the case, your doctor may consider the following approach.

MONTHLY

❐ Take 300 milligrams of ferrous sulfate daily for seven days during menstruation only. (Check with your doctor before doing so to make sure that taking extra iron is appropriate for you.) Ferrous sulfate (an inexpensive supplement available without a prescription) ensures that you get the iron you need when you need it most, without risking toxic buildup, says Allan Erslev, M.D., professor of medicine at Thomas Jefferson University Hospital in Philadelphia.

NIGHTTIME

❐ Take iron tablets on an empty stomach with orange juice at bedtime. Taking them with milk or food inhibits iron absorption, says Dr. Skikne.

❐ If you take both iron and calcium supplements, space them three hours apart. Calcium supplements taken in combination with iron pills may impede iron absorption, says Dr. Clydesdale.

Medical **Alert**

See a doctor immediately if you have abnormal blood loss for any reason, such as blood in your stool or urine, which may indicate a more serious condition than anemia, says Dr. Skikne.

Also, consult your doctor if you are taking iron supplements for fatigue or other symptoms of anemia and your energy levels don't improve within two to three months, says Dr. Skikne.

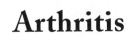

Arthritis

Arthritis has a reputation as an age-related disease. While it does seem to favor the senior set, it also affects people who are years younger. In one survey of 24,000 women, nearly 9 percent of those between the ages of 15 and 44 reported arthritis symptoms. Nearly every one of us will suffer some degree of arthritis by the time we reach 65, predicts Doyt Conn, M.D., senior vice president of medical affairs for the Arthritis Foundation in Atlanta.

Arthritis takes more than 100 different forms. The two most common—and the two we are usually referring to when we use the word *arthritis*—are osteoarthritis and rheumatoid arthritis.

Osteoarthritis, or degenerative joint disease, affects about 16 million people in the United States, according to Dr. Conn. The condition is characterized by the gradual breakdown of cartilage, the soft, spongy material that cushions joints. Eventually, joint pain and stiffness set in.

Osteoarthritis typically affects the finger joints as well as weight-bearing joints such as the knees and hips, and the lower back and neck. The condition can result from an injury, overweight, or simply years of routine wear and tear. Osteoarthritis develops slowly and, in some cases, can progress for years without noticeable symptoms.

Rheumatoid arthritis isn't nearly so subtle. Medically speaking, it is classified as an autoimmune disease. In effect, the body's immune system turns on itself—in this case, causing the synovial membrane, which lubricates each joint, to become inflamed. The inflammation damages cartilage and bone, producing swelling, redness, warmth, and pain in the joints, along with fever, fatigue, and loss of appetite.

Rheumatoid arthritis affects about 2.5 million people in the United States—mostly women in their thirties, forties, and fifties. In fact, almost three times as many women as men develop rheumatoid arthritis.

Thanks to advances in treatment, a diagnosis of osteoarthritis or rheumatoid arthritis no longer means a lifetime of pain. By eating right, exercising regularly, and adopting a few essential lifestyle changes, you can learn to manage your arthritis symptoms and perhaps even slow or stop the progression of the disease, says Dr. Conn.

Rx — *Prescriptions*
TO SUBDUE SYMPTOMS

For either type of arthritis, nonsteroidal anti-inflammatory drugs (NSAIDs) may be used to help control the symptoms. But other, nondrug remedies can also help ease the ache and improve joint mobility. Try the following for prompt relief.

TIME IT RIGHT   ❐ Apply cold to the affected joint for 10 to 15 minutes at a time, two or three times a day. Continue the treatment for a few days until the flare-up subsides. Cold works best for reducing inflammation, notes Philip J. Mease, M.D., a rheumatologist at Minor and James Medical Clinic in Seattle. Use a bag of frozen peas if you have one handy. It conforms to the shape of the joint. And remember to wrap the bag in a towel so that the ice doesn't damage your skin.

MORNING   ❐ Take a warm bath or shower for 10 to 15 minutes first thing in the morning. Heat relaxes tense muscles and improves circulation, says Dr. Conn.

NIGHTTIME   ❐ On cold nights, sleep between flannel sheets covered by an electric blanket, recommends the Arthritis Foundation. Then turn on the blanket for 20 minutes before getting up in the morning. This bedtime technique helps ease the morning stiffness associated with arthritis.

❏ For osteoarthritis, try an over-the-counter cream formulated with TIME IT RIGHT capsaicin, like Zostrix and Menthacin. Capsaicin is a chili pepper extract. It reduces pain by depleting a chemical in the nerves called substance P, which is responsible for sending pain messages to the brain. The cream usually begins to work within two to four weeks, but it must be applied three to four times a day, every day. If the product is not used in this way, pain may recur in a few days or weeks.

When you first apply a capsaicin cream, you may feel a burning sensation on your skin, according to Jaya Rao, M.D., a rheumatologist at the Roudebush Veterans Affairs Medical Center in Indianapolis. It should subside within a few weeks.

❏ For rheumatoid arthritis, take 400 milligrams of curcumin TIME IT RIGHT three times a day until the flare-up subsides. Curcumin—the yellow pigment that gives turmeric its color—may be nature's most potent anti-inflammatory agent, according to Joseph E. Pizzorno Jr., N.D., a naturopathic doctor and founding president of Bastyr University in Seattle and author of *Total Wellness*. Studies of people with rheumatoid arthritis have shown that curcumin improves mobility, morning stiffness, and joint swelling. Curcumin capsules are available at health food stores.

❏ Drink a cup of ginger tea before going to bed. Like curcumin, NIGHTTIME ginger has anti-inflammatory properties. Those with rheumatoid arthritis who have tried the herb report less-intense pain, improved joint movement as well as decreased swelling and morning stiffness, according to Dr. Pizzorno.

To make ginger tea, slice a piece of fresh ginger and put a few shavings or slivers of it in a tea ball. Put the tea ball in a cup, pour freshly boiled water over it, and allow the ginger to steep for 10 minutes. Make sure the tea has cooled off before sipping it.

Prescriptions
TO FEND OFF FLARE-UPS

NUTRITION
Rx

Beyond short-term pain relief, you can actually reduce the frequency and severity of arthritis flare-ups with a few basic lifestyle changes. Take your diet, for instance: By consuming more of some foods and less of others, you may be able to keep your arthritis symptoms in check. Here's what experts recommend.

❒ Eat at least one three-ounce serving of fish each day. In some studies, the omega-3 fatty acids found in abundance in certain species of fish have helped to reduce the inflammation associated with rheumatoid arthritis. Just three ounces of Atlantic salmon, canned anchovies, or Atlantic herring contain 1.6 grams of omega-3's, the amount linked to lower risk of rheumatoid arthritis.

❒ Eat at least one serving of a vitamin C–rich fruit or vegetable each day. Vitamin C may help slow the progression of osteoarthritis, according to Dr. Conn. For starters, the nutrient plays a role in the manufacture of collagen, a connective tissue that your body uses to repair cartilage. In addition, vitamin C is an antioxidant. That means it helps neutralize free radicals, unstable molecules that occur naturally in the body and that appear to worsen arthritis inflammation. Excellent sources of vitamin C include guava (165 milligrams per one whole fruit) and fresh-squeezed orange juice (106 milligrams per eight-ounce serving).

❒ Follow an elimination diet to isolate those foods that may trigger symptoms of rheumatoid arthritis, says Dr. Pizzorno. Research has established a link between flare-ups of rheumatoid arthritis and the consumption of certain foods. Among the most common offenders: milk, wheat, sugar, corn, soy, and all members of the nightshade family (including tomatoes, potatoes, peppers, and eggplant). Try giving up these foods for at least three months. Then reintroduce one food each week to determine which, if any, may aggravate your symptoms. If you find a potential culprit, drop it from your diet completely. You may notice that you have fewer flare-ups.

Rx ——— *Prescriptions*
FOR STAYING ACTIVE

Along with proper nutrition, regular exercise figures prominently in any arthritis treatment plan. Of course, when your joints hurt, you probably don't feel much like working out. But physical activity can actually prevent swollen or stiff joints from becoming even more painful, according

Virtually Vegetarian

Can a very low fat, almost meatless diet minimize the symptoms of rheumatoid arthritis? At least one study suggests that it can.

Researchers at Loma Linda University in California placed 45 people with rheumatoid arthritis on a diet of mostly vegetarian meals. The participants were allowed three ounces of fish or chicken each day. Their daily fat intake was limited to just 10 percent of calories.

After three months, the participants reported half as many painful and tender joints and one-quarter as many swollen joints. Morning stiffness decreased by half, and walking times improved by 30 percent.

Why does following a semivegetarian diet help ease rheumatoid arthritis? The researchers have come up with a couple of theories. First, this type of diet restricts the consumption of animal protein, which may trigger symptoms in some people. Second, it shifts the nutrition focus to fruits and vegetables. Produce has an abundance of antioxidant nutrients, which may help prevent inflammation.

If you decide to give an almost meatless diet a try, make sure that you fill your plate with plenty of whole grains, legumes, and soy foods (for example, low-fat tofu), and at least five servings of fruits and vegetables a day, says Edwin H. Krick, M.D., associate professor of medicine at Loma Linda University. (A serving is one medium fruit, one cup raw leafy vegetables, one-half cup chopped vegetables or fruit, or three-quarters cup juice.) Eliminate most animal products, except for fish such as Atlantic salmon, canned anchovies, and Atlantic herring, which are high in omega-3 fatty acids (omega-3's help reduce inflammation); skim milk; and nonfat yogurt (both are important calcium sources).

to Dr. Rao. "When a particular joint aches, you tend to avoid using it," she explains. "But if you don't use it, regaining normal function is that much harder."

Exercise eases arthritis in other ways, too. It helps you maintain a healthy weight, and it builds muscle strength and tone. "Muscle takes pressure off the joints, so you feel more comfortable," explains James M. Fox, M.D., senior partner with the Southern California Orthopedic Institute and Medical Group in Van Nuys.

To develop a joint-friendly exercise routine, follow this advice from the experts.

❒ Schedule your workout for the time of day when you tend to have the least pain, says Dr. Fox. If you have rheumatoid arthritis, for instance, you may be most comfortable exercising later in the day. That way, any morning stiffness has a chance to subside.

TIME IT RIGHT

❒ Swim or cycle for 30 minutes every day. Both activities strengthen muscles while placing minimal stress on the joints, notes Dr. Fox. Swimming has another plus: The warm water relaxes muscles and eases pain.

❒ Practice tai chi or yoga. The slow, flowing movements of tai chi and the poses of yoga build strength and improve flexibility. They also relax the body as well as the mind, says Dr. Mease.

❒ If arthritis has affected your hands, do hand and wrist exercises after washing dishes or during a bath. The warm water leaves your hands and wrists relaxed and limber, so moving them is more comfortable.

One exercise that arthritis experts recommend, the thumb walk, is helpful for improving your wrist flexibility. Holding your wrist straight, form the letter O by touching your thumb to each fingertip. After making each O, spread out your fingers. Use your other hand to help, if necessary.

NIGHTTIME

❒ Stretch before you sleep. Performing light flexibility exercises prior to going to bed can head off morning stiffness, explains Dr. Fox. For example, if your knees are stiff, sit with your legs stretched out in front of you. Place a rolled towel under your knee to keep the joint straight. Tighten the muscles in your leg, but don't move your knee. Hold the contraction, then relax and repeat up to 25 times. Work up to where you can keep the muscles taut for 30 seconds.

Prescriptions
FOR PAIN-FREE LIVING

Rx

Besides proper nutrition and regular exercise, other strategies can help minimize the impact that arthritis has on your life. Consider making the following part of a joint-friendly lifestyle.

❒ Watch your weight. Carrying extra pounds puts stress on joints and aggravates arthritis symptoms, says Dr. Fox. In fact, being overweight may contribute to the development of osteoarthritis in the first place.

While there are a number of complex formulas for calculating your ideal weight, one simple formula used by some experts can let you know if you're close: If you are five feet tall, you should weigh 100 pounds. If you're taller, add 5 pounds for each additional inch of height. Then to that number, add 10 percent if you have a large frame, or subtract 10 percent if you have a small frame.

❒ Meditate every day. Meditation helps to ease arthritis pain by deeply relaxing your body. This releases tension in your muscles and causes subtle changes in your central nervous system that lower pain. "Find a quiet place where you can sit or lie still and collect your thoughts," suggests Dr. Mease. "Meditation doesn't have to be mystical or religious. Just take a moment to focus inward."

❒ Maintain an active sex life with your partner. Experts say that sexual arousal prompts your body to produce cortisone and other natural painkillers, which help ease arthritis symptoms.

Medical **Alert**
If you suspect that you have arthritis, you should see your doctor for a proper diagnosis, says Dr. Conn. Any of the following symptoms also warrant prompt medical attention: severe joint pain that doesn't respond to ice packs, heat, or pain relievers; persistent joint stiffness after an injury; or persistent joint swelling accompanied by fever or chills.

Asthma

You love cats. From afar. But get anywhere near a feline, and suddenly you start to wheeze, cough, and gasp for air.

That's asthma—when breathing suddenly becomes difficult, thanks to some trigger, usually an allergy to something in your environment. Other triggers can include respiratory infections, colds, laughter, crying, anger, exercise, and stress.

NIGHTTIME

Scary. Even scarier is that the majority of asthma attacks occur in the middle of the night, says Neil Feldman, D.O., an asthma and allergy specialist in Allentown, Pennsylvania. Why? Allergies are the most common risk factor for asthma, and one of the most common allergens, dust mites, thrive in your bedroom. The dander found in pet fur is also a very potent allergen. So if your cat sleeps with you, you are spending hours exposed to her dander. Scarier still is that asthma attacks often are most severe at night because we breathe more shallowly in the predawn hours.

MORNING

Other common allergens that trigger asthma include molds, pollens, chemicals, and cigarette smoke. If you are sensitive to these allergens, you will be most susceptible when you wake up.

"If you wake up at 2:00 or 3:00 A.M. with asthma, it's a bad sign—you know that your asthma is active and your preventive measures are not working as they should," Dr. Feldman says.

MONTHLY

In women, asthma often gets worse before or during menstruation, says Steven Kagen, M.D., founder and director of the Kagen Allergy Clinic in Appleton, Wisconsin. A week or so before menstruation, women produce more mucus in their nose, throat, and lungs, he says.

The mucus that ends up in the lungs may cause more-than-usual constriction and difficulty breathing, says Richard J. Martin, M.D., professor of medicine at the University of Colorado Health Sciences Center and head of the pulmonary division and vice chairman of the department of medicine at the National Jewish Medical and Research Center, both in Denver.

Some women are more sensitive to hormonal fluctuations than others—and it is these women who are most likely to experience heightened asthma symptoms during menstruation or pregnancy, Dr. Kagen says. "Any small change in hormone level, and such women will feel it big time."

Asthma tends to worsen in the late-second and early-third trimesters, but some women actually experience less asthma in the last month of pregnancy, says Leonard Bielory, M.D., director of the Asthma and Allergy Research Center at the New Jersey Medical School in Newark.

Prescriptions
FOR ASTHMA RELIEF

Rx

Asthma is a chronic disease that can't be cured but can be controlled. If you know that you have asthma, chances are that your doctor has prescribed preventive medicines, such as inhaled steroids or oral medications. These will reduce inflammation and swelling and slow your body's reaction to allergens and irritants. When an asthma attack strikes, other medications may be used to open up your bronchial passages. But medication alone isn't enough.

You can talk to your doctor about using a peak flow monitor at home to measure how well your lungs are functioning. "This device can give you important information when you are starting to have problems, and your

ASTHMA EMERGENCIES AND YOUR MENSTRUAL CYCLE

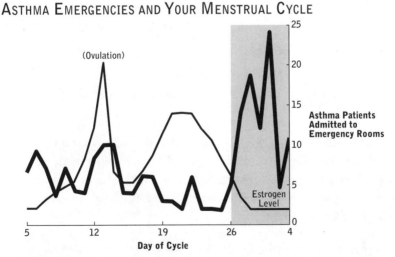

Menstruating women are more likely to experience an asthma attack that leads to a trip to the emergency room three days before the start of their periods and then during their periods. Tracking your menstrual cycle may help you to anticipate — and control — attacks.

doctor can help you adjust your preventive medications before your symptoms get really bad," explains Daryl R. Altman, M.D., director of Allergy Information Services, a consulting service in Hewlett, New York. "There are also lifestyle changes that can help minimize attacks and their intensity." To cut down on attacks, however, you have to know what causes them. So pay attention to when your asthma strikes.

Though you can't control everything in your environment that might bring on an asthma attack, you can make changes in your home, which can lessen the possibility of an asthma attack, doctors say.

❏ If possible, get rid of carpeting, which harbors dust mites. Or spray a 3 percent solution of tannic acid on your carpet every 60 days, suggests Dr. Altman. Because tannic acid may discolor your carpet, spot-test a small area first to see what the finished result will be. If you don't like the color, you may want to try one of the many other spray products designed to control dust mites. All are available through mail-order allergy suppliers.

❏ Wash your bedding twice a week in hot water to kill dust mites, Dr. Martin says.

❏ Delegate dusting, vacuuming, mopping, and other dusty indoor chores. Otherwise, says Dr. Martin, trying to clean up may stir up dust mites and dander, triggering an attack.

❏ Recruit someone else to mow the lawn and rake the leaves. Outdoor chores stir up pollen, which will irritate overreactive airways, says Dr. Bielory.

TIME IT RIGHT ❏ If you must exercise outside, do it in the early afternoon, not the morning, so that you are outside when pollen and mold levels are at their lowest. Grass pollinates between 5:00 and 10:00 A.M., says Dr. Kagen. Weeds pollinate at sunrise and sundown. If you are allergic to weed pollen, midday activities are best.

❏ If it is windy outside, stay indoors. Pollen counts—and allergic responses—rise on windy days, says Dr. Kagen.

❏ Run the air conditioner in your car so that pollen doesn't fly in open windows, says Dr. Kagen.

PRESCRIPTION FOR AN ALLERGY-FREE BEDROOM

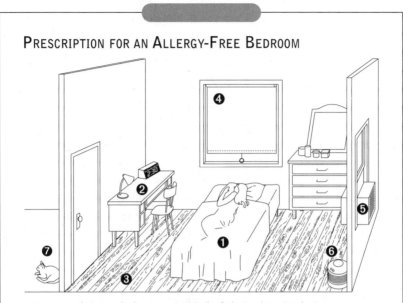

Most people spend about one-third of their time in their bedrooms. And asthma attacks more frequently occur at night, between 2:00 and 3:00 A.M. So the more you can allergy-proof the room in which you sleep, the less likely you will be to wake up in the middle of a night with breathing trouble.

1. Encase your mattress in vinyl or a combination vinyl-and-cotton casing, available from mail-order allergy suppliers.

2. Remove as much clutter as you can to give dust and mold less of a chance to collect. Plus, an uncluttered surface is easier to wipe clean.

3. If you can, go with bare wood or tile floors. Carpeting collects mites and molds, which trigger asthma.

4. Replace curtains with shades or vertical blinds—they collect much less dust than curtains or horizontal blinds.

5. Environmental irritants also can provoke asthma. When possible, close the windows, turn on the air conditioner, and use a high-efficiency particulate (HEPA) filter.

6. Run a dehumidifier at all times. Humidity breeds mold, which breeds dust mites, which increases the intensity of your allergies and asthma.

7. Shut the door on your pets. Most people would no sooner get rid of Fido or Fluffy than they would their children, so compromise. Keep your cat or dog out of your bedroom.

❏ Clean your air conditioner (including the air filter) every week. If you don't, dust mites and mold will congregate there, says Dr. Feldman. Portable air conditioners are easier to clean than the vents in central air conditioners.

❏ If you can, time your vacations for the height of the pollen season. Then go to the beach or other pollen-free destinations, says Dr. Bielory.

❏ Be especially careful to avoid asthma triggers during pregnancy, says Dr. Bielory.

MONTHLY

❏ If you are prone to heartburn, try to eat four to six small, frequent meals, with your last meal no later than four hours before bedtime. That way, your body has time to digest your food, explains Dr. Bielory. Aside from hormonal changes, gastroesophageal reflux—which causes heartburn and belching and is especially common during pregnancy—can make asthma worse.

❏ If you smoke, quit. And don't let others smoke in your house. Cigarette smoke is one of the worst triggers of asthma, and that goes double when you are pregnant, says William Storms, M.D., associate clinical professor of medicine at the University of Colorado Health Sciences Center and an allergist in Colorado Springs.

NUTRITION
Rx

Prescriptions
FOR ASTHMA

Some vitamins and minerals have been found to lessen symptoms associated with asthma, says Elson Haas, M.D., director of the Preventive Medical Center of Marin in San Rafael, California, and author of *Staying Healthy with Nutrition*. He recommends talking with your doctor about adding the following to your individual treatment plan.

❏ Take 1,000 milligrams of vitamin C four times a day. Vitamin C may help to reduce the coughing and wheezing associated with asthma.
Note: Taking more than 1,200 milligrams of vitamin C a day has been known to cause diarrhea in some people. If this happens to you, reduce the dosage until your symptoms subside.

❏ Take 250 milligrams of quercetin a day. A bioflavonoid (plant compound), quercetin is thought to ward off asthma by inhibiting the mast cells, a component of your immune system that causes allergic reactions by releasing histamines. Quercetin can be purchased in health food stores.

❐ Take 240 milligrams of fish oil twice a day. Available in capsule form from health food stores, fish oil can help reduce the inflammation associated with asthma.

❐ Take two 500-milligram capsules of evening primrose oil three times a day. Available in health food stores, evening primrose oil may also reduce the effects of inflammation.

❐ Take 100 to 500 milligrams of magnesium one to three times a day, says Kendall Gerdes, M.D., allergist and director of Environmental Medicine Associates in Denver. Many people with asthma don't have enough magnesium in their diet. Extra magnesium may help to decrease the muscle tension and spasms of the airways that are associated with asthma, he explains. Because high doses of magnesium (350 milligrams or more) can cause cramps, gas, or diarrhea for some people, Dr. Gerdes suggests starting with the lowest dosage and increasing it gradually until you experience symptoms. Then cut back the dosage until your symptoms subside. To get the most benefit, you should take as much magnesium as your system can tolerate, advises Dr. Gerdes.

Note: If you have heart or kidney problems, talk to your doctor before taking supplemental magnesium.

❐ If your asthma symptoms are worsened by your menstrual cycle, try taking 100 to 400 milligrams of vitamin B_6 for a day or two before you anticipate a flare-up, Dr. Gerdes says. Vitamin B_6 may help your body adjust better to the hormonal swings of your menstrual cycle. The recommended dosage is not intended for daily use, however. Taken for a prolonged period of time, high doses of B_6 (50 milligrams to 2 grams daily) can cause numb feet and unstable gait.

Monthly

Medical Alert

If you are having an asthma attack, use a doctor-prescribed inhaler immediately, says Dr. Storms. Then get away from what triggered your asthma, if possible. Sip a cup of warm water or tea and try to breathe slowly and deeply. If you still can't breathe easily, call 911 or have someone drive you to the emergency room immediately.

Cancer Prevention

It's probably the last thing in the world anyone wants to think about. But we still do every now and then, particularly when someone we know gets cancer. Each of us wonders, could cancer be silently growing somewhere inside *my* body?

But is worrying about cancer so bad if it induces us to take action to avoid it, perhaps even prevent a recurrence?

In fact, the major cancer killers of women—lung, breast, and colon cancers—are pretty much avoidable. "People need to realize that cancer is a preventable illness, just like heart disease," says Graham Colditz, Dr.P.H., associate professor of medicine at Harvard Medical School. "Nearly two-thirds of cancer deaths in the United States can be linked to tobacco use, diet, and lack of exercise. If people simply applied in their own lives the knowledge that we now have about preventing cancer, we could cut its incidence way back."

Some people, apparently, are confused about the best ways to prevent cancer. Should they eat that carrot, even if it's not organically grown? Drink only bottled water? And what about things like green tea and ginseng?

"The truth is that although these things may one day prove to be helpful, there are a lot more prosaic things already proven to help prevent cancer," says Dr. Colditz. So we are listing them here—the things that experts say every woman should do, all the time, to reduce her risk for cancer.

Rx

Prescriptions
FOR A CANCER-COMBATING LIFESTYLE

These cancer-dodging tactics offer the most protection in exchange for your efforts, experts say.

MONTHLY

❒ If you smoke, quit. Cigarette smoking causes nearly all cases of lung cancer, the current top cancer killer in women. It has also been directly linked to one-third of all other cancers, including cancers of the throat, mouth, cervix, colon, bladder, kidney, and pancreas, says Peggy O'Hara, Ph.D., associate professor of epidemiology and public health at the University of Miami School of Medicine. Once you stop smoking, your risk for many of these cancers begins to drop until, in 10 to 15 years, it's comparable to the cancer risk of someone who has never smoked.

The best time to kick the habit is during the first half of your menstrual cycle. That's when high levels of female hormones can counterbalance withdrawal symptoms such as irritability and depression, recommends Dr. O'Hara.

❏ Limit your alcohol consumption to no more than one drink a day. "Consuming more than that increases your risk for esophageal cancer and, possibly, breast cancer," Dr. Colditz says. A drink, by the way, is one 12-ounce beer, one 5-ounce glass of wine, or a mixed drink made with 1½ ounces of liquor.

❏ Maintain a healthy weight. If you exceed your optimum weight by 35 percent or more, you raise your risk for cancer of the breast, cervix, endometrium, uterus, and ovaries, Dr. Colditz says. So for a woman whose optimum weight is 135 pounds, for instance, carrying an extra 47 pounds—or 182 pounds total—would put her in the danger zone. While there are a number of complex formulas for calculating your ideal weight, one simple formula used by some experts can let you know if you're close: If you are five feet tall, you should weigh 100 pounds. If you are taller, add 5 pounds for each additional inch of height. Then to that number, add 10 percent if you have a large frame, or subtract 10 percent if you have a small frame.

❏ Exercise for at least 30 minutes every day. "Even moderate levels of activity, such as brisk walking, for a total of three hours a week could substantially lower your risk of cancer," Dr. Colditz says. "So figure on a half-hour almost every day." More active women—those who run or jog for a total of five hours or more a week—probably cut their risk by more than half, he adds.

"Exercise decreases bowel transit time, so it reduces the amount of time that potential carcinogens in the stool may be in contact with the intestines," explains David P. Rose, M.D., D.Sc., Ph.D., chief of the division of nutrition and endocrinology at the Naylor Dana Institute of the American Health Foundation in Valhalla, New York.

TIME IT RIGHT

It also reduces insulin levels, "and there's some evidence that high circulating levels of insulin promote tumor growth," Dr. Colditz says. In the case of breast cancer, exercise may change levels of hormones, such as estrogen, in a way that makes them less cancer-promoting.

❏ Identify all of the hazardous materials that you are exposed to at work and learn how to handle them safely. If you are a hairdresser, electronics assembler, or x-ray technician, for instance, or if you are exposed to glues, solvents, paints, radioactive materials, wood dust, pesticides, or other chemicals, know the names and chemical compositions of all potentially hazardous substances with which you work, Dr. Colditz recommends. "Get a copy of the 'Material Safety Data Sheet' for the material you're handling and read it," he says. By law, your employer is obligated to provide this to you. Wear personal protective equipment where indicated. Insist that your work environment be designed and ventilated to prevent exposure to toxic substances.

NUTRITION Rx

Prescriptions
FOR SHORING UP YOUR DEFENSES

Good nutrition is absolutely essential to a cancer-combating lifestyle. In fact, certain foods contain nutrients and other compounds that appear to reduce cancer risk. Based on what research has shown so far, experts suggest the following guidelines for creating your own anti-cancer eating plan.

MEALTIME

❏ Eat a cup or two of dark green, leafy vegetables each day. Kale, spinach, mustard greens, beet greens, and romaine lettuce are your best sources of folate, a B vitamin that helps protect cells against cancer-inducing genetic damage from chemicals and viruses. In fact, folate gets its name from foliage. To prepare greens, try lightly steaming or braising them, then sprinkling them with olive oil and sesame seeds.

❏ Eat at least half a cup of orange-colored produce every other day. Try rich sources such as carrots, sweet potatoes, and pumpkin to boost your intake of carotenoids, which have shown promise as cancer-fighting compounds. Research has suggested that carotenoids may slow the development of precancerous lesions and even reverse precancerous cell changes. Try adding shredded carrots to tomato sauce and meat loaf, serving mashed sweet potatoes or baked sweet potato fries, or baking a low-fat pie using pumpkin and evaporated skim milk.

❒ Eat cruciferous vegetables such as broccoli, brussels sprouts, cabbage, and cauliflower at least every other day. Crucifers contain compounds that stimulate your body's production of cancer-blocking enzymes. Enjoy low-fat coleslaw or steamed broccoli in garlic sauce.

❒ Eat tomatoes every day. Tomatoes are rich in lycopene, a member of the carotenoid family with similar cancer-fighting properties. Italian researchers found that people who ate seven or more servings of tomatoes a week were 60 percent less likely to develop cancer of the stomach, colon, and rectum than were people who ate two or fewer servings a week. If tomatoes don't tempt your tastebuds, then try red grapefruit and sweet red peppers, which also have abundant supplies of lycopene.

❒ Eat a clove of garlic at least once a week. Research suggests that garlic and other members of the onion family, known as alliums, cut your odds of developing cancer. In one study, women who ate garlic at least once a week cut their colon cancer risk by one-third as compared with women who never ate the stuff.

❒ Replace at least a portion of the red meat that you eat with fish and seafood. These rich sources of omega-3 fatty acids have been shown in clinical and epidemiological studies to decrease the incidence of both colon and breast tumors.

❒ Try substituting some vegetables for meat, too, recommends Dr. Rose. Vegetables also provide a healthy dose of cancer-fighting compounds such as genistein and other isoflavones.

❒ As for red meat, reduce your intake and try to limit yourself to just MONTHLY one serving a month. Harvard University researchers have shown that restricting your consumption of red meat in this way can cut your risk for colon cancer in half as compared with that of women who normally eat beef, pork, or lamb every day.

❏ Substitute olive oil for saturated fats, such as butter and lard. Scientists have yet to establish a definite link between a high-fat diet and cancer. But they do know that eating more monounsaturated fats, such as olive oil, and fewer saturated fats can protect against breast cancer, according to Dr. Colditz.

❏ Take a daily multivitamin that contains 500 to 1,000 milligrams of vitamin C, 200 to 400 international units of vitamin E, and 800 micrograms of folic acid (the supplement form of folate), along with other essential nutrients. "I believe that women need this extra protection against cancer—even if they eat healthfully," says Dr. Rose.

Note: Doses of folic acid exceeding 400 micrograms per day should be taken only under the supervision of a doctor. In large amounts, the nutrient can mask signs of a vitamin B_{12} deficiency.

Medical **Alert**

Cancer takes many forms, and so do its symptoms. The American Cancer Society recommends that you see a doctor promptly if you have any of these symptoms: a persistent cough, bloody phlegm, chest pain, recurring pneumonia, or bronchitis; rectal bleeding or a change in bowel habits; a lump, thickening, dimpling, or irritation in a breast, or nipple tenderness or discharge; enlarged lymph nodes, itching, fever, night sweats, anemia, and weight loss; fatigue, repeated infections, frequent bruising, and nosebleeds; abdominal pain or swelling or jaundice; headaches, nausea, and vomiting; vision or hearing loss; difficulty speaking or swallowing; or a change in the shape, color, or size of a mole.

Chronic Fatigue

Energy is hard to describe but easy to achieve—for most people. Step into a shower in the morning, and your whole body wakes up. Grab a cup of coffee in the middle of the afternoon, and you get a second wind. Get a good night's sleep after a trying day, and you're ready to get back into the fray.

Now, imagine never getting a good night's sleep. Never feeling fully awake and energized, no matter how many showers you take or cups of java you drink. You have entered the Chronic Fatigue Zone.

Four out of five people in the United States who enter the Chronic Fatigue Zone are women—women who are bone-crunchingly tired almost all the time, often for no apparent reason. No one knows what causes chronic fatigue, though experts say that it probably stems from any number of factors, including poor diet, viral illnesses, weak immune systems, stress, or even sinus problems.

For years, doctors distinguished between simple chronic fatigue and outright chronic fatigue syndrome. Now, it seems, you qualify as chronically fatigued with or without some or all of the classic chronic fatigue syndrome symptoms: faulty memory and poor concentration, constant sore throat, joint and muscle pain, headaches, and poor sleep.

So far, no one has a cure for chronic fatigue. Doctors say that most people recover eventually, but that may take as long as five years. The encouraging news is that by making some changes in your routine—what you eat and when, for example, or timing forays outdoors just right—you can regain some of your lost energy.

Prescriptions
FOR BUILDING STAMINA

EXERCISE
Rx

Experts say that exercise is a major force in launching out of the Chronic Fatigue Zone. You might feel as though you can't lift a finger, let alone a dumbbell. But, in fact, moving your body—and establishing an exercise routine—can help you regain physical and mental pizzazz. Women with chronic fatigue become deconditioned when they don't do any exercise and they spend a lot of time lying down, explains Daniel Hamner, M.D., physiatrist in private practice in New York City.

The same thing happens to astronauts, says Nelson Gantz, M.D., chief of the department of medicine and the division of infectious diseases at Pinnacle Health System in Harrisburg, Pennsylvania. Remember Shannon Lucid? After 188 continuous days in space, she could barely walk away from the space shuttle under her own power. Many astronauts are so deconditioned after even a few days in space that they have to be carried off, Dr. Gantz explains.

The key to exercise is to think small, experts say.

TIME IT RIGHT

❐ Today, walk five minutes at a moderate pace, then take a day off, says Dr. Hamner. As you grow comfortable with that amount of exercise, try to increase your walking time by two to three minutes a week. Or, if you prefer, ride a stationary bicycle for five minutes or go swimming.

MORNING

❐ Exercise in the morning. Most people with chronic fatigue find that exercise is best done first thing in the morning, says Dr. Hamner. And don't be afraid that you will use up the energy that you need to do housework or other activities. "Exercise really gives more energy in the long run," he says.

WINTERTIME

❐ Take advantage of sunny days. Lack of sunlight seems to lead to more fatigue, especially during the winter months when there are fewer hours of daylight, says Allan Magaziner, D.O., president of Magaziner Medical Center in Cherry Hill, New Jersey. Your pineal gland, a pea-size organ in your brain, needs natural light to secrete melatonin, a hormone that helps you sleep and makes you feel better. So, try to take your five-minute walk first thing in the morning to take advantage of the sun's rays when you can.

❐ Keep an exercise diary. Write down how you feel right after exercise, later that morning or afternoon, that evening, and the next day. Over the weeks, refer to your notes. In time, you should note an improvement in your energy levels.

Some fatigue is normal for the first couple of weeks. If you experience unrelenting or recurring joint pain, though, see a doctor before continuing, says Dr. Gantz.

❐ Expect some limitations. A lot of people with chronic fatigue were once very active, says Dr. Hamner. "If they don't exercise the way they used to, they feel that they're not really exercising, so they get discouraged and think, 'Why do it?' Don't defeat yourself before you start," he says. Even a few minutes of exercise will lessen fatigue.

NUTRITION
Rx

Prescriptions
TO BEAT TIREDNESS

Not surprisingly, women with chronic fatigue can no sooner prepare full-course meals from scratch than they could fly to Mars under their own power. The natural tendency is to rely on frozen pizza, canned spaghetti, and other processed foods, says Dr. Magaziner. The problem is that a diet built on convenience foods skimps on beans, fruits, vegetables, whole grains, and other foods rich in vitamins and minerals. Without energy-building nutrients, he says, you will be tired all the time. Here's his nutritional prescription for beating chronic fatigue.

❐ Start your day with fruits and grains. A healthy breakfast is crucial for anyone, and that goes triple if you have chronic fatigue, says Dr. Magaziner. You don't have to make pancakes from scratch; quick-cooking or microwaveable oatmeal and a sliced apple will do the trick. Oatmeal is a good source of magnesium, which the body needs to get energy from food. One sign of magnesium deficiency is muscle weakness.

MORNING

❐ Have a cup of soup for lunch. Everyone knows that homemade soup is best, but when you're pinched for time, look for instant soups featuring beans or grains (like split pea or barley soup) in supermarkets and health food stores. Beans and grains provide B vitamins that shore up your immune system, says Dr. Magaziner. Just add boiling water to the ingredients and let the mix sit for a few minutes, according to the package directions.

DAYTIME

❐ Have beans and grains with dinner, too. You can choose any kind of beans or grains you like, says Dr. Magaziner. Lima beans or chickpeas, for example, or rice or couscous will do.

MEALTIME

❐ Snack on pumpkin and sunflower seeds. They provide zinc, a trace mineral that can help restore energy by boosting the immune system and reducing the risk of infection, says Dr. Magaziner. And seeds take no time to prepare. The same goes for nuts, another reliable source of zinc.

❐ Try coenzyme Q_{10}, a natural compound that's available in supplement form in health food stores. Taking 30 milligrams a day improves the body's ability to use oxygen efficiently and ultimately gives you more energy, says Dr. Magaziner.

❐ Supplement your diet with malic acid. Taking 300 milligrams a day in pill form helps feed the energy-producing cycles of the body, says Dr. Magaziner. Malic acid is available in health food stores.

❐ Take a daily multivitamin/mineral supplement that includes 400 milligrams of magnesium and up to 25 milligrams of each B vitamin, says Dr. Magaziner. Your body needs magnesium in order to get energy from food. Deficiencies of B vitamins—especially B_{12}—have been linked to fatigue and memory loss, among other symptoms.

Clear Your Sinuses, Escape Fatigue

Who would have thought that there might be a link between sinus trouble and chronic fatigue? Yet an enormous number of people with chronic fatigue also have chronic sinus problems, says Alexander C. Chester, M.D., clinical professor of medicine at the Georgetown University Medical Center in Washington, D.C.

"A lot of chronic fatigue relates to sinusitis," Dr. Chester says. Sinusitis is often a systemic illness, one that affects the entire body. People who suffer from sinusitis can feel sick all over, and extreme fatigue or malaise may be the chief complaint.

When your head is stuffed up and heavy with congestion all the time, and on top of that you have a pounding headache that won't go away, it's no surprise that you feel exhausted, says Dr. Chester. Those with mild sinusitis symptoms can also feel quite tired. A study in two Boston otolaryngologists' offices that compared the general health of people with chronic sinusitis with that of the general population found chronic sinusitis to be much more debilitating than angina, congestive heart failure, chronic obstructive pulmonary disease, and chronic back pain or sciatica. The people with chronic sinusitis described having intense body pain, physical limitations, and decreased energy that affected their everyday activities, and at surprisingly high levels. If you have chronic fatigue *and* sinusitis, here's some advice on how to keep your sinuses clear—and maybe lessen your chronic fatigue in the bargain.

Note: If you have heart or kidney problems, check with your doctor before taking supplemental magnesium. Supplemental magnesium may cause diarrhea in some people. Also, doses of folic acid exceeding 400 micrograms per day should be taken only under the supervision of a doctor. In large amounts, the nutrient can mask signs of a vitamin B_{12} deficiency.

❒ Avoid alcohol. Beer and wine in particular contain sulfites and other substances that may aggravate your sinuses by provoking an allergic reaction. Alcohol in general may dehydrate you and clog your sinuses, says Dr. Chester.

❒ Avoid milk and wheat, too. Milk and, less often, wheat products often provoke allergic responses in women with chronic fatigue and sinus conditions, says Dr. Chester.

❒ Steam out your sinuses. Breathing dry air clogs your sinuses in the worst way. Old-fashioned nasal treatments four times a day—like breathing in the steam from a steaming pot of hot water for 5 to 10 minutes—will shrink and moisturize your nasal membranes, Dr. Chester says. Take care not to burn yourself—keep your face at a comfortable distance from the hot steam.

❒ Stay wet. Nasal saline sprays are often helpful in moistening dry, inflamed nasal membranes and sometimes can have a decongestant effect. Spray your nose four times a day, says Dr. Chester. If your nose feels swollen, try a decongestant spray, he suggests.

Caution: Decongestant sprays should be taken no more often than three times a day for three days, or you may actually end up feeling more congested than before, says Dr. Chester.

Nasal steroid sprays or nasal antihistamine sprays can also be helpful, but you will need to see your doctor first because they are available by prescription only.

Rx ——— ## *Prescriptions*
TO BREATHE BETTER

In some people, chronic fatigue has been tied to allergies, especially to the dust, molds, and mold spores that develop in unused heating ducts and unventilated homes. The problem is most likely to occur during the winter months, when you keep your windows shut all the time, says Dr. Magaziner. His advice follows.

❏ If possible, have good ventilation and air filters installed in your home.

❏ Have the heating and ventilation system cleaned every one to two years. And don't forget to change the furnace air filters every month or so.

❏ If possible, and even in the wintertime, open your windows an inch if you are going out for an hour or so to allow for some fresh air exchange.

Rx ——— ## *Prescriptions*
FOR GET-UP-AND-GO

Nature's anti-fatigue prescription involves just the right amount of rest. Try these tips to feel refreshed and invigorated each morning.

TIME IT RIGHT ❏ Don't spend too much time in bed. Sleeping too much can make you feel more, rather than less, fatigued, says Alexander C. Chester, M.D., clinical professor of medicine at the Georgetown University Medical Center in Washington, D.C. Most people need seven to eight hours of sleep a night, no more.

MORNING ❏ If you feel tired when you get up, try a hot bath. It might refresh you in ways that a shower can't, says Dr. Chester.

Medical **Alert**

If you have unexplained severe fatigue for a month, see your doctor. Also, consult your doctor if you are still tired no matter what strategies you try to regain energy, says Dr. Chester.

Diabetes

What do prosciutto and melon, a walk in a rose garden, and vitamin E have in common? They are all natural prescriptions for diabetes.

Diabetes affects more than eight million American women. Surprisingly, half of them don't even know that they have the disease.

About 90 percent of women with diabetes have Type II, in which the body creates enough insulin but can't use it effectively. (Insulin is a hormone that helps the body to use blood sugar, or glucose, to fuel cells.) This results in hyperglycemia, or too much sugar in the bloodstream. Extended periods of high blood sugar damage the heart, kidneys, and eyes.

Type II diabetes usually shows up in women over age 40. It is caused primarily by overweight and a sedentary lifestyle, although heredity plays a role, too. Sometimes Type II is preceded by a condition called impaired glucose tolerance. In this condition, which affects 11 percent of adults, blood sugar levels are higher than normal, but they are not high enough to be classified as diabetes. Impaired glucose tolerance is considered a major risk factor for Type II diabetes and complications such as heart attack and stroke.

Another form of diabetes, Type I, usually shows up in childhood. People who have Type I can't produce enough insulin because certain cells in the pancreas have been destroyed. These folks require insulin injections to manage their condition.

Another form of diabetes—called gestational diabetes—occurs during pregnancy. So doctors routinely order a glucose tolerance test midway through pregnancy to check women for abnormally high blood sugar, says Elizabeth Livingston, M.D., assistant professor of obstetrics/gynecology in the department of maternal and fetal medicine at Duke University Medical Center in Durham, North Carolina. Gestational diabetes tends to favor women who exceed their ideal weight by more than 20 percent—say, 25 pounds or more—before they get pregnant. Women over 30 years old and women with a family history of diabetes are also at risk.

Gestational diabetes is an early warning sign—about 50 percent of women who have diabetes while pregnant end up with Type II diabetes

LIFETIME

within 10 years, says Dr. Livingston. If you don't lose the "baby fat" after childbirth or if your child weighed more than nine pounds at birth, you may be at higher risk of developing Type II diabetes in later life, she says.

Pregnant or not, if you are overweight and have a family history of diabetes, your doctor may prescribe diet and lifestyle changes that can delay the onset of Type II diabetes for years, says Denise Faustman, M.D., Ph.D., associate professor of medicine at Harvard Medical School.

SELF-CARE
Rx ———— *Prescriptions*
FOR DIABETES

Whether you have diabetes or are just at risk for the condition, self-care is part of smart treatment, doctors say.

Dietary Prescription for Diabetes

If you have diabetes—or you're at risk for developing diabetes—chances are that your doctor has recommended some kind of meal plan based on an optimal combination of carbohydrates and protein, plus a small amount of fat, says Stanley Mirsky, M.D., associate clinical professor of metabolic diseases at the Mount Sinai School of Medicine of the City University of New York in New York City and co-author of *Controlling Diabetes the Easy Way.* He suggests aiming for 40 to 50 grams of carbohydrates at each meal.

Here's what an optimal diet might look like for someone who is eating approximately 1,500 to 1,800 calories a day, based on Dr. Mirsky's recommendation.

BREAKFAST

Three ounces orange juice or eight ounces tomato juice (10 grams carbohydrates)

Two slices toasted oat bran bread, one English muffin, two

❏ If you have diabetes, ask your doctor to teach you how to monitor your own blood sugar levels during the day, every day. Your doctor can then advise you on how to adjust your diet and exercise levels accordingly to keep your internal systems running smoothly, says Dr. Faustman.

❏ Eat three meals a day. Instead of eating little or no breakfast, a fast lunch, and a big dinner—the usual pattern for many women—it's important to have three adequate meals, advises Stanley Mirsky, M.D., associate clinical professor of metabolic diseases at Mount Sinai School of Medicine of the City University of New York in New York City and co-author of *Controlling Diabetes the Easy Way*. For breakfast, have cereal, milk, and orange juice. For lunch, have a sandwich with turkey, romaine lettuce, tomato, and mustard. For dinner, have six ounces of chicken, fish, or meat; a salad; one-half cup of vegetables; one dinner roll; and a piece of fruit.

MEALTIME

small corn muffins, four four-inch pancakes, two slices of French toast, or three-quarters cup cold cereal with eight ounces milk (30 grams carbohydrates)

LUNCH
Sandwich made with three ounces turkey breast and mustard on two slices oat bran bread (30 grams carbohydrates)
Salad made with one cup lettuce, one-half cup tomatoes, and one tablespoon Italian dressing (10 grams carbohydrates)
Two-thirds cup cantaloupe cubes (10 grams carbohydrates)

DINNER
Three to six ounces chicken, fish, or other lean meat
One medium ear corn (15 grams carbohydrates)
One-half cup peas (15 grams carbohydrates)
One-half cup sliced peaches, packed in juice (15 grams carbohydrates)

MORNING

❐ Stock up on high-fiber breakfast cereal. A study conducted at the Harvard School of Public Health found that diets low in fiber can significantly increase women's risk of Type II diabetes. In this study, women who consumed the most high-glycemic foods (the glycemic index is an indicator of a food's ability to raise blood sugar levels) and the least fiber from cereal were 2½ times more likely to develop Type II diabetes than those who ate the fewest high-glycemic foods and the most fiber from cereal. Cereal fiber was associated with a 28 percent reduction in diabetes risk, though fruit and vegetable fiber made no difference.

❐ Use oat bran bread for toast and sandwiches. Bread is a substantial source of carbohydrates, a cornerstone of meal plans to manage diabetes. But oat bran seems to have an edge: A study at the University of Alberta in Canada found that the blood sugar levels of men who ate oat bran bread rather than white bread over a six-month period were much better controlled.

NIGHTTIME

❐ Have a bedtime snack of two graham crackers with one tablespoon peanut butter and eight ounces skim milk. This can help keep your blood sugar level on an even keel while you sleep, says Dr. Faustman.

❐ Take a multivitamin with E. Vitamin E may help deter diabetes complications such as heart disease, stroke, kidney, and nerve disease, says Aaron Vinik, M.D., Ph.D., director of the Diabetes Research Institute in Norfolk, Virginia. He recommends taking 400 to 800 international units (IU) daily. But get clearance from your physician before self-prescribing amounts higher than 30 international units, the Daily Value for vitamin E, he adds.

WEIGHT-LOSS Rx ——— *Prescriptions* FOR DIABETES

If you lose weight, you may be able to stop diabetes in its tracks before you get so much as a symptom, doctors say.

Your personal weight-loss prescription for diabetes will depend on how much you weigh now and how much you should weigh. Figuring out your ideal weight is simple: If you are five feet tall, you should weigh 100 pounds, with 5 pounds allowed for each extra inch of height. So if you are five feet, four inches tall, you should weigh 120 pounds, says Dr. Vinik. To that number, add 10 percent if you have a large frame, or subtract 10 percent if you have a small frame.

Next, figure out how many calories you should eat on average per day. If you don't get any exercise, figure 10 calories per pound, says Dr. Vinik. (If you weigh 120 pounds, that's 1,200 calories a day.) For every 100 calories you burn through exercise, you can consume another 100 calories a day. But if you are taking in 2,000 calories and burning only 1,300, you need to either cut 700 calories a day from your diet or burn up additional calories by exercise, he says.

❏ Lose 10 pounds, and keep it off. According to Dr. Vinik, unless you are severely overweight, that's all it may take to bring your insulin and blood sugar levels under control. "Usually, it's the first 10 pounds that count the most," he says.

❏ Measure your waist and hips. To reduce your risk of cardiovascular disease, the number one killer of women with diabetes, you need to make sure that your waist is considerably smaller than your hips. Research says that in women, the ideal waist-to-hip ratio is 0.8 or less, says Dr. Vinik. You may not be able to judge your waist-to-hip ratio visually. So measure your waist, and then measure your hips at their widest point. Then simply divide your waist measurement by your hip measurement to give you your waist-to-hip ratio.

❏ Reduce your fat intake so that less than 30 percent of your diet comes from fat, Dr. Vinik says. Cut out saturated fats and polyunsaturated fats such as butter and corn, safflower, and soybean oils. Instead, use small amounts of oils high in monounsaturated fats, such as peanut, canola, and olive oils. "Use these oils to cook with, grease pans, and so forth," he says.

Prescriptions
FOR BLOOD SUGAR CONTROL

EXERCISE
Rx

"A major cause of diabetes is remote control," says Dr. Vinik. In other words, he says, if you don't even get up to change the channels on your television set, let alone to try to stay physically fit, you are at greater risk for diabetes than if you move around. "Studies show that exercise will prevent the development of diabetes or prevent complications in those diagnosed with diabetes," he says.

❒ For best results, exercise daily. So says Kay McFarland, M.D., endocrinologist and professor of medicine at the University of South Carolina School of Medicine in Columbia. "For some people, skipping a day may make it easier not to exercise the next day."

TIME IT RIGHT

❒ Start small. If you are not used to exercising, any amount of activity can seem daunting. "I recommend starting with five minutes a day and increasing that by five minutes a week, until you are up to 30 minutes," says Dr. McFarland. "Once you're at 30 minutes, walk farther to improve your speed."

MORNING

❒ Walk early. Walk when you can, but exercising well before supper time is best, says Dr. McFarland. Walking in the morning or early afternoon will give you more energy during the day and help you get to sleep at night, she says. When you exercise late in the day or evening, you may feel too energized to fall asleep.

❒ Before you exercise, eat some fruit or crackers. That will give your blood sugar the lift needed to work out. Give yourself time to digest your food—no less than 20 minutes—and then get out there, says Dr. Mirsky. For people who take insulin, the best time to exercise is in the morning after breakfast, to keep blood sugar levels even.

TIME IT RIGHT

❒ While exercising, sip or snack every hour on the hour. Exercise quickly depletes your blood sugar. So if you are going to exercise for an hour or more—say, hiking or bicycling—Dr. Mirsky suggests drinking three ounces of orange juice or eating two graham crackers or four small hard candies every hour to keep your blood sugar up to par.

Medical **Alert**

In an effort to identify those people with undiagnosed diabetes, the American Diabetes Association recommends that all adults ages 45 and over be tested for the disease. Women of any age who are pregnant should be tested for gestational diabetes, or temporary high blood sugar, says Dr. Faustman.

In addition, if you experience possible symptoms of diabetes—blurry vision, frequent urination, dizziness, or infections that don't heal—see your doctor.

Fibromyalgia

The word *myalgia* means muscle pain. With fibromyalgia, what hurts are the fibrous tissues of the body: muscles, ligaments, tendons, and fasciae. (Fasciae are sheets of connective tissue.)

People diagnosed with fibromyalgia—mostly women—have pain at 11 or more specific tender points around their bodies. "It hurts when a doctor applies moderate pressure that normally wouldn't cause pain," explains Norman Harden, M.D., director of the pain clinic at the Rehabilitation Institute of Chicago. These tender points often include the inside edges of the shoulder blades, the base of the head, the outer forearms just below the elbows, and the insides of the knees—places that don't usually hurt from simple wear and tear.

But the symptoms of fibromyalgia extend beyond mere soreness, Dr. Harden says. People who have the condition seem to be extra-sensitive to pain. They hurt even when they are not moving. In fact, they may feel worse when they are sedentary—and especially when they first wake up in the morning.

Fibromyalgia disrupts normal sleep patterns, too. "People have trouble reaching the deep stages of sleep, when tissue repair takes place," Dr. Harden explains. And because they lack deep, restful sleep, they feel very tired—perhaps even anxious or depressed.

What makes fibromyalgia so difficult to treat is that scientists have yet to figure out what causes it. In fact, doctors often make a diagnosis of fibromyalgia when physical exams, blood tests, and x-rays fail to turn up an obvious reason for pain. "Research has shown microscopic damage in muscle cells, although these findings have not been reliable or consistent across investigations," notes Laurence A. Bradley, Ph.D., director of the Fibromyalgia Study Group at the University of Alabama School of Medicine in Birmingham.

Research has also shown that people with fibromyalgia have high levels of the chemical pain messenger substance P, which may help explain their increased sensitivity to pain.

Still, "we have a lot to learn about fibromyalgia," says Jennifer Brett, N.D., a naturopathic doctor in private practice in Stratford, Connecticut. While the future may hold a cure for the condition, for now, at least, the most effective treatment focuses on managing symptoms.

Rx — *Prescriptions*
FOR PROMPT PAIN RELIEF

If you have fibromyalgia, you can do things for yourself that will help you feel better, reduce your soreness, and regain your energy. You will have to stick with them, though, to keep symptoms at bay, says Dr. Harden. "The more you do them, the better you'll feel," he adds.

To help minimize pain, experts recommend the following tactics.

TIME IT RIGHT

❏ Engage in some form of aerobic exercise for at least 30 minutes every day. Many women with fibromyalgia are seriously out of shape, according to Dr. Harden. "We don't know if lack of physical conditioning causes symptoms, but it certainly contributes to symptoms," he says. In several studies, aerobic exercise (the huff-and-puff kind that increases your heart rate) has provided dramatic pain relief.

If you haven't been physically active, you may need to start working out at a snail's pace. Some women can manage no more than 5 minutes at a time at first, but the goal is to improve. Try to increase the amount of time you spend exercising by no more than 5 minutes each week, suggests Dr. Harden. "I like to get my patients to the point where they hit their target heart rates for at least 30 minutes a day—and twice a day is even better." (See "Aim for Your Target.") Any type of aerobic exercise can do the job: swimming, bicycling, jogging, walking, inline skating, or country-western line dancing.

❏ For short-term relief, try massage. People with fibromyalgia tend to tighten their muscles and hold their breath to brace themselves against their pain. Over time, the muscles become tight and breathing becomes shallow and rapid. Tense, tight muscles and rapid, shallow breathing patterns intensify the pain, says Susan Middaugh, Ph.D., a research psychologist in the department of physical medicine and rehabilitation at

Aim for Your Target

To determine whether you are getting the most from an aerobic workout, use your target heart rate range as a gauge. To figure out what your target is, experts recommend this formula: Subtract your age from 220, then multiply the remainder by 0.6 and 0.85. The two answers you get establish your target heart rate range.

Let's use a 45-year-old woman as an example. To determine the low end of her target heart rate range, she would subtract 45 from 220, then multiply the remainder (175) by 0.6, which equals 105. For the high end, she would multiply 175 by 0.85, which equals about 149. So her target heart rate range is 105 to 149 beats per minute. When she works out, she wants to be sure that her heart rate falls somewhere within that range.

To check your heart rate, use your index and middle fingers to take your pulse at your wrist. Count the number of beats for 10 seconds, then multiply by six—but be quick. Your heart rate drops immediately when you stop exercising for as little as 10 seconds.

the Medical University of South Carolina College of Medicine in Charleston.

A gentle massage relaxes tight muscles and keeps them flexible. It works wonders for aching muscles, especially if you feel sore after exercising, Dr. Harden says.

You can schedule an appointment with a professional massage therapist or simply enlist the services of a spouse or friend. Or you can give yourself some relief with a long-handled, handheld vibrating muscle massager, says Dr. Middaugh.

❐ Practice deep breathing for five minutes several times a day. "You want to slow your breathing, but not so much that you find yourself gasping for air," Dr. Middaugh says. She suggests aiming for

TIME IT RIGHT

eight breath cycles per minute. You should feel the area below your rib cage expand as you inhale and contract as you exhale. "This technique, also called diaphragmatic breathing, relaxes tightened muscles, improves circulation to the muscles, and calms the central nervous system," she says.

TIME IT RIGHT

❐ Practice progressive muscle relaxation for 10 to 15 minutes twice a day, recommends Dr. Middaugh. This technique involves gently contracting and then relaxing every muscle in your body. Why contract already-tight muscles? "People often don't realize that their muscles are tight until they contract them," she explains. "By first contracting and then relaxing their muscles, people with fibromyalgia are able to relieve some of the tightness."

To try progressive muscle relaxation, begin by clenching your fists gently until you can feel the muscles tensing, says Dr. Middaugh. Hold for three seconds, then release. Repeat, working your muscles in the following sequence: arms, shoulders, neck, face, abdomen, lower back, buttocks, thighs, calves, and feet.

To maximize the benefits of progressive muscle relaxation, you may want to get some training in the technique. Both Dr. Middaugh and Dr. Bradley recommend training sessions with a licensed psychologist, psychiatrist, or similar health professional.

NUTRITION Rx

Prescriptions
TO MANAGE SYMPTOMS

Certain dietary strategies appear to reduce the frequency and severity of fibromyalgia flare-ups. Some doctors recommend the following to their patients.

❐ Take a combination of magnesium and malic acid (found in apples). Researchers at the University of Texas Health Science Center at San Antonio found that people with fibromyalgia who followed this regimen experienced welcome reductions in muscle pain and tenderness. "We theorize that people with fibromyalgia have a problem with energy metabolism in their muscles—that they don't produce enough ATP (adenosine triphosphate), which is the basic fuel for muscle cells," says I. Jon Russell, M.D., Ph.D., the study's main researcher. "The combination of magnesium and malic acid may facilitate the production of ATP." The researchers could not be sure that an ATP shortage exists in fibromyalgia, but evidence from several studies in the United States and Europe support that conclusion. The supplements containing magnesium and malic acid did seem to help fibromyalgia symptoms when the total dosage was greater than 300 milligrams of magnesium and 1,200 milligrams of malic acid per day.

To try this regimen, begin with 150 milligrams of magnesium and 600 milligrams of malic acid in supplement form twice daily. Continue at this dosage for one to two weeks, says Dr. Russell. After that, gradually increase the dosage every two to three days until you reach a maintenance dosage of 300 milligrams of magnesium and 1,200 milligrams of malic acid twice daily.

Some drugstores and health food stores carry combination magnesium/malic acid supplements. If the stores you frequent don't stock these products, you can order them by mail. One brand, Super Malic, is available from Optimox. You can write to the company at P.O. Box 3378, Torrance, CA 90510.

Note: High doses of magnesium can cause diarrhea in some people. If it happens to you, reduce your dosage to one that does not cause diarrhea, Dr. Russell says. Also, if you have heart or kidney problems, you should check with your doctor before taking magnesium supplements.

❏ Take a high-quality multivitamin/mineral supplement every day. Make sure that it contains all the trace minerals, including tongue twisters like molybdenum, Dr. Brett says. "Even with a fairly decent diet, you would have a hard time getting all the nutrients you need in the right amounts—especially the trace minerals," she notes. And vitamin and mineral deficiencies, in general, make it hard for the body to repair tissues, subdue harmful unstable molecules called free radicals, and respond to inflammation, she adds.

❏ Consume a tablespoon ground flaxseed (available in health food stores) every day, recommends Dr. Brett. Flaxseed contains the fatty acids found in flaxseed oil. These fatty acids can act as an anti-inflammatory. Flaxseed is also rich in a fiber called lignan. "Flax fiber helps balance a woman's estrogen levels," she says. "Fluctuating estrogen levels can exacerbate the perception of pain's intensity."

Flaxseed has a nutty flavor and tastes good sprinkled on hot cereal or added to rice or pasta. Just don't cook flaxseed—always add it *after* cooking the cereal, rice, or pasta, Dr. Brett says. The reason: The heat from cooking destroys the fatty acids.

MEALTIME

❐ Eat at least two three-ounce servings of fatty fish such as mackerel, salmon, and tuna each week, recommends Dr. Brett. These types of fish are rich in omega-3 fatty acids, which have anti-inflammatory properties.

❐ Limit your daily intake of saturated fat to 7 percent of calories. "Getting more than 7 percent of your calories from saturated fat interferes

Herbal Prescriptions to Alleviate the Ache

If you rely on an over-the-counter pain reliever to ease your fibromyalgia symptoms, you may want to consider an herbal alternative. "I choose the herb that best matches a woman's particular symptoms," says Jennifer Brett, N.D., a naturopathic doctor in private practice in Stratford, Connecticut. She often prescribes the following herbal remedies to her patients. (All of the doses are for the tincture form of the herbs in amounts appropriate for a 150-pound woman. You can buy these herbs in health food stores.)

❐ For aching joints and an upset stomach, take 30 drops of black cohosh three times a day.

❐ For muscle cramps and tightness, take 10 to 20 drops of cramp bark two times a day.

❐ For muscle spasms with fatigue and coughing, take 10 drops of skunk cabbage three times a day.

❐ For muscle twitching and pain accompanied by insomnia, nervousness, and restlessness, take 10 to 30 drops of skullcap two times a day.

with the action of the omega-3 and omega-6 oils in fish and flaxseed," says Dr. Brett.

❐ Also limit your consumption of red meat. Besides being a source of saturated fat, red meat contains inflammation-causing oils called arachadonic acid, explains Dr. Brett.

❐ Eliminate—or at least cut back on—alcohol and caffeinated beverages. "Both make sleeping problems worse," Dr. Harden says. "And that's the last thing someone with fibromyalgia needs." If you must imbibe, hold yourself to no more than three drinks a week and no more than two cups of coffee a day, he suggests. (A drink is defined as one 12-ounce beer, 5-

❐ For muscle spasms accompanied by insomnia, depression, and distress, take 15 to 30 drops of valerian three times a day.

❐ For spasmodic pain, nightmares, and swelling around the joints, take 10 to 30 drops of peony two times a day.

If you are already taking over-the-counter pain relievers as directed by your doctor, you should check with your doctor before switching to an herbal remedy, advises Dr. Brett. Also, women who are pregnant should consult with their doctors before taking any herbs.

In fact, Dr. Brett suggests that all women consult an herbalist or a naturopathic doctor to make sure that they are taking the right herb for their symptoms. To find a qualified herbalist in your area, contact the American Herbalists Guild at P.O. Box 746555, Arvada, CO 80006. Also, the American Association of Naturopathic Physicians offers a directory of naturopathic doctors. You can order one for a nominal charge by writing to the organization at 601 Valley Street, Suite 105, Seattle, WA 98109.

ounce glass of wine, or a mixed drink made with 1½ ounces of liquor.) Also, be sure to avoid caffeine past noon, he adds. That means no cola, coffee, tea, or chocolate after lunchtime.

TIME IT RIGHT

❐ Keep a food diary to pinpoint possible symptom-triggering foods. For two weeks, write down everything you eat and when as well as any symptoms you have. Then review your notes at the end of the two weeks, looking for foods that seem to instigate flare-ups. A food doesn't have to be "junk" to cause symptoms. "It could be something that's perfectly healthy," Dr. Brett notes. Different foods bother different people, but according to Dr. Brett, the most common culprits are wheat, dairy, eggs, alcohol, soy, corn, shellfish, tomatoes, potatoes, eggplant, and peppers. These problem foods may intensify the pain or make it more frequent.

Not everyone with fibromyalgia has food sensitivities. But those who do might notice hip and lower back pain and stiffness 12 to 24 hours after eating their trigger foods, Dr. Brett says. "Some people also complain of mental fogginess—they feel that they have hangovers, even though they have had nothing to drink," she adds.

Medical Alert

Don't self-diagnose fibromyalgia. If you think that you have it, see your doctor. The symptoms of fibromyalgia can mimic those of other, potentially serious conditions, including inflammatory muscle or joint diseases (arthritis is one), thyroid disorders, and polymyalgia rheumatica, a rare autoimmune disease that usually strikes people over age 55.

Food Allergies

Most women who think that they have food allergies probably don't. In fact, less than 2 percent of the entire U.S. population has true food allergies.

TIME IT RIGHT

If you eat a food to which you are allergic, you will know within 15 minutes—two hours at the very most, according to Stephen Wasserman, M.D., professor of medicine at the University of California, San Diego,

School of Medicine. Typically, your tongue will swell or itch, and your skin may break out in hives or a rash. You may also experience a headache or digestive upset in the form of extreme flatulence, stomach cramps, or diarrhea.

On rare occasions, an allergic reaction may progress to anaphylaxis, a potentially fatal condition in which the throat swells shut, blood pressure drops, wheezing sets in (which can possibly lead to an asthma attack), and the body ultimately goes into shock, says Sandra Gawchik, D.O., co-director of the division of allergy and clinical immunology at Crozer Chester Medical Center in Chester, Pennsylvania.

How could something as harmless as food trigger such a severe physical response? Believe it or not, it's all a case of mistaken identity. The first time you eat a certain food, your immune system flags a protein in that food as an invader, much like a virus or bacteria. Then whenever you eat that food, your immune system overreacts by flooding your body with antibodies—specifically, immunoglobulin E (IgE) antibodies. These antibodies fuel the physical symptoms of a food allergy.

Peanuts and shellfish—especially shrimp, crab, and lobster—often cause allergic reactions in adults, notes Robert J. Dockhorn, M.D., chairman of the food allergy committee and professor of medicine and pediatrics at the University of Missouri—Kansas City School of Medicine. Other common allergens include wheat, eggs, milk, corn, and soy.

Prescriptions
TO OUTFOX FLARE-UPS

If you suspect that you have a food allergy, schedule an appointment with an allergist. She will most likely ask you about your medical and dietary history, then do simple blood tests or skin-prick tests to confirm your suspicions. And if you are diagnosed with a food allergy, your doctor will most likely tell you to avoid the problem food. Take her advice, says Dr. Dockhorn.

To reduce your risk of experiencing a negative reaction to a particular food, heed this advice.

❒ Carefully read the ingredient lists on the labels of packaged foods and beverages. Food allergens often show up in unexpected places, notes Dr. Gawchik. For instance, you will find peanuts not only in peanut butter but also in ice cream, candy bars, meatballs, breads, and pastries. And foods whose labels mention emulsifiers or flavorings may contain ingredients derived from peanuts or soy. Similarly, wheat is used to make breads as well as beer, wine, and processed meats such as hot dogs, she says.

❏ If you are allergic to wheat or eggs, switch to baked goods made without these ingredients. Most health food stores carry a selection of wheat-free and egg-free breads, cookies, and cakes, says Dr. Gawchik. Check the labels.

MEALTIME

❏ When you eat out, ask your server specific questions about the ingredients in a dish. This is especially important if you have a food allergy. If you feel as though you are wasting the server's time, remember that eating a food to which you are allergic could trigger a potentially life-threatening reaction. In fact, Dr. Gawchik suggests letting your server know this, too. Tell her, "If I eat anything with peanuts, I could die." And if your server isn't sure of the ingredients, order something else.

❏ Also ask your server how a dish is prepared. A restaurant may fry your husband's popcorn shrimp and your french fries in the same oil. If you are allergic to shellfish, this could be dangerous, says Dr. Gawchik.

❏ Check out the ingredients in beauty products. These items may contain food allergens. For instance, cosmetics manufacturers sometimes use milk to make lipstick, according to Dr. Gawchik.

❏ Contact the Food Allergy Network for educational materials. You can write to the organization at 10400 Eaton Place, Suite 107, Fairfax, VA 22030.

Rx

Prescriptions
TO FOIL FOOD INTOLERANCE

What most of us refer to as a food allergy is more accurately described as food *intolerance*, according to Daryl R. Altman, M.D., director of Allergy Information Services, a consulting service in Hewlett, New York. Like a food allergy, food intolerance may leave you with a headache, extreme flatulence, stomach cramps, or diarrhea—but unlike allergy, intolerance is never life-threatening, explains Dr. Gawchik.

Also, while a minuscule amount—sometimes literally just a whiff—of a food that you are allergic to can cause a severe reaction, you may be able to eat a small portion of a food that you have an intolerance to without problems, notes Dr. Dockhorn. For example, in a study conducted by the University of Minnesota in St. Paul and the Minneapolis Veterans Affairs Medical Center, people who described themselves as lactose intolerant—meaning that they have difficulty digesting lactose, a sugar found in milk—could actually drink an eight-ounce glass of low-fat (2%) milk every day with no ill effects. Because food allergy and food intolerance produce such similar symptoms, only your doctor can say for sure which condition you have. Don't attempt to self-diagnose—especially since an undetected food allergy can have such serious consequences.

If your doctor confirms that you have a food intolerance, you can narrow down the problematic food or foods by doing one, or both, of the following "tests" on your own.

TIME IT RIGHT

❐ Write down everything you eat for two weeks. You don't need an actual diary; a notebook or a sheet of paper will do. Draw a line down the center of the page to divide it into two columns. In the left-hand column, document your diet. Include details—not only what you eat but how much and at what time. Make note of any beverages you drink as well as any medications you take. In the right-hand column, list any symptoms you experience, along with the time they occur. After two weeks, look for a pattern to your symptoms, Dr. Altman says. You may notice that you consistently feel sick after eating a certain food.

❐ Give up suspected offending foods for two weeks. During this time, suggests Dr. Gawchik, build your diet around five or six foods that you know you can tolerate. Typical choices include lamb, rice, sweet potatoes, squash, and applesauce. Divide these foods among five or six small meals spread over the course of the day. Try to avoid eating the same food at three or more meals in a row. Drink lots of water, too.

At the end of two weeks, says Dr. Gawchik, add one of the banished foods back into your diet for two or three consecutive meals to see if you have a reaction. Continue reintroducing these foods, one at a time, until you have tested them all and isolated the culprit (or culprits).

Prescriptions for Living with Lactose Intolerance

Does drinking milk make your stomach do the samba? You may have lactose intolerance—in other words, your small intestine doesn't produce enough lactase, an enzyme that breaks down lactose, a sugar in milk. That doesn't mean that you should just give up the white stuff. Milk is one of the best sources of calcium, the mineral that women need to keep their bones strong and prevent osteoporosis. (Women between ages 19 and 50 should consume 1,000 milligrams of calcium a day. If you are pregnant, lactating, or menopausal, you need 1,500 milligrams of calcium a day, according to current federal government guidelines.)

Lactase supplements, such as Lactaid and Dairy Ease, help milk go down easier by subsidizing your supply of the digestive enzyme. If you can't tolerate the supplements or you would rather not take them, try these alternatives.

❒ Buy lactose-free or lactose-reduced dairy products, says Lana Miller, R.D., of Mead Johnson Nutritionals in Littleton, Colorado.

❒ Get your calcium from an eight-ounce serving of nonfat or low-fat yogurt (447 milligrams per serving) or a one-ounce serving of naturally aged, hard cheese (177 milligrams per serving). "Many people who develop gastrointestinal symptoms, such as gassiness and bloating, from milk can eat other dairy products without problems," says Miller.

❒ If you find that you can't tolerate any dairy products, be sure to take a daily calcium supplement, suggests Sandra Gawchik, D.O., co-director of the division of allergy and clinical immunology at Crozer Chester Medical Center in Chester, Pennsylvania.

❐ Once you identify a problem food, try rotating it into your diet on a weekly basis. You may be able to manage your symptoms by reducing how much or how often you eat the food rather than cutting it out completely, says Dr. Dockhorn.

MEALTIME

If you have trouble with eggs, for instance, eat them for breakfast only once a week rather than every day. You may discover that you can eat eggs on occasion without experiencing digestive upset or other symptoms of intolerance, says Dr. Gawchik.

❐ If you do have to give up a problem food altogether, take the same precautions as someone with a food allergy. Read the ingredients lists on packaged foods and beauty products. And when you eat out, be sure to ask your server what is in a particular dish and how it is prepared.

Medical **Alert**

If you have a severe, potentially life-threatening food allergy, your doctor will probably give you a prescription for an injectable form of epinephrine, such as EpiPen. Keep this medication with you at all times and use it at the first sign of an allergic reaction, recommends Marianne Frieri, M.D., Ph.D., director of the allergy/immunology training program at Nassau County Medical Center and North Shore University Hospital in East Meadow, New York. Epinephrine stops the reaction from progressing to full-scale anaphylaxis.

If you are inadvertently exposed to a food allergen and you don't have your medicine at hand, you must get to a hospital emergency room without delay.

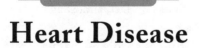

Heart Disease

Thanks to the hormone estrogen, women rarely develop heart disease as early in life as men. Estrogen helps keep female arteries clear and healthy by regulating the amounts of low-density lipoprotein, or LDL, cholesterol (the "bad" kind that clogs) and high-density lipoprotein, or HDL, cholesterol (the good kind that cleans up) floating around in the bloodstream.

LIFETIME

But all that changes once a woman enters menopause, when estrogen production begins to slow down. "After menopause, a woman's risk of heart disease rises each year. By the time she reaches age 65, her risk is about equal to a man's," says Elizabeth Ross, M.D., a cardiologist at Washington Hospital in Washington, D.C., and author of *Healing the Female Heart*. "Heart disease ends up killing more women than all cancers combined."

Any number of factors can boost your odds of developing heart disease. Some of them, such as age and family history, you can't do anything about, notes Marianne Legato, M.D., associate professor of clinical medicine at Columbia University College of Physicians and Surgeons in New York City and author of *The Female Heart*. But others you can change. Why not start now?

Rx

Prescriptions
FOR A HEALTHY HEART

Heart disease doesn't happen overnight. The artery-clogging process begins long before symptoms appear. Fortunately, you can minimize and even reverse any existing damage by living a heart-friendly lifestyle that includes the following. (For tips on managing high blood pressure and high cholesterol—both leading risk factors for heart disease—see pages 204 and 209.)

❒ If you smoke, quit. For women, smoking stands head and shoulders above other risk factors for heart disease. A woman who smokes is two to six times more likely to experience a heart attack than a woman who has never smoked, and her risk increases with the number of cigarettes she smokes each day. In fact, almost all women who have heart attacks before age 50 are smokers.

Smoking undermines a woman's natural protection against heart disease, explains Ruth Marlin, M.D., staff physician and head of medical education at the Preventive Medicine Research Institute in Sausalito, California. It does this by somehow negating the positive effects of estrogen. It also speeds the buildup of artery-clogging plaque, reduces the amount of oxygen in your blood, causes arteries in your arms and legs to constrict, and increases your heart rate. "Nothing else you do to prevent heart disease will make as much of a difference as giving up smoking," Dr. Marlin says.

❐ Take charge of your weight. Carrying a little extra body fat is okay as long as it congregates on your hips, thighs, and butt. But if you are more than 20 percent above your ideal weight, or if body fat takes up residence around your waist, your risk for heart disease edges upward, explains Dr. Marlin. So for a woman whose ideal weight is 140 pounds, an extra 28 pounds puts her in the cardiac danger zone.

While there are a number of complex formulas for figuring out your ideal weight, one simple formula used by some experts can tell you if you are close: If you are five feet tall, you should weigh 100 pounds. If you are taller, add 5 pounds for each additional inch of height. To that number, add 10 percent if you have a large frame, or subtract 10 percent if you have a small frame.

❐ Engage in aerobic exercise for at least 30 minutes every day. "Aerobic exercise (the kind that pumps up your respiration and heart rates) helps prevent heart disease by raising the level of HDL cholesterol in your blood," says Dr. Marlin. It also strengthens and tones your heart muscle so that your heart pumps more blood with each beat. And it reduces the stickiness of blood platelets, making them less likely to form clots. Time it right

Compared with active women, "sofa slugs" have double the risk of a fatal heart attack, all other factors being equal. So get out and walk, swim, bicycle—whatever you enjoy, as long as you are on the move. If you have been inactive, however, you should get your doctor's okay before trying anything more strenuous than walking, advises Dr. Ross.

❐ Minimize stress as much as possible. Your body responds to stress by releasing a cascade of hormones. One thing that these hormones do is raise your blood level of fibrinogen, a biochemical that makes blood clot, according to Dr. Marlin.

How you cope with and control the stress in your life really depends on your needs, interests, and lifestyle. One technique that Dr. Legato suggests to her patients is to put the problem on paper. "First, they explain to themselves what is causing their stress, in their own words," she says. "Then they list all the positives and negatives that the situation presents, highlighting those negatives that they find absolutely intolerable." This

Strike a Pose, Strike Out Heart Disease

At the Preventive Medicine Research Institute in Sausalito, California, yoga plays an important part in nursing hearts back to health. "Yoga relieves stress and anger, both of which contribute to heart disease," says Ruth Marlin, M.D., staff physician and head of medical education at the Institute. It also offers a very gentle workout that helps relax and strengthen muscles throughout your body.

Try taking a class in integral yoga, the type used at the Institute, recommends Dr. Marlin. To find an instructor in your area, write to Satchidananda Ashram–Yogaville, Route 1, Box 1720, Buckingham, VA 23921.

exercise enables people to examine their problems more objectively and to brainstorm realistic solutions. In fact, Dr. Legato has her patients write down their solutions as well, to encourage them to follow through.

"I consider stress reduction very important for women," says Dr. Legato. "Developing workable solutions to unresolved personal problems can do a lot to relieve stress."

❐ If you have diabetes, do what you can to keep it under control. Diabetes can increase your risk for heart disease fourfold. "Women who have diabetes need to acknowledge the seriousness of this risk," Dr. Legato says. "And they need to work closely with their doctors to develop a diabetes-management plan that they are comfortable with."

NUTRITION Rx

Prescriptions

TO PRIME YOUR PUMP

Your eating habits play an important role in your heart health, too. Plenty of attention has been given to the relationship among dietary fat, cholesterol, and heart disease. While keeping a lid on your daily fat intake is important (many experts suggest getting no more than 25 percent of your calories from fat), it is not the only nutrition strategy that helps. The following may also reduce your risk of heart disease.

❑ Eat a broad-ranging diet that includes a wide variety of fruits and vegetables. Focus on produce that has an abundant supply of the antioxidant nutrients—vitamins C and E and beta-carotene, says Dr. Marlin. Antioxidants protect "bad" LDL cholesterol from undergoing oxidation, which contributes to the artery-clogging process. Dr. Marlin suggests consuming at least five servings of antioxidant-rich fruit and vegetables each day, such as broccoli, carrots, collards, Swiss chard, citrus fruits, papaya, and cantaloupe. One serving of a vegetable is equal to one cup raw leafy vegetables, one-half cup any other kind of vegetable, or three-quarters cup vegetable juice. One serving of fruit is equivalent to one medium apple, banana, or orange; one-half cup chopped, cooked, or canned fruit; one-half cup berries; or three-quarters cup fruit juice.

❑ Take a daily multivitamin/mineral supplement. Even if you eat healthfully, you may not get enough of certain nutrients to protect against heart disease, says Dr. Marlin. A multivitamin can help you get those preventive amounts.

❑ Eat one or two three-ounce servings of fatty fish each week, suggests Dr. Ross. Fish such as herring, salmon, tuna, and mackerel contain omega-3 fatty acids, a heart-friendly fat that helps prevent the formation of blood clots.

MEALTIME

❑ Consume 20 to 25 grams of soy protein a day, says Dr. Ross. In studies, soy has demonstrated a remarkable ability to disrupt the chain of events that leads to high cholesterol levels and, ultimately, to blocked arteries. These days you can choose from an array of soy products, such as tofu (about 8 grams of soy protein per three-ounce serving), tempeh (about 19 grams per three-ounce serving), and soy milk (about 3 grams per three-ounce serving). You can also try soy-filled veggie burgers—but check the label for soy protein content, which can vary greatly from product to product.

Medical Alert

Women who have heart disease often do not develop chest pain, the classic symptom of a heart attack. As a consequence, other symptoms of heart attack may not be recognized by women or their doctors as serious, says Dr. Ross. If you experience severe breathlessness, nausea, fatigue, or back, jaw, or arm pain while you are engaging in physical activity, you should consult your doctor without delay. These are warning signs of heart disease and could signal a heart attack. Also, if any of these symptoms occurs suddenly or is severe and unremitting, head for the nearest emergency room immediately.

High Blood Pressure

High blood pressure doesn't hurt. In fact, it doesn't produce any noticeable symptoms. What makes this stealthiness so scary is that high blood pressure is a leading risk factor for two of America's top three killers: heart disease and stroke.

For a woman over the age of 18, a blood pressure reading of 120/80 mm Hg (millimeters of mercury) is considered normal, while a consistent reading of 140/90 mm Hg is considered high. A woman who has high blood pressure is $3\frac{1}{2}$ times more likely to develop heart disease and $2\frac{1}{2}$ times more likely to experience a stroke than a woman who has normal blood pressure. With statistics like these, you have every reason to want to rein in high blood pressure, even if you feel perfectly healthy.

Scientists have yet to figure out exactly how high blood pressure happens. (If you have been told that you have essential hypertension, it means that you have high blood pressure with no identifiable cause.) But they do know that certain factors raise a woman's risk. If you are African-American, Puerto Rican, Cuban, or Mexican-American, for instance, you have a much higher risk of developing high blood pressure. Being overweight or having diabetes can also make you more vulnerable to the condition.

Stress can temporarily spike your blood pressure, too, according to Lauren Zoschnick, M.D., assistant professor in the department of obstetrics and gynecology in the division of women's health at the University of Michigan in Ann Arbor.

In terms of gender, high blood pressure plays no favorites. Women and men are equally susceptible. "The difference is that women are more likely to know that they have high blood pressure and to be doing something about it," says Ellen Cohen, M.D., associate professor of internal medicine at Albert Einstein College of Medicine of Yeshiva University in Bronx, New York. That's because women tend to visit doctors more often and have their blood pressures checked routinely.

Prescriptions
TO PARE POINTS

NUTRITION
Rx

Doctors prescribe a variety of medications to treat high blood pressure. Certain foods may help as well. If you prefer to go the nondrug route, give these remedies a try. (If you are already taking blood pressure medicine, be sure to consult your doctor before making any changes in your dosage.)

❒ Try eating four stalks of celery a day. In his book *The Green Pharmacy*, James A. Duke, Ph.D., notes that studies have shown celery to be effective in lowering blood pressure. It acts as a mild diuretic, much like many commonly prescribed blood pressure medications.

❒ Eat one clove of garlic a day. Garlic contains allicin, a compound that appears to lower not only blood pressure but also cholesterol. In his book, Dr. Duke suggests meeting your daily garlic requirement by using the herb to flavor salads and cooked dishes.

❒ Eat enough magnesium- and potassium-rich foods to meet their respective Daily Values of 400 milligrams and 3,500 milligrams. Magnesium and potassium work with a third mineral, sodium, to regulate your blood pressure. It was long believed that an excessive sodium intake would drive a person's blood pressure reading through the roof. But the latest research suggests that consuming as much as 4,000 milligrams of sodium a day doesn't affect blood pressure all that much—as long as you are also consuming adequate amounts of magnesium and potassium, says David McCarron, M.D., head of the division of nephrology, hypertension, and clinical pharmacology at Oregon Health Sciences University in Portland.

MEALTIME

You can make sure that you are getting enough magnesium and potassium simply by following a healthy diet that includes plenty of whole grains, beans, fruits, and vegetables. Good sources of magnesium include broccoli (47 milligrams per 3½ ounces cooked), bananas (41 milligrams in one medium fruit), dry-roasted soybeans (228 milligrams per one-half cup), and barley (133 milligrams per one-half cup). Good sources of potassium include baked potatoes (239 milligrams per one medium potato), cantaloupe (247 milligrams per one-half cup), spinach (283 milligrams per one-half cup boiled), and oats (429 milligrams per one-half cup).

LIFETIME

❐ If you are pregnant, get 1,200 to 1,500 milligrams of calcium a day from foods, supplements, or a combination of both. Research suggests that calcium can help prevent pregnancy-induced high blood pressure, says Dr. McCarron. In a 14-study analysis conducted at Chinese University in Hong Kong, researchers found that moms-to-be who supplemented their diets with calcium cut their risk of high blood pressure by 38 percent.

Some of the best sources of calcium are milk and milk products. One cup skim milk, for instance, contains 302 milligrams of the mineral. And one cup plain yogurt made from skim milk contains 452 milligrams.

Rx — *Prescriptions*
FOR A LOW-PRESSURE LIFESTYLE

Dietary remedies can do wonders to whittle points from your blood pressure reading. But to control blood pressure permanently, you must identify and change those risk factors that drove your reading upward in the first place. Use the following strategies to shape your own blood pressure management plan.

❐ Lose superfluous poundage. "If you are overweight, dropping those extra pounds is the single most effective thing that you can do to control your blood pressure," says Dr. Zoschnick. "In studies, losing an average of 10 pounds and maintaining the loss over several years consistently produces significant drops in blood pressure—even to the point where drug treatment can be stopped."

While there are a number of complex formulas for figuring out your ideal weight, one simple formula used by some experts can tell you if you are close: If you are five feet tall, you should weigh 100 pounds. If you are taller, add 5 pounds for each additional inch of height. To that number, add 10 percent if you have a large frame, or subtract 10 percent if you have a small frame.

The Pill That Pumps Up Pressure

If you are on oral contraceptives, you should know that the Pill can greatly increase your risk of high blood pressure. The Nurses Health Study—a large, long-term study designed to examine associations between lifestyle, diet, and the occurrence of major illnesses—has shown that women who take oral contraceptives are 1½ to 2 times more likely to develop high blood pressure than women who don't, says Ellen Cohen, M.D., associate professor of internal medicine at Albert Einstein College of Medicine of Yeshiva University in Bronx, New York. What's more, the risk is greatest among women in their midthirties and older. Women on estrogen-progestin pills experience average increases of five to seven points systolic (the top number in a blood pressure reading) and one to two points diastolic (the bottom number).

This doesn't mean that you should stop taking oral contraceptives, since high blood pressure in younger women is still relatively rare. "It does mean that you should have your blood pressure checked before you start on the Pill and then again a few months after you start," Dr. Cohen says. If your blood pressure is going to rise, it usually happens relatively early in the course of oral contraceptive use.

If screenings indicate that your blood pressure has gone up, you should consider a different form of birth control—especially if you are a smoker or if you have a family history of high blood pressure and stroke, advises Dr. Cohen.

Interestingly, hormone-replacement therapy, which also involves supplemental estrogen, has none of the blood pressure—elevating tendencies of oral contraceptives.

Slimming down is especially important for women who carry their excess body fat around the middle rather than on the hips, butt, and thighs. "In terms of fat distribution, having an apple-shaped body instead of a pear-shaped body puts women at increased risk for heart attack, stroke, and diabetes," notes Dr. Zoschnick.

TIME IT RIGHT

❏ Work out aerobically for 30 to 45 minutes at least four times a week. "Independent of its important role in weight loss, aerobic exercise (the kind that increases your respiration and heart rates) helps lower blood pressure," says Dr. Zoschnick. "Women who are in good cardiovascular shape experience smaller increases in blood pressure in response to physical or emotional demands."

If you have already been diagnosed with high blood pressure, get your doctor's okay before you begin a new exercise program. Your blood pressure naturally rises when you work out.

❏ Limit your alcohol consumption to two drinks a day, recommends the National Heart, Lung, and Blood Institute. (A drink is defined as one 12-ounce beer, one 5-ounce glass of wine, or a mixed drink made with 1½ ounces of liquor.) Alcohol's effects on blood pressure are significant. In a four-year study at Harvard Medical School, nurses between ages 34 and 59 who consumed two or three alcoholic beverages daily increased their risk of high blood pressure by 40 percent.

Rx

Prescriptions
TO SHORT-CIRCUIT STRESS

Research suggests that people who react poorly to chronic or habitual stress experience lasting adverse effects on their blood pressure. Those who learn how to change their reactions to stress and how to regulate the body's response to stress may lower their blood pressure readings, says Peter Parks, Ph.D., a psychophysiologic (biofeedback) therapist with the Menninger Clinic in Topeka, Kansas.

Even if stress isn't chronic or habitual, it can at times cause your blood pressure reading to shoot up briefly. You can prevent these spikes first by becoming aware of your body's stress response, then by practicing skills that defuse the response, says Dr. Parks. Make the following tactics part of your own antistress arsenal.

❒ Practice relaxation. Techniques such as meditation, visualization, progressive muscle relaxation, deep breathing, and self-massage can help you deal more effectively with various types of stress. They do this by relieving some of the immediate pressure of situations that habitually evoke feelings of apprehension, anger, or depression, says Debra R. Judelson, M.D., senior partner with the Cardiovascular Medical Group of Southern California in Beverly Hills and immediate past president of the American Medical Women's Association. These techniques may also help you change your body's response to stress (tense muscles, racing heartbeat, headache, stomach cramps, and clammy hands) as well as the thought patterns that prevent you from constructively dealing with the situation that has caused stressful feelings. They can calm and focus your mind, she notes.

❒ When you feel yourself becoming stressed, stop for a minute, take a breath, and relax. Then do something constructive. For instance, if you are angry or upset about a situation that you can't change or control, work out your feelings by engaging in a vigorous physical activity such as running or racquetball, suggests Dr. Judelson. If you are just having a bad day, soothe your stress by listening to quiet, peaceful music or taking a long walk.

Medical **Alert**
Because high blood pressure has no outward symptoms, it's good to have your blood pressure checked at least once a year, advises Dr. Zoschnick.

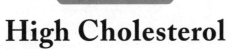

High Cholesterol

High cholesterol isn't a disease. It's a risk factor. Like obesity and high blood pressure, it ups your odds of developing atherosclerosis, a condition in which fatty deposits build up on the walls of your arteries. Eventually, an artery can become completely blocked, causing a heart attack or stroke.

Traditionally, a diagnosis of high cholesterol has meant that your total cholesterol equals or exceeds 240 milligrams per deciliter of blood. A reading of less than 200 is desirable, and anything in between is considered borderline high.

But many doctors now believe that total cholesterol may not be the best indicator of a person's risk for atherosclerosis. More significant, they say, are the levels of "bad" low-density lipoprotein (LDL) cholesterol and "good" high-density lipoprotein (HDL) cholesterol. LDL is the stuff that clogs your arteries. Doctors like to see an LDL reading of 130 milligrams per deciliter of blood or less. HDL escorts LDL out of your body and helps keep your arteries clean. An HDL reading of 60 milligrams per deciliter or more is considered healthy.

LIFETIME

Before menopause, women tend to have slightly higher cholesterol levels than men, mostly because their HDL cholesterol levels are higher. "Women average HDL levels of 55, while men average only 45," states Marianne Legato, M.D., associate professor of clinical medicine at Columbia University College of Physicians and Surgeons in New York City and author of *The Female Heart.* "So unless she smokes or has diabetes, a premenopausal woman has less chance of developing heart disease than a man does."

That begins to change at menopause, however, as levels of heart-protective estrogen drop. Estrogen helps keep arteries supple and dilated and increases substances that sweep cholesterol from the bloodstream. So as a woman's supply of the hormone dwindles, her risk of cardiovascular disease increases.

Ultimately, cardiovascular disease kills more than 500,000 women a year—that's more than all types of cancer combined. So you have good reason to keep your cholesterol levels in check.

NUTRITION
Rx

Prescriptions
FOR MANAGING CHOLESTEROL

What you eat plays an important role in whether or not you develop high cholesterol. The high-fat, meat- and dairy-rich diet that many Americans favor can load your bloodstream with LDL cholesterol and pave the way to heart disease. To swing your eating habits in your arteries' favor, adopt the following nutrition strategies.

❒ Consume 25 to 30 grams of fiber a day, according to American Heart Association guidelines. A specific type of fiber, called soluble fiber, forms a gel that binds with cholesterol in your gut, explains Ruth Marlin, M.D., staff physician and head of medical education at the Preventive Medicine Research Institute in Sausalito, California. The fiber escorts the cholesterol out of your body. That way, the cholesterol can't be reabsorbed into your bloodstream.

People eat, on average, about half the recommended amount of fiber each day, according to the American Heart Association. To boost your intake, select high-fiber foods such as fresh fruits (like apples, oranges, and grapefruit), vegetables (like brussels sprouts, broccoli, and spinach), grains (like oatmeal, brown rice, and whole-wheat bread), and legumes (like kidney or navy beans).

MEALTIME

❒ Eat a three-ounce serving of fish such as mackerel, salmon, or tuna at least once a week, says Dr. Marlin. These species are rich in omega-3 fatty acids. Research suggests that omega-3's may help sustain heart-friendly HDL cholesterol at a healthy level even as the heart-damaging LDL cholesterol level falls. There is also evidence that replacing saturated fat with omega-3-rich fish oil can decrease LDL levels.

If you are not a fish fan, you can get your omega-3's from other sources. Try whole grains, beans, soybeans, and seaweed.

❒ Eat about four cloves of garlic a day. Research has shown that this regimen can cut total cholesterol by about 7 percent, a significant reduction for some people. If you like the taste of garlic, try to eat it fresh or lightly cooked, since a long cooking time reduces some of its cholesterol-lowering potency. Add sliced garlic to salad dressings or sliced or crushed garlic to a stir-fry or marinara sauce at the end of the cooking time.

❒ As an alternative to fresh garlic, try a garlic supplement. "There is some evidence that garlic supplements such as Kyolic and Madaus Murdock Garlicin Pro reduce cholesterol, too," says Mary Bove, N.D., a naturopathic doctor and director of the Brattleboro Naturopathic Clinic in Brattleboro, Vermont. "I'll recommend a supplement to people who don't like the taste of fresh garlic." You can buy garlic supplements in health food stores and some drugstores. For the proper dosage, follow the directions on the label.

Low Fat, Healthy Heart

If your doctor has already told you that you have high cholesterol, you can significantly lower your reading within six to eight weeks by following the Ornish diet, according to Ruth Marlin, M.D., staff physician and head of medical education at the Preventive Medicine Research Institute in Sausalito, California.

The Ornish diet was developed by renowned internist Dean Ornish, M.D., for patients with coronary artery disease at the Preventive Medicine Research Institute. It slashes total fat intake to just 10 percent of calories. How? By focusing on foods of plant origin—grains, fruits, vegetables, and beans. You use egg whites and nonfat dairy products instead of whole eggs and full-fat dairy products. And you completely eliminate poultry, fish, and meat. (If your goal is to prevent high cholesterol rather than treat it, you can have three servings of lean poultry or fish per week, but absolutely no red meat.)

"If a doctor recommends cholesterol-lowering drugs, we believe this diet is worth a try first," Dr. Marlin says. "But we do consider it a medical treatment, and we think that people do best with it when they get a nutritionist's help right from the start." Your doctor can refer you to a nutritionist.

❏ Take 500 to 1,000 milligrams of vitamin C a day, suggests Dr. Bove. Even in people with healthy intakes of vitamin C, additional vitamin C seems to help increase HDL levels. In one study at the Jean Mayer USDA Human Nutrition Research Center on Aging at Tufts University in Boston, men and women with low blood levels of vitamin C who took 1,000 milligrams of supplemental vitamin C a day for eight months averaged a 7 percent increase in their HDL readings.

Prescriptions
FOR KEEPING ARTERIES CLEAR

HERBAL
Rx

Just as certain foods can improve your cholesterol profile, certain herbs can help, too. Consider adding these two herbal remedies to your personal cholesterol-reduction program.

❒ Consume one to two tablespoons ground fenugreek seeds three or four times a day, suggests Dr. Bove. In one study at the National Institute of Nutrition in India, people who ingested roughly three-quarters cup of the herb every day for 20 days cut their LDL levels by one-third. Even better, their HDL levels remained unchanged.

Fenugreek has a bittersweet taste. Try sprinkling some of the ground seeds on food. Or make a tea by steeping one teaspoon ground seeds in one cup freshly boiled water.

❒ If the taste of fenugreek doesn't appeal to you, take one or two 580-milligram capsules of the herb three or four times a day, advises Dr. Bove. You can buy the capsules in most health food stores.

❒ Season foods with turmeric, says Dr. Bove. Researchers in India—where turmeric is a staple ingredient—have found that the herb enhances your body's ability to process cholesterol. She recommends using turmeric to flavor poultry, fish, beans, and curry and tomato sauces.

❒ As an alternative to ground turmeric, take 150 milligrams of the herb in capsule form three times a day, suggests Dr. Bove. Turmeric capsules are available in most health food stores.

Prescriptions
FOR LIFETIME CHOLESTEROL CONTROL

Rx

Once you achieve a healthy cholesterol reading, you can sustain it for the long term. Simply follow a heart-friendly lifestyle that includes the following strategies.

❒ Control your weight once and for all. If you exceed your ideal weight by more than 20 percent, you increase your chances of developing heart disease, according to Dr. Marlin. So let's say that your ideal weight is 135 pounds. Carrying more than 27 extra pounds—or more than 162 pounds total—puts you at risk for heart problems.

While there are a number of complex formulas for figuring out your ideal weight, one simple formula used by some experts can tell you if you are close: If you are five feet tall, you should weigh 100 pounds. If you are taller, add 5 pounds for each additional inch of height. To that number, add 10 percent if you have a large frame, or subtract 10 percent if you have a small frame.

As you lose body fat through diet and exercise, you will see improvement in your cholesterol profile. Your HDL level will rise, while your total cholesterol and LDL cholesterol levels drop. How much of a change you see will depend on how many pounds you lose.

TIME IT RIGHT

❏ Exercise for at least 30 minutes every day. Physical activity elevates your HDL level. Try bicycling, swimming, gentle weight training, or even brisk walking—anything that gets your heart pumping, says Dr. Marlin. But build up to the recommended 30 minutes a day gradually—especially if you have been inactive.

Medical **Alert**

Many physicians recommend that all women get their cholesterol checked at least once a year. If you have high cholesterol, you should get it checked twice a year until it returns to a healthy reading. You should also get it checked more than once a year if one of the following applies.

✓ You have recently gained a lot of weight.

✓ You are on cholesterol-lowering medication.

✓ You have diabetes or kidney disease.

✓ You have had your ovaries removed.

✓ You have recently gone through menopause.

✓ You have heart disease or symptoms of heart disease.

The National Cholesterol Education Committee of the National Institutes of Health has issued guidelines to doctors regarding the treatment of high cholesterol, taking into consideration other risk factors for heart disease. You may want to ask your doctor if she follows these guidelines.

Irritable Bowel Syndrome

Call it the case of the grumbly gut. Scientists have not yet solved the mystery of what causes irritable bowel syndrome, or IBS. Nor can they explain why IBS affects twice as many women as men.

They do know that IBS is a chronic condition in which the muscular lining of the intestines twitches, spasms, and cramps uncontrollably, says Ralph Giannella, M.D., professor of medicine and director of the division of digestive diseases at the University of Cincinnati College of Medicine. As a result, you experience constipation, diarrhea, gas, or abdominal pain—or more than likely, a combination of all four symptoms.

Irritable bowel syndrome usually develops when you are in your twenties or thirties, and the symptoms sometimes worsen with age, says Sheila Rodriguez-Stanley, Ph.D., gastrointestinal laboratory director for the Oklahoma Foundation for Digestive Research in Oklahoma City. For some women, IBS becomes so disruptive that they pare down their daily routines just to stay close to a bathroom.

MONTHLY

Stress ranks high on the list of potential triggers for an IBS flare-up, according to Dr. Rodriguez-Stanley. A woman's menstrual cycle appears to provoke symptoms as well—though again, scientists have yet to figure out why.

MONTHLY

It could be that monthly hormonal changes affect the movement of stool through the intestines, says Gerard Guillory, M.D., assistant clinical professor of medicine at the University of Colorado Health Sciences Center in Aurora and author of *IBS: A Doctor's Plan for Chronic Digestive Troubles*. Or it could be that the fatty, sugary foods women tend to crave during their periods irritate the intestines.

Prescriptions
to Dodge Intestinal Distress

NUTRITION
Rx

Even though IBS is a chronic condition, you can do a lot to reduce the frequency of flare-ups and to ease your symptoms when a flare-up does occur. Your first assignment is to take a good, hard look at your dietary habits. What you eat and when you eat it can influence your symptoms for

Prescriptions for Relaxing Relief

While doctors don't yet know what causes irritable bowel syndrome (IBS), they do know that stress can provoke a flare-up. The following relaxation techniques can help short-circuit your body's stress response before it has a chance to get your gut grumbling, says Gerard Guillory, M.D., assistant clinical professor of medicine at the University of Colorado Health Sciences Center in Aurora and author of *IBS: A Doctor's Plan for Chronic Digestive Troubles.*

❐ Breathe deeply for two to three minutes (or as long as your time will allow) when tension sets in. Begin by placing your hands on your abdomen. Inhale slowly and deeply through your nose, feeling your abdomen expand as you do. Hold your breath for a second or two, then exhale very slowly through your mouth. Repeat this cycle several times until you feel at ease.

❐ Take a mental vacation from a stressful situation. Visualize yourself lying on a sun-drenched beach. Feel the sun's warm rays caressing your skin as a cool breeze gently blows over you. With each breath you take, your body feels invigorated by the clean, fresh air. You hear waves splashing against the shore and seagulls calling in the distance. Continue this imagery until you feel completely calm and relaxed.

❐ Practice progressive muscle relaxation for 15 minutes whenever you feel tense. If you can, find a quiet room or an outdoor setting where you can sit or lie down. Once you are in a comfortable position, begin by contracting the muscles around your eyes, as if you were squinting in bright sunlight. Hold for a few seconds, then relax. Repeat three times. Continue moving down your body, contracting and then relaxing the muscles in your shoulders, hands, hips, knees, and feet. By the time you reach your toes, all of your muscles should feel warm and relaxed.

better or for worse. To make your diet more bowel-friendly, try these tips from the experts.

❒ Eat your meals at the same time every day. If you are like most women, a hectic daily routine dictates when—or maybe even if—you have your mealtimes. Eating "on the fly" throws off your body's circadian rhythms (its internal clock), so it doesn't know when to void. This can lead to constipation or to cycles of constipation and diarrhea, both of which are characteristic of IBS, says Dr. Giannella. Establishing regular mealtimes, on the other hand, cues your body to void at certain times of the day. You don't have to eat breakfast at precisely 7:00 A.M. and lunch precisely at noon. Choose times that work for you and stick with them, he says.

❒ Eat at least one serving of a grain, a fruit, and a vegetable at each meal. These foods have plenty of fiber, which not only keeps you regular but also eases your symptoms during an IBS flare-up, says Dr. Giannella. If you have constipation, for instance, fiber makes your stool retain water so that it softens and passes more easily. And if you have diarrhea, fiber gives your stool bulk. Good sources of fiber include brown rice, split peas, blackberries, and avocado.

Increasing your fiber intake may seem to worsen your symptoms at first—especially if your diet has consisted primarily of processed foods. But within a few weeks, your body will adjust, says Dr. Giannella. To minimize your discomfort, try phasing in fiber slowly. One suggestion is to add 5 grams a day the first week, then another 5 grams a day the next week, and so on until you reach the Daily Value of 25 grams. Five grams is roughly the amount in one-half cup high-fiber cereal.

❒ If eating whole fiber-rich vegetables makes your IBS symptoms intolerable, try their juices for a week or two. Four ounces of carrot, celery, or parsley juice at lunch and dinner provides all the vitamins and minerals you need without aggravating your bowel, says Eve Campanelli, Ph.D., a practitioner of holistic medicine in Beverly Hills, California. You can buy these juices ready-made at the grocery store, or you can make your own concoctions at home with a juicer.

❒ Take a natural fiber supplement two or three times daily for up to four days. You can make your own by adding one-quarter teaspoon powdered psyllium seed, one-quarter teaspoon whole flaxseed, and one-half teaspoon slippery elm bark powder to an eight-ounce glass of water. (Unlike the powders, the flaxseed won't dissolve, but it does wash down easily.) This combination of ingredients supplies both soluble and insoluble fiber, which work together to move stool through your bowels, according to Mitchell Fleisher, M.D., assistant clinical professor of family medicine at the University of Virginia Health Science Center in Charlottesville and a family-practice and homeopathic physician in Nellysford, Virginia. You will find all three ingredients in health food stores. He suggests squeezing a slice or two of lemon into the mix before drinking it.

❏ Add spices to your food after cooking—for instance, sprinkle crushed red pepper flakes or black pepper over your cooked eggs. Seasoning your food after it is prepared makes the spices less irritating to your digestive tract, according to Dr. Campanelli.

❏ Curtail your consumption of coffee, black tea, and alcohol. These beverages act as stimulants, making stool move through your bowels too quickly, says Dr. Campanelli. Also, alcohol is acidic, which can upset your stomach.

❏ Identify foods and beverages that may be aggravating your IBS symptoms by tracking your diet for two weeks. Simply write down what you eat and drink as well as when you experience symptoms. Then after two weeks, look over your notes for potential triggers. Keep in mind that up to five hours may elapse between when you consume something and when you develop symptoms, says Dr. Giannella.

Once you have identified a potential trigger, eliminate it from your diet for a week. Notice whether the frequency or severity of your symptoms decreases. If so, you may have found your culprit—and you may want to eliminate it from your diet for good, says Dr. Rodriguez-Stanley.

HERBAL
Rx

Prescriptions
TO SHORT-CIRCUIT SYMPTOMS

When IBS does flare up, you want relief—fast. Certain herbs can help ease your symptoms and nurse your intestinal tract back to pain-free functioning. Give the following herbal remedies a try.

❐ During a flare-up, take one to three capsules of the herb cramp bark 15 minutes before each meal. When your symptoms subside, cut your dosage to one or two capsules only before your largest meal. Cramp bark relaxes tension in your bowels and allows stools to pass without spasms, explains Dr. Campanelli. You can buy cramp bark capsules in health food stores. How many capsules you need depends on your height and weight, she says. A woman who is five feet, four inches tall and weighs 120 pounds should take one capsule, while a woman who is six feet tall and weighs 200 pounds should take two or three. Each company dilutes its product differently, so be sure to follow the dosage directions on the package.

❐ Before each meal, add 5 to 10 drops each of peppermint oil and caraway seed oil to an eight-ounce glass of warm water and drink it, says Dr. Fleisher.

German researchers found that a combination of peppermint oil and caraway seed oil reduced IBS-related abdominal pain in 90 percent of people taking the herbs. While the study was small and lasted only four weeks, the researchers concluded that the herbs are an appropriate alternative to the medications traditionally prescribed to manage IBS symptoms. You'll find peppermint oil and caraway seed oil in health food stores.

Note: Women who are pregnant should not use caraway seed oil. In large dosages, the herb can harm a developing fetus. Also, be aware that taking peppermint oil for long periods of time can cause serious stomach upset and inflammation. Give your stomach "time off" every so often, or use only as needed, not continuously.

Prescriptions
TO RIDE OUT A FLARE-UP

Rx

Besides dietary changes and herbal remedies, a couple of other strategies can help you through an IBS flare-up. Many doctors agree that the following are essential to managing IBS symptoms.

❐ Drink at least ½ ounce of water for each pound of body weight every day. A woman weighing 140 pounds, for instance, should aim for 70 ounces of H_2O—almost nine 8-ounce glasses—a day. Water helps regulate your bowel movements, explains Dr. Fleisher. If you are constipated, it softens your stools. If you have diarrhea, it works with fiber to bulk up your stools.

TIME IT RIGHT

❐ Engage in aerobic exercise for at least 20 minutes, three times a week. The word *aerobic* refers to any activity that gets your heart pumping—not just aerobic dance but also running, swimming, and even brisk walking. Scientists can't yet explain why, but exercise seems to reduce the frequency of both constipation and diarrhea, says Joel Mason, M.D., associate professor in the divisions of gastroenterology and clinical nutrition at Tufts University School of Medicine in Boston.

Medical **Alert**

If you have IBS and you notice blood in your stool or experience unexplained weight loss, see your doctor right away. These symptoms may indicate a more serious underlying health problem. You should also see your doctor if constipation, diarrhea, or abdominal pain becomes so severe that it disrupts your daily routine, says Dr. Rodriguez-Stanley.

Osteoporosis

Medical experts have dubbed osteoporosis a silent disease. It takes years to develop, yet during that time, it never shows any outward symptoms. Women seldom realize that they have it until they sustain fractures from incidents as minor as bumping against a kitchen table or lifting a grocery bag.

In osteoporosis, bones become fragile and prone to breaking. More than 28 million Americans either have the disease or are at risk for it, according to the Washington, D.C.–based National Osteoporosis Foundation. Of that number, 80 percent are women.

LIFETIME

Why the gender gap? For starters, women have about 25 percent less bone mass than men. And while both sexes lose about 1 percent of their bone mass each year, the rate for women jumps to 2 to 3 percent during and after menopause. After menopause, the female body's production of the hormone estrogen, which helps bones absorb and retain calcium, sharply declines.

That is why now is the time for you to start taking care of your skeleton. You can build bone into your thirties, and thereafter, you can preserve the bone you have. "At any stage of your life—whether you are premenopausal or postmenopausal—you can slow and stop bone loss," says Kendra Kaye Zuckerman, M.D., assistant professor of medicine and director of the osteoporosis program at Allegheny University Hospitals in Philadelphia.

In her practice, Dr. Zuckerman has noticed an increase in the number of women seeking preventive care for their bones. "It's a trend that we want to promote, to get more women to think about osteoporosis long before they might suffer their first fractures," she says.

Prescriptions
FOR A STURDY SKELETON

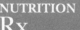

Safeguarding your bones begins with calcium. The mineral is so important to skeletal health that the National Institutes of Health advises all women between ages 25 and 49 to consume 1,000 milligrams of calcium a day. (If you are pregnant or breastfeeding, you need a little more—1,200 to 1,500 milligrams a day.) Unfortunately, the average American woman gets less than half this amount.

To increase your intake of calcium and other nutrients essential to a strong skeleton, consider these dietary changes, recommended by osteoporosis experts.

❐ Drink at least eight ounces of skim or low-fat (1%) milk each day. Milk has few peers in the calcium department. Yet many women shy away from the beverage because of its high fat content. If you are among them, you should know that both skim and low-fat (1%) milk have slightly more calcium than the full-fat variety, according to Dr. Zuckerman. In fact, you get about 350 milligrams of calcium in an eight-ounce glass of skim milk, which covers about one-third of your daily requirement. A same-size glass of low-fat (1%) milk supplies 300 milligrams of the mineral; whole milk, just 291 milligrams.

❏ Eat three to four servings of calcium-rich dairy foods per day, says Dr. Zuckerman. While plain old milk is a top-notch calcium source, other "moo foods" provide healthy doses of the mineral, too. You get at least 300 milligrams of calcium in one cup nonfat or low-fat yogurt, two one-ounce slices of Cheddar or Muenster cheese, or one-half cup part-skim ricotta cheese. As you choose from among these foods, be sure to keep in mind your individual calcium requirement, based on the guidelines cited earlier.

❏ Eat at least one cup broccoli, collard greens, or turnip greens each day, says Dr. Zuckerman. While these vegetables contain less than one-third as much calcium per serving as milk, they still help you meet your daily requirement of the mineral.

❏ Eat canned pink salmon with bones, recommends the National Osteoporosis Foundation. The bones in three ounces of the fish contain calcium—approximately 180 milligrams per serving.

❏ Look for processed foods that have been fortified with calcium. Manufacturers often add the mineral to cereals, breads, and orange juice. For example, eight ounces of calcium-fortified orange juice supplies 300 milligrams of the mineral.

❏ Try sprinkling nonfat dry milk into soups and casseroles, says the National Osteoporosis Foundation. Dry milk gives foods an extra calcium boost—one-third cup contains 300 milligrams.

❏ Consider taking a daily calcium supplement to reach your recommended intake. Whichever brand you choose, check the label for the amount of elemental calcium it contains. (Look for the words *elemental calcium* or for a percentage of calcium.) This figure shows how much of the calcium your body can actually absorb and use, says Dr. Zuckerman. A 1,000-milligram supplement, for example, may supply only 500 milligrams of absorbable calcium.

MEALTIME

❏ If you choose a calcium carbonate supplement, take it at mealtime with a full glass of water. Food improves the absorption of this form of calcium, according to Dr. Zuckerman.

An Exercise Rx for Your Bones

Exercise plays a crucial role in the prevention and treatment of osteoporosis. It builds bone mass early in life and prevents bone loss in later years. And as a bonus, it improves strength and coordination, reducing the likelihood of fractures caused by slips and falls.

For optimum bone health, you should engage in 30 minutes of weight-bearing exercise at least five days a week, advises Kendra Kaye Zuckerman, M.D., assistant professor of medicine and director of the osteoporosis program at Allegheny University Hospitals in Philadelphia. Weight-bearing means that you are on your feet, letting your skeleton support the weight of your body. Walking, running, tennis, and aerobic dance are just some of the activities that fill the bill.

Exercise does have a catch, however: For its skeleton-saving effects to last, you must engage in it regularly. "If you work out for six months and then stop, you lose what you had gained," says Dr. Zuckerman.

If you have already been diagnosed with osteoporosis or another health problem, you should consult your physician before starting an exercise program.

❒ If you choose a calcium citrate supplement, take it on an empty stomach, says Dr. Zuckerman. It's better absorbed that way.

❒ Consider taking a daily multivitamin that contains 400 international units of vitamin D. Vitamin D supports the bone-building process by helping your body absorb calcium, says Dr. Zuckerman. Normally, your body uses sunlight to manufacture its own supply of the vitamin. But if you wear sunscreen—as experts advise you to—or get limited exposure to the sun, you may not have as much vitamin D as you need. Also, your body's ability to produce the vitamin declines with age. Besides supplements, you can get vitamin D from fortified foods such as milk.

❒ Eat enough magnesium-rich foods to meet the Daily Value of 400 milligrams, experts say. Magnesium works double duty in the bone-building process. It helps calcium get into your bones, and it converts vitamin D to its active form in your body. Excellent food sources of magnesium include almonds (84 milligrams in one ounce), toasted wheat germ (90 milligrams in one-quarter cup), and spinach (78 milligrams in one-half cup).

❒ Eat enough vitamin C–rich foods to meet the Daily Value of 60 milligrams. One theory holds that vitamin C plays a role in the manufacture of collagen, a connective tissue that provides the framework for bones. Oranges are perhaps the best-known source of vitamin C, with 70 milligrams in one fruit. But don't overlook sliced strawberries (94 milligrams per cup), kiwifruit (75 milligrams per fruit), and red bell peppers (142 milligrams per one-half cup chopped).

❒ Consume 30 to 50 milligrams of isoflavones each day, experts recommend. Isoflavones are weak, plant-derived forms of estrogen that are found in abundance in soybeans. Researchers at the University of Illinois have suggested that these compounds may help stave off bone loss in the same way that estrogen-replacement therapy does. To meet the recommended daily intake of isoflavones, choose soy foods such as tofu (35 milligrams in one-half cup) and roasted soy nuts (60 milligrams in one-quarter cup).

Rx ——— *Prescriptions*
to Stop the Bone Robbers

Just as certain foods protect against bone loss, others speed up the process. To make your eating habits more bone-friendly, heed this advice.

MEALTIME

❒ Limit your red meat consumption to one three-ounce serving per week. Researchers at the Harvard School of Public Health studied the effects of protein on bone health and concluded that meat-based protein can increase the amount of calcium excreted in urine as well as the risk of bone fractures. Women in the study who ate five or more servings of red meat per week had a significantly increased risk of forearm fractures compared with women who ate less than one serving per week.

❐ Limit your sodium intake to 2,400 milligrams a day. Too much dietary sodium can contribute to bone loss by causing more calcium to be excreted in the urine, says Bess Dawson-Hughes, professor of medicine and chief of the calcium and bone metabolism laboratory at the Jean Mayer USDA Human Nutrition Research Center at Tufts University in Boston.

❐ Limit your coffee consumption to two cups a day. Like sodium, the caffeine in coffee increases the amount of calcium that is excreted in the urine, says Dr. Zuckerman.

Prescriptions — Rx
FOR BREAKING BAD-TO-THE-BONE HABITS

To round out your skeleton-supporting lifestyle, doctors recommend the following strategies.

❐ Quit smoking. Smoking reduces estrogen production in pre-menopausal women, explains Clifford Rosen, M.D., chief of medicine at St. Joseph Hospital in Bangor, Maine. As a result, these women have a more difficult time maintaining their bone mass. A woman who smokes one pack of cigarettes a day may have 5 to 10 percent lower bone density than a nonsmoker by the time they reach menopause. Smoking may also cause more rapid bone loss in the early post-menopausal years.

❐ Give up alcohol—but if you must imbibe, limit yourself to three drinks per week. (A drink is defined as one 12-ounce beer, one 5-ounce glass of wine, or a mixed drink made with 1½ ounces of liquor.) Alcohol interferes with your body's ability to absorb and use calcium and vitamin D. It also impairs your balance, which could lead to a fall and a fracture, notes Dr. Zuckerman.

Medical **Alert**
Major risk factors for osteoporosis include a thin or petite frame, a family history of osteoporosis, early menopause, a calcium-poor diet,

use of certain medications (such as corticosteroids and anticonvulsants), inactivity, cigarette smoking, and abnormal absence of periods. If any of these apply to you, talk to your doctor about whether you should have a bone-density test, says Dr. Zuckerman. Such a test can help determine your risk for experiencing an osteoporosis-related fracture.

Overweight

Every year, more than half of all Americans are either dieting or trying to keep off pounds that they have already lost. For too many of us, weight wars wage on and on. Why do we have so little success when it comes to weight loss?

"I think it's because we want a quick fix rather than a long-term cure," says Cheryl Norton, Ed.D., professor of human performance, sport, and leisure studies at the Metropolitan State College of Denver. "Once typical Americans pass age 20, they gain about a pound a year because they live sedentary lifestyles. So they try all sorts of diets and even starve themselves to take off the weight fast." Sure, the extra pounds disappear . . . for a while. But inevitably, they creep back on.

Make no mistake: If you are overweight, you will do yourself a world of good by aiming for a healthier weight—one that's right for your age and your size, says G. Michael Steelman, M.D., a physician in Oklahoma City and chairman of the board of the American Society of Bariatric Physicians. To figure out your healthy weight, use the following guideline recommended by Dr. Steelman: Start at around 100 pounds if you are five feet or taller. Then add 5 pounds for every inch that you are over five feet. To that number, add 10 percent if you have a large frame, or subtract 10 percent if you have a small frame.

Carrying extra pounds is much more than a cosmetic issue. It is associated with numerous health problems, including heart disease, diabetes, and cancers of the breasts, ovaries, and uterus.

Overweight affects your emotional health as well, notes Dr. Steelman. While some women feel completely comfortable with their bodies, others experience dips in their self-confidence and self-esteem.

Outgrow That Baby Fat

Canadian researchers at McGill University in Montreal found that women who gain a lot of weight early in their pregnancies tend to retain those extra pounds long after their babies are born. The researchers' findings suggest that women—especially those who are overweight—should defer most of their weight gain until they are at least 20 weeks into their pregnancies. This strategy should help keep those postpartum pounds to a minimum.

If you want to slim down sensibly and permanently, there is only one "secret formula" that works: You must burn more calories than you consume. You can do that by eating healthfully and exercising regularly.

Prescriptions
FOR LASTING WEIGHT LOSS

Most of us have no problem starting a weight-loss program. Sticking with it is a whole other ball game. To shape a program that you can live with, experts suggest the following tactics.

❏ Begin your weight-loss program in the spring or summer. You naturally tend to eat more during the fall and winter months, when the weather turns cold. That undermines your chances for success from the get-go. Warm weather, on the other hand, encourages you to head outdoors and get active. SPRINGTIME

❏ Strive for gradual weight loss—no more than two pounds per week. Take off more than that, and your metabolism (your body's calorie-burning mechanism) will slow down in an effort to conserve energy. "It's your body's way of protecting you from starvation," explains Dr. Norton. Your weight loss will taper off, and you'll regain those pounds quite easily.

TIME IT RIGHT

❏ Make only one or two minor changes at a time in your eating and exercise habits. For example, look for ways that you can cut your calorie intake by roughly 125 calories a day, says Dr. Steelman. You might try putting mustard instead of mayonnaise on your sandwich or using low-fat (1%) milk instead of cream in your coffee. Same goes for exercise: Start with a 10-minute workout and gradually build from there, he suggests. By going slowly and giving yourself time to adjust to the lifestyle changes you make, you set yourself up for lasting weight loss.

TIME IT RIGHT

❏ If you use a scale to monitor your progress, weigh yourself at the same time every day. Your weight fluctuates over the course of 24 hours. Stepping on the scale in the morning one day and at bedtime the next can leave you with an inaccurate (and discouraging) picture of how you are doing.

NUTRITION
Rx

Prescriptions
to Trim the Fat

Weight-loss programs sometimes get stuck in a nutrition rut, focusing primarily on dietary fat. For the record, many experts advise limiting your daily fat intake to 25 percent of calories—for a variety of health reasons. You can make other, equally important changes in your eating habits to support your weight-loss goals. Start with these dietary strategies.

❏ Measure serving sizes. "Many women have cut way back on dietary fat but overcompensate with too-large portions of nonfat or low-fat foods," says Dr. Steelman. "These foods can be quite high in calories."

❏ Consume at least 25 grams (the Daily Value) of fiber each day. Fiber, which is found only in plant foods, acts as a natural appetite suppressant. It fills you up, so you feel less hungry, explains Ingrid Lofgren, R.D., of the University of Massachusetts Medical Center in Worcester. To ensure that you are meeting your daily fiber quota, build your meals around grain products, beans, vegetables, and fruits. One-half cup chickpeas provides 7 grams of fiber, one-half cup kidney beans provides 6.9 grams, one cup raspberries provides 6 grams, one cup cooked whole-wheat spaghetti provides 5.4 grams, and one pear (with the skin) provides 4.3 grams.

❒ Drink eight ounces of water 15 minutes before a meal. Water literally drowns your appetite, so you eat less, notes Lofgren.

TIME IT RIGHT

❒ Divide your usual three meals a day into five or six "mini-meals." By eating smaller meals more often, you stave off hunger and prevent yourself from overeating when you finally do sit down at the table, says Dr. Steelman.

❒ Eat breakfast every morning. Breakfast jump-starts your metabolism and keeps calories burning efficiently throughout the day, says Dr. Steelman. Plus, by filling up first thing in the A.M., you are less likely to overindulge at lunch or dinner.

MORNING

❒ For breakfast, choose healthful foods such as toast with all-fruit preserves, nonfat or low-fat yogurt, or nonfat or low-fat cottage cheese with fruit. Fatty, sugary foods such as doughnuts and Danish send your blood sugar for a roller-coaster ride. That pumps up your appetite and sparks sugar cravings, according to Dr. Steelman.

MORNING

❒ If you work in an office, stock your desk with low-fat foods such as single-serving cans of tuna and dehydrated soups. Then on days when you don't have time to pack your lunch, you have a fast and healthful meal right at your fingertips. You won't be as tempted to head for the nearest vending machine or fast-food outlet for a bite to eat, says Lofgren.

DAYTIME

❒ Stash healthful snacks such as dried fruit, single-serving cans of vegetable juice, and low-fat granola bars in your purse, briefcase, or car. These foods make great antidotes for between-meal munchies. They satisfy your hunger without a lot of calories or fat, notes Lofgren.

❒ Eat your meals at the kitchen or dining-room table rather than in front of the TV. People who watch TV during meals tend to eat significantly more food than people who don't, according to Dr. Steelman. That means TV-watchers are likely taking in more calories and fat.

MEALTIME

❒ Eat dinner at least three hours before going to bed. Based on his patients' experience, Dr. Steelman has concluded that people who eat the majority of their calories close to bedtime have a harder time losing

NIGHTTIME

weight. Blame it on your body's metabolism: It slows down at night, so your body stores fat more easily.

NIGHTTIME

❐ If you must eat less than three hours before hitting the sack, choose fruits, vegetables, whole grains, and lean proteins such as nonfat or low-fat dairy products. These foods supply the most vitamins and minerals in exchange for a modest number of calories, explains Dr. Steelman.

❐ Keep a food diary, writing down not only what you eat but also how much you eat, when you eat it, and what you're doing at the time. This process helps you shape healthier dietary habits by uncovering hidden sources of calories and fat, notes Dr. Steelman. It also identifies situations that switch on your appetite—for instance, you may realize that you consistently turn to food when you are bored or stressed-out.

EXERCISE
Rx

Prescriptions
to Shape Up and Slim Down

Exercise is an essential component of the weight-loss equation. Remember that to slim down, you need to burn more calories than you consume. And the best way to burn more calories is to work out regularly. To develop a more physically active lifestyle, give these tips a try.

TIME IT RIGHT

❐ Help yourself to at least 30 minutes of aerobic exercise five to seven days a week, suggests Dr. Steelman. *Aerobic* means that the activity makes you breathe faster and your heart beat faster. Walking, running, and bicycling all qualify.

❐ Choose an aerobic activity that you enjoy. The more you like what you're doing, the more you will want to stick with it, notes Dr. Steelman.

❐ Add strength training to your workout. Strength training increases your lean body mass, or muscle. Since muscle burns more calories than fat, your metabolism speeds up. And it stays up, whether you are active or at rest. "That's an extremely big plus when you are talking about weight loss or maintenance," says Dr. Steelman.

You can do a combination of strength training and aerobic exercise on the days you work out or alternate between aerobic exercise one day and strength training the next. Just be sure to substitute strength training for aerobic exercise on no more than three of your workout days, Dr. Steelman adds.

❏ Find little ways to increase your physical activity throughout the day. If you walk to work, for example, tack an extra block onto your route. You will burn 10 more calories per day, or roughly 3,500 more calories per year—the number of calories in one pound of fat, says Dr. Norton. Some other strategies are to take the stairs instead of the elevator, go for a brisk walk at lunch, and park your car at the far end of the parking lot when you go to the supermarket.

Daytime

❏ Establish exercise goals and reward yourself for meeting them. If you walk for 30 minutes every day this week, for instance, treat yourself to a movie or a relaxing bubble bath.

Medical **Alert**

If you exceed your healthy weight by 20 percent or more, you have a higher-than-average risk for developing health problems such as heart disease, diabetes, and some forms of cancer. You should see your doctor for a checkup and for assistance in developing a weight-management program that works for you.

Poor Resistance

Wintertime

Ah, flu season—the time of year when microscopic malcontents reduce full-grown women to achy, nauseous, bedridden bundles of misery. The only thing that stands between you and a week of chicken soup is your immune system.

The immune system is a complex network of organs, glands, and cells that work together to protect your body against infection and disease. It seeks out and destroys harmful substances that invade your body, such as viruses and bacteria.

Most of the time, the immune system does a fine job of keeping you healthy. But sometimes it weakens—the result of poor nutrition, lack of exercise, lack of sleep, or excessive stress. That is when an opportunistic intruder can gain a foothold and make you sick.

Can you do anything to bolster the immunity troops? Absolutely, says Sandra McLanahan, M.D., medical director of the Integral Health Center in Buckingham, Virginia. You know the drill: Eat right, exercise regularly, get plenty of rest, and manage stress. Together, these strategies keep your immune system strong.

Rx ———— *Prescriptions*
FOR A DISEASE-DEFYING LIFESTYLE

To fortify your body's immune power, start with the basics. The following tactics lay the foundation for a robust and resilient immune system.

❏ Eat five to seven servings of fruits and vegetables every day. These foods contain phytochemicals, compounds that bolster your immunity, according to Dr. McLanahan. Produce also supplies healthy doses of the antioxidant nutrients—vitamins C and E and beta-carotene. The antioxidants neutralize free radicals, unstable molecules that occur naturally in your body and that weaken and impair your immune system.

One cup leafy greens counts as a serving, as does one-half cup cooked or raw chopped vegetables, one medium-size whole fruit, and one-half cup canned or fresh chopped fruit.

❏ Reserve sugary, processed foods for a once-in-a-while treat—and when you do indulge, make sure that it is after a nutritious meal. If you fill up on foods that are high in calories but low in nutrients, you cheat your body out of important nutrients and weaken your immune system, observes Dr. McLanahan.

TIME IT RIGHT ❏ Walk for 30 minutes at least five days a week. Moderate exercise such as walking boosts the activity of your immune system's infection-fighters, including natural killer cells, B-cells, and T-cells, says Gregory Heath, D.Sc., an epidemiologist and exercise physiologist for the Centers for Disease Control and Prevention in Atlanta.

❏ Refrain from super-strenuous workouts. Or, provide a sufficient amount of time for recovery following such workouts. For example, alternate more-moderate workouts with more-strenuous workouts. Research has shown that exercising intensely (30 minutes of continuous or inter-

Herbal Prescriptions for Optimum Immunity

Do you feel as if you get more than your fair share of colds and flu? Try giving your immune system a natural boost with the following herbal remedies, suggests Sandra McLanahan, M.D., medical director of the Integral Health Center in Buckingham, Virginia. You can buy the herbs in capsule, tablet, or tincture form in health food stores.

❏ Eat two cloves of fresh garlic every day. Garlic enhances immune function by recharging your natural killer cells, white blood cells that seek out and destroy disease-causing invaders. The pungent bulb also has antibiotic properties. Worried about garlic breath? Chew on some parsley to mask the odor.

❏ Take two capsules or tablets of ginseng twice a day, unless otherwise noted on the label. Russian cosmonauts and Asian Olympic athletes use ginseng to enhance their resistance to the physical effects of stress. The herb also protects against free radicals, those renegade molecules that harm healthy cells.

❏ Take two tablets of echinacea three times a day for up to two weeks, unless otherwise noted on the label. Echinacea has won widespread praise for its immunity-enhancing and antibiotic properties. Research suggests that the herb is most effective when taken in small doses for short periods of time.

❏ Take astragalus capsules or tincture as recommended on the product label. The root of the astragalus plant strengthens immunity by boosting the activity of several types of white blood cells. It also increases production of disease-fighting antibodies.

mittent exercise at 90 percent or greater of your aerobic capacity) actually suppresses immune function, according to Dr. Heath. So does exercising too long (more than one hour of sustained exercise at greater than 80 percent of aerobic capacity).

NIGHTTIME

❐ Get at least seven hours of sleep each night. Research suggests that too little shut-eye impairs your immune system, leaving you more susceptible to colds and perhaps even to certain cancers. In fact, when researchers at the University of California in San Diego deprived 23 men of four hours of sleep for four nights in a row, the men's natural killer cells showed a 30 percent reduction in activity. Natural killer cells are white blood cells that search for and destroy viruses and tumors.

NUTRITION
Rx

Prescriptions
FOR ENHANCING IMMUNITY

Eating healthfully plays an important part in maintaining a strong immune system. Foods supply nutrients, the raw materials that your body uses to manufacture cells and perform other essential tasks related to immune function. The following tips can help ensure that your body gets the disease-fighting vitamins and minerals it needs most.

TIME IT RIGHT

❐ Take 1,000 milligrams of vitamin C three times a day, preferably with meals, says Dr. McLanahan. Vitamin C prompts your immune system to react more aggressively to viruses, bacteria, and cancer cells. It also prevents inflammation, reducing the congestion that goes along with colds and infections.

Note: Some people develop diarrhea when they take more than 1,200 milligrams of vitamin C a day. If you're one of them, simply cut back your dose to a more tolerable level.

❐ Take 300 international units of vitamin E every day, preferably with a meal. In a study at the Jean Mayer USDA Human Nutrition Research Center on Aging at Tufts University in Boston, people who took this dosage of vitamin E for close to eight months showed the greatest improvements in immune function. Pairing off the vitamin with food enhances its absorption.

❐ Consume enough iron- and zinc-rich foods to meet their respective Daily Values of 18 milligrams and 15 milligrams. Iron and zinc work to ensure that lymphocytes—the white blood cells that make up your body's first line of defense against disease—are ready to take on invading viruses and bacteria. One baked potato and one-half cup of Raisin Bran provide 2.75 and 4.5 milligrams of iron, respectively. One-half cup lima beans and three ounces of chicken respectively contain 1.7 and 2.5 milligrams of zinc.

❐ If you are over age 60 (or hope to be some day), take a daily multivitamin/mineral supplement. A study conducted at the New Jersey Medical School in Newark found that people age 60 or older who took a multivitamin every day for 12 months scored significantly better in tests of their immune function than people who took a placebo (a pill that looked like the real thing but did nothing) for the same amount of time.

LIFETIME

Prescriptions
TO SHORT-CIRCUIT STRESS

Rx

Stress can really do a number on your immune system. Research suggests that women who experience chronic stress are especially vulnerable to colds and other infectious diseases, says Bert Uchino, Ph.D., assistant professor in the department of psychology at the University of Utah in Salt Lake City. To make sure that stress doesn't get the best of you, heed this advice from the experts.

❐ Practice deep breathing twice each day. Begin by sitting in a chair with your back straight. Inhale slowly, filling your lungs from bottom to top. Focus on your belly as it expands with your breath. Then exhale slowly while saying the word *relax* aloud, emptying your lungs from top to bottom. Continue this pattern of deep breathing for five minutes. At the end of the session, you should feel calm and relaxed, says Dr. Uchino.

TIME IT RIGHT

❐ Humor yourself with a funny movie, *I Love Lucy* reruns, or a CD of your favorite comedian. Laughing not only buoys emotions but also boosts immunity. Research at Loma Linda University School of Medicine in California has shown that laughter activates T-cells (which direct your immune system's attack on an invader) and stimulates production of B-cells (which manufacture disease-fighting antibodies).

❏ Diversify your personal relationships. Scientists at Carnegie Mellon University in Pittsburgh have found that people with more varied ties to family, friends, work, and community are less susceptible to the common cold than people with less varied ties. Cultivating different types of relationships matters more to your emotional health than having a large number of people in your social universe.

❏ Address marital conflicts with calm reasoning rather than finger-pointing and name-calling. In a study at Ohio State University in Columbus, women who were engaged in heated discussions with their spouses experienced greater surges in their stress hormone levels than the men. The women also showed declines in their white blood cell counts. Both of these physical changes indicate a suppressed immune response. In other words, high-voltage bickering with your spouse makes you more prone to colds and other illnesses.

Rx ——— *Prescriptions*
FOR A PRO-IMMUNITY ENVIRONMENT

While you can control some factors that influence your immunity, such as what you eat and how often you exercise, you are more or less at the mercy of other factors. The environment is one. Air pollution, pesticides, and other toxins can lower your resistance and make you more susceptible to disease, says Martha H. Howard, M.D., medical director for Wellness Associates in Chicago.

Even your home and office can play host to immune-system offenders. Formaldehyde in fabrics and upholstery, glues in carpeting and wallboard, aerosols, and mold spores all conspire to undermine your immunity. And because newer buildings are tightly sealed and have internal ventilation systems, they keep fresh air out and chemical poisons in, says Dr. Howard.

Under such circumstances, your best bet is to change what you can in your immediate environment to make it as health-supporting as possible. According to Dr. Howard, the following strategies can minimize the external assault on your immune system.

❐ Install an air purifier in your home. Choose one that has both charcoal and high-efficiency particulate air (HEPA) filters.

❐ Choose hardwood or tile flooring over carpeting.

❐ If you must have carpeting, make sure that it is made from un-treated natural fibers.

❐ Limit your contact with people who have colds. If you are the family caregiver, you may find this challenging. But keep in mind that you can greatly reduce your risk of colds just by avoiding exposure to cold-causing viruses.

❐ Wash your hands often, especially in winter. Cold and flu bugs lurk everywhere at this time of year. Wash your hands immediately after contact with someone who has a cold, and always wash before every meal.

WINTERTIME

❐ Keep your hands away from your mouth, nose, and eyes. Even if you do pick up a virus, at least you can foil its efforts to get inside your body and start doing its dirty work.

Medical **Alert**

If you frequently get sick despite your best preventive efforts, see your doctor for a thorough exam. This is especially important if you are prone to bacterial infections such as sinusitis and bacterial pneumonia. You or someone in your family may have allergies, which are often the root cause of recurrent sinusitis or ear infections.

Repetitive Strain Injury

When he could no longer push his child's stroller or open a jar of peanut butter, Doug Ross, D.C., finally acknowledged the truth. The in-tense pain in his wrists and arms signaled a repetitive strain injury, the ironic result of treating patients in his practice at Rockridge Family Chi-ropractic in Oakland, California.

"I had gone through all the denials," says Dr. Ross. "I kept telling myself that the pain would go away on its own."

But as anyone with a repetitive strain injury knows, the pain lingers. It can affect not only the hands, wrists, and forearms but also the shoulders and neck. And it may be accompanied by other symptoms, including tingling, numbness, decreased dexterity, and fatigue.

As the name suggests, repetitive strain injuries can develop as the result of performing the same motion over and over again, usually with force or while in an awkward posture. Your tendons become swollen from overuse and impinge upon nearby nerves. That's when you feel pain.

Perhaps the best-known form of repetitive strain injury is carpal tunnel syndrome. In this condition, the median nerve, which runs through the bony carpal tunnel in your wrist, becomes compressed by swollen tendons. Other common forms of repetitive strain injuries include bursitis, tendinitis, and de Quervain's disease (which produces pain in the thumb side of the wrist).

Certain occupations seem to predispose people to repetitive strain injury. Among those at high risk are data-entry clerks, secretaries, cashiers, musicians, electricians, cake decorators, postal workers, and assembly-line workers. Hobbies such as knitting and woodworking can also lead to injury, especially in combination with high-risk jobs, says Dr. Ross.

LIFETIME

Pregnancy increases your likelihood of developing carpal tunnel syndrome, as fluid retention causes swelling of the carpal tunnel and pressure on the median nerve. In most cases, the condition subsides after you give birth.

Rx

Prescriptions
FOR OUTSMARTING INJURY

Experts agree that for repetitive strain injury, prevention is the best medicine. That means scrutinizing your lifestyle and work-style to identify and change those practices that may be putting you at risk. Start with the following strategies.

TIME IT RIGHT

❒ When you are engaged in a repetitive activity, take breaks every 20 to 30 minutes. Roll your shoulders, stretch your wrists, massage your hands and fingers—anything to stimulate blood flow, says Dr. Ross.

❒ Alternate tasks whenever possible to avoid sequences of activities that use the same muscles and tendons. For example, if you spend most of your day in front of a computer or doing intensive filing or photocopying, break up this time with meetings or a walk down the hall. "This forces you to move and stretch your body," notes Ira Janowitz, P.T., a certified professional ergonomist for the ergonomics program at the University of California, San Francisco/Berkeley. "The human body is designed for movement, not for sitting still longer than an hour at a time."

❏ Sit so that you maintain the normal curvature of your spine in your lower back and neck. Slouching damages the disks and ligaments in your spine, according to Dr. Ross. Over time, your spine weakens, and your spinal nerves and associated soft tissues may become damaged.

❏ Correct any habits that contribute to repetitive strain injury. For example, if you use a computer, refrain from resting your wrists on the desk or wrist pad, suggests Dr. Ross. "Play" the keyboard as you would play a piano, moving your arms as well as your wrists. Rest on the wrist pad only when you are not typing.

Also, check your grip on your mouse. It should be comfortable and relaxed rather than tight, with your wrist parallel to the ground, not tipped up or back. Position the mouse near the keyboard and the keyboard at a level where your elbows are at about a 90-degree angle. Placement is important because repeatedly reaching for the mouse can hurt your elbows and shoulders over time. If using the mouse continues to bother you, replace it with a trackball or another type of pointing device.

❏ Choose tools that fit your hands. From staplers to wrenches to wire cutters, many gadgets are too big or too heavy for the average woman's grip. "Just as you try on shoes for size, you should try out tools before buying them," says Janowitz.

❏ If you sit for long periods of time, make sure that you have a chair that is properly proportioned for your body. Furniture is not one-size-fits-all. A chair with a too-deep seat presses against your calves, obstructing your blood flow, says Janowitz. A chair with a too-small seat, on the other hand, presses against the backs of your thighs, impeding circulation there.

When you are sitting, your knees should bend at close to a 90-degree angle, and your feet should be flat on the ground. The back of the chair should firmly hold you upright and not allow you to slouch back as the day wears on and you get tired. And don't forget to get up and stretch every 20 to 30 minutes, advises Dr. Ross.

❏ If your job requires moderate to heavy phone use, wear a headset. Refrain from pinning the receiver between your shoulder and chin, which could leave you with a pain in the neck—literally.

❏ Rearrange your work areas to reduce repetitive reaching. At home, for example, store the dishes you use every day on cupboard shelves between waist- and shoulder-height so that you can easily retrieve them. The same rule applies at work: Keep the supplies that you use most often at your fingertips.

Repetitive reaching is responsible for a variety of musculoskeletal problems, but primarily ones at the shoulder. Whenever you stretch your arm straight out, you create pressure inside your shoulder equal to about 90 percent of your body weight, says Janowitz. If you happen to have something in your hand, such as a stapler, it adds to the force and puts additional strain on your wrist and elbow. By keeping things you use often close at hand, you can avoid the problems that may come with over-reaching.

TIME IT RIGHT

❏ Exercise for at least 30 minutes every day. People who stay in shape through regular aerobic exercise are less likely to develop repetitive strain injuries than those who don't, according to Dr. Ross. Aerobic exercise, the kind that elevates your heart and breathing rates, helps to decrease stress by increasing blood flow to constricted body tissues, he adds. And by getting the large muscle groups—namely your arms and legs—moving, you can relax the little muscle groups, including your fingers.

Rx — *Prescriptions*
FOR SENDING PAIN PACKING

If, despite your best efforts at prevention, you suspect that you have a repetitive strain injury, Dr. Ross urges you not to ignore it. "When you have to modify your daily activities because of pain, discomfort, or weakness for more than a few days or on a repeated basis, then you have a medical problem that requires treatment," he says. First and foremost, you should schedule an appointment with your doctor so that she can make

Sitting Smart

Perching in front of a computer all day could qualify you as a prime candidate for repetitive strain injury. In fact, reported cases of repetitive strain injury have increased sixfold in the past decade, making it the unofficial health complaint of the modern age. You can help protect yourself from pain if you set up your workstation as shown here.

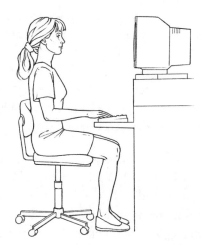

Your head is directly over your shoulders, about an arm's-length from the screen. You should be looking straight ahead at the monitor.

✓ Your neck is stretched upward and relaxed.
✓ Your shoulders are pulled down and relaxed.
✓ Your elbows are at your sides, bent at about a 90-degree angle.
✓ Your wrists are straight and level. Avoid resting them on the keyboard.
✓ Your fingers are in straight lines with your forearms, gently curving onto the keyboard.
✓ Your knees are slightly lower than your hips.
✓ Your feet are flat on the floor.
✓ Your chair is inclined slightly forward.
✓ Your keyboard is flat, at or just below elbow level.

an official diagnosis. Then try the following tips to help manage your pain.

❏ For acute pain, or within one to three days of the onset of pain, apply ice to the painful area for 15 to 20 minutes, five to six times throughout the day. Cold treatments help reduce inflammation and swelling, explains Dr. Ross. Remember to wrap the ice in a towel before putting it on your skin, to protect your skin from the extreme cold. And use common sense: If your pain gets worse, stop the ice applications and try something else.

❏ For chronic pain, or pain that persists for more than three days, lay a hot pack or hot-water bottle over the affected area six to seven times a day for no more than 15 to 20 minutes at a time. Heat relaxes and soothes deep-seated aches and increases blood flow to speed healing, according to Dr. Ross. Be careful not to overheat your body or fall asleep on the pad. A heating pad could also be used, but since hot packs and hot-water bottles lose heat over time, they are safer.

❏ For carpal tunnel syndrome, practice acupressure for on-the-spot pain relief, says David Nickel, O.M.D., a doctor of Oriental medicine in Santa Monica, California, and author of *Acupressure for Athletes*. "Acupressure works by activating the pituitary gland to release endorphins, which are strong, painkilling, opiate-like chemicals," he explains.

If both wrists are affected, begin by treating the most sensitive side first. If most of the pain is on your left side, for example, place the thumb of your right hand on the inside of your left wrist crease or a few inches above, toward the elbow. Then place your right index finger on the back of your left wrist, opposite your right thumb. Probe for the most sensitive area, then apply firm pressure to both sides of your wrist, alternating five seconds on and five seconds off. At the same time, gently move your left hand from side to side. To increase the pain-reducing effect, exhale or blow through your mouth when you apply pressure. Continue the on-and-off applications for one minute. Repeat on the opposite wrist, if necessary.

When used correctly, this acupressure technique significantly reduces pain within minutes, says Dr. Nickel. You can expect to feel tenderness, soreness, or an aching sensation in your wrist, under the thumb or finger, during treatment. But if the pain is worse after using this technique, apply less pressure or discontinue treatment.

❏ Practice yoga. Certain forms of hatha yoga can help a woman develop an awareness of her body's messages, including pain, according to Marian Garfinkel, Ph.D., a health educator and certified senior Iyengar yoga teacher in Philadelphia. "The more aware you are of your body, the more you may be able to treat and prevent injuries, including repetitive strain injuries," explains Dr. Garfinkel. Yoga helps put you in tune with your posture and how you use your arms and legs. "Yoga can't 'cure' a repetitive strain injury on its own. But it can help when used in combination with other therapies, like acupuncture," says Dr. Garfinkel.

❏ Resist the temptation to self-prescribe a splint for carpal tunnel syndrome or another repetitive strain injury. If you think you need one, consult your doctor. Wearing a splint improperly can aggravate your injury and slow the healing process, says Dr. Ross.

❏ If your doctor prescribes a splint, wear it only as prescribed and discontinue its use as soon as you can. Overuse of a splint can make you dependent on it, causing your muscles to atrophy. "Splints are meant to act as extra ligament support while you are healing, not to replace your own strength. You wouldn't want to wear a cast forever, would you?" asks Dr. Ross.

❏ Cut back on physical activities that may reinjure the affected area. While exercise can help prevent a repetitive strain injury, a strenuous workout can make an existing injury worse, says Dr. Ross. Any exercise or repetitive movement breaks down muscle, tendon, and ligament cells.

"You need to rest your body so that the protein and nutrients from your diet can speed up the healing process. This advice is especially important for repetitive strain injury," says Dr. Nickel. He suggests light walking (not uphill), yoga, riding an exercise bike, tai chi, and other low-impact activities for the time being.

❏ Minimize stress as much as possible. Stress can aggravate a repetitive strain injury by increasing muscle tension, explains Dr. Ross. As the muscles contract, they pull even tighter over the affected area, worsening the pain.

❐ Rest as much as possible. Tissue healing takes place while you sleep, explains Dr. Ross.

❐ Once you feel better, seek out a training routine that builds good posture and strengthens your back and arms. This can help prevent future injury, says Dr. Ross.

Medical **Alert**

If you suspect that you have a repetitive strain injury, seek out a health-care professional who has a proven track record in treating this type of condition. Don't settle for "It'll go away." The sooner you receive treatment, the better your chances are for recovery, says Dr. Ross.

Until your appointment, write down any symptoms you experience as well as what you are doing when the symptoms arise. This diary will provide you and your doctor with vital clues about the nature of your injury and how it should be treated.

Chapter 3

PRESCRIPTIONS

FOR HORMONAL AND

REPRODUCTIVE PROBLEMS

Some folks like to blame Eve. If she hadn't taken a bite of the apple, they say, womankind would not have to deal with "female problems" such as menstruation and menopause.

Scientists, of course, may debate this point. No matter. The fact remains that women spend the better part of their lives trying to maintain a peaceful coexistence with their reproductive systems.

Granted, some women breeze through their menstrual cycles and even menopause without so much as a cramp or a hot flash. But others experience symptoms so severe that they are unable to carry out their day-to-day routines.

By the same token, some women have easy pregnancies, short labor, and trouble-free breastfeeding. Others are not so fortunate.

Why the same basic physical processes affect women so differently is anyone's guess. But when menstruation, pregnancy, or menopause has you feeling less than your best, you could probably care less where the symptoms come from. You just want relief.

And you can get relief—without drugs. Caught in the throes of a hot flash? Practice deep breathing to cool down quickly. Got menstrual cramps that won't quit? Press a point on the crease between your leg and the trunk of your body for a couple of minutes. Suffering from menopause-related vaginal dryness? Take ginseng supplements to restore moisture.

For the mom-to-be, our experts have recommended self-care measures for a healthful and comfortable pregnancy and delivery. If you and your partner are trying to conceive, our natural prescriptions may help increase your chances of success.

Sure, menstruation, pregnancy, and menopause are facts of life. That doesn't mean that you should suffer through them. The natural prescriptions in the pages that follow can help you get an upper hand on your reproductive health.

Burning Mouth Syndrome

Burning mouth syndrome has the experts stumped. They have yet to come up with an explanation for the stinging, tingling, agonizing sensation that affects the tip of the tongue, the roof of the mouth near the front teeth, and sometimes the inside of the lower lip. Even tissue samples from these parts of the mouth look pretty much normal under a microscope, with none of the usual signs of disease.

For this reason, some scientists theorize that burning mouth syndrome may be a form of neuralgia—that is, it has something to do with the inappropriate stimulation of nerves. In fact, burning mouth responds nicely to medications prescribed for other forms of neuralgia, such as lingering shingles pain (called postherpetic neuralgia).

LIFETIME

Burning mouth syndrome may have a hormonal link as well. Among people who have the condition (it affects as many as 3 of every 100 people), most are women past menopause, according to April Mott, M.D., director of the Taste and Smell Clinic at the University of Connecticut Health Center in Farmington. Interestingly, though, burning mouth does not seem to respond to hormone replacement therapy

(HRT). "HRT may help some women who develop burning mouth in the early stages of menopause," says Craig Miller, D.M.D., associate professor of oral medicine at the University of Kentucky College of Dentistry in Lexington. "But it seldom benefits women who are 10 to 15 years past menopause when they develop the condition."

If you have burning mouth syndrome, you may notice that the burning sensation sets in after the first meal of the day and gets worse as the day goes on. "Actually, most women report that their symptoms improve while they're eating," says Miriam Grushka, D.D.S., Ph.D., associate in dentistry at the University of Toronto School of Dentistry. "Symptoms seem most severe immediately after meals." What's more, some women say that they feel better when they eat hot foods, while others say they feel worse. Same goes for cold foods—though usually cold foods, such as ice cream or ice cubes, are more soothing than hot foods.

TIME IT RIGHT

One good thing about burning mouth syndrome is that for about 30 percent of the cases, the syndrome disappears within six to seven years, even without treatment. And another 30 percent progress from constant to occasional pain. "Here again, we do not know why this happens," says Dr. Grushka.

Prescriptions
TO EXTINGUISH THE FIRE

NUTRITION
Rx

Of course, if you have burning mouth syndrome, you probably don't want to wait six to seven years for the pain to go away. The following two remedies may help relieve your symptoms sooner.

❏ **Season your meals with hot peppers.** Researchers in British Columbia found that capsaicin—the stuff that puts the heat in hot peppers—completely relieved symptoms in one-third of a group of people with burning mouth syndrome. Another one-third reported partial relief of their symptoms.

MEALTIME

"Capsaicin depletes substance P, a neurotransmitter involved in the transmission of pain messages," explains Joel B. Epstein, D.M.D., professor in the department of oral medicine at the University of British Columbia in Vancouver. "Over time, capsaicin decreases the nerves' abilities to send messages of burning, stinging pain to your brain."

"At the very least, if you enjoy hot and spicy foods, you now know that you don't necessarily have to avoid them," adds Dr. Mott. "You may find that eating them improves your symptoms." Of course, if the burning sensation increases after you eat hot peppers, you may be among those for whom capsaicin is not effective.

❒ Take flaxseed oil, evening primrose oil, and fish oil daily, each in a dosage of 1,000 to 3,000 milligrams. These oils contain essential fatty acids that may help reduce inflammation, according to Craig Zunka, D.D.S., a dentist in Front Royal, Virginia, and president of the Holistic Dental Association. They work quite slowly, however. "You may have to wait six months or longer before you see any change in your symptoms," he says. All three of these oils are sold at health food stores in 500-milligram capsules.

Rx —— *Prescriptions*
TO UNCOVER THE CAUSE

While relieving your pain is important, you also want to find out what's behind it. Remember that a burning sensation in your mouth doesn't necessarily mean that you have burning mouth *syndrome.* Your symptoms may result from diabetes, an oral yeast infection, irritation caused by dentures or a denture adhesive, or sensitivity to certain foods or certain ingredients in dental products. You and your dentist or doctor should work together to rule out these potential culprits. Here's how to go about it.

❒ Get checked for deficiencies of vitamin B_6, vitamin B_{12}, and folate. Running low on any one of these nutrients could lead to burning mouth symptoms—although this seldom happens. "I think a shortage of B_6 is most likely to produce burning mouth, although a shortage of any B vitamin could have the same effect," says Dr. Zunka.

How do you know if you are deficient? Your doctor may prescribe a blood test to measure levels of the B vitamins. Or she may ask you to complete a seven-day food diary that is then analyzed by a computer to pinpoint possible dietary problems, says Dr. Zunka.

If you don't have enough of a particular B vitamin in your blood, your doctor may recommend taking a B-complex supplement to correct it. Expect to see improvements in your symptoms in three to four months.

❐ Avoid cinnamon-flavored products for one month to see if your symptoms subside. Cinnamon often shows up on the ingredient lists of toothpastes, mouthwashes, and chewing gums. "Some people have true allergic reactions to the spice, developing ulcers (similar to canker sores) in their mouths within 72 hours of exposure," says Michael A. Siegel, D.D.S., associate professor at the University of Maryland School of Dentistry in Baltimore. "Other people simply become sensitive to it over time. They use cinnamon for so long that it becomes caustic. That's when they start noticing a burning sensation in their mouths."

❐ If you use a tartar-control toothpaste, switch to a non-tartar-control formula or plain baking soda for four weeks to see if your symptoms subside, says Dr. Siegel. Tartar-control toothpastes contain pyrophosphate, a compound that has been linked to burning mouth conditions.

Switch back to the tartar-control toothpaste once your symptoms improve, suggests Dr. Mott. If the burning sensation recurs, you know that you have found your culprit.

Medical **Alert**

If you can't figure out why your mouth burns, see your doctor. Burning mouth sometimes signals the onset of diabetes, a thyroid problem, or Sjögren's syndrome (a connective tissue disorder that can cause dry eyes and dry mouth), according to Dr. Grushka.

You should also consult your doctor if self-care measures fail to ease your symptoms. Your doctor may prescribe klonopin (Clonazepam), a drug used to treat stubborn nerve pain. Often klonopin is combined with a small amount of a tricyclic antidepressant, says Dr. Grushka.

Difficulty Conceiving

It's something that most women take for granted. Some even spend most of their reproductive years trying to avoid it. So imagine the irony and despair, the frustration and sense of loss that comes when a woman finally decides to have kids—and then just can't make it happen.

Technically, a couple is considered infertile when they have tried for a year or more to produce a baby, without success. This happens to about one in six couples. And the problem seems to be equally divided between men and women, says Marc Goldstein, M.D., director of the Center for Male Reproductive Medicine and Microsurgery at New York Hospital/Cornell Medical Center in New York City.

Often the problem can be figured out and fixed. A woman's fallopian tubes may be blocked with scar tissue, for instance. Or a man may have a varicose vein (called a varicocele) in his scrotum that slows blood flow and raises the temperature too high for sperm production. Surgery can correct such problems.

But sometimes the cause of infertility is not so obvious and seems to be related to hormonal or metabolic imbalances. True, just getting older slows the productivity of a woman's ovaries. (Men, by comparison, can go strong into their midsixties with little effect on their fertility, says Dr. Goldstein.)

The stressful part of infertility is the uncertainty of it all. Is it me? Is it him? Is it just bad timing? Do we try harder? Do we try less? Stop trying to guess the answers. Science has gotten a whole lot smarter about this stuff. If you sense there is a problem, both you and your partner should get your reproductive gear checked out. That said, there is much that you can do on your own to increase the chances of conceiving. That's what we'll explore here.

Rx

Prescriptions
TO GET PREGNANT

All else being equal, the healthier you are, the more likely you are to conceive easily. Here is what fertility experts recommend.

❐ Take a folic acid supplement each day. A study by researchers in Budapest, Hungary, found that women who took daily prenatal supplements containing 800 micrograms of folic acid got pregnant slightly faster than women who were not taking prenatal supplements.

Note: Doses of folic acid exceeding 400 micrograms per day should be taken only under the supervision of a doctor. In large amounts, the nutrient can mask signs of a vitamin B_{12} deficiency.

❐ Limit your consumption of caffeinated beverages. You may not have to give up caffeine for good. But one study conducted by researchers from the Johns Hopkins University School of Hygiene and Public Health in Baltimore found that women who got more than 300 milligrams of caffeine a day from coffee, cola, or tea were 26 percent less likely to get pregnant over the course of a year than women who avoided the stuff, says Chris Meletis, N.D., a naturopathic doctor at the National College of Naturopathic Medicine in Portland, Oregon. If you are monitoring your caffeine consumption, keep in mind that 6 ounces of coffee supplies 103 milligrams; 12 ounces of cola, 37 milligrams; and 6 ounces of tea, 36 milligrams.

❐ Take time to get turned on. The vaginal lubrication that occurs TIME IT RIGHT with sexual arousal is slightly more alkaline than normal vaginal secretions. This creates a more hospitable environment for sperm during the short time that they may be in the vagina, explains Niels Lauerson, M.D., Ph.D., a fertility specialist in New York City and author of *Getting Pregnant.*

Also, while orgasm is not necessary for conception, it does help semen move upward in the female reproductive tract, says Jacqueline Gutman, M.D., clinical associate professor of reproductive endocrinology at the University of Pennsylvania School of Medicine in Philadelphia and a staff doctor at the Philadelphia Fertility Institute.

❐ Learn to nurture yourself. "Trying to conceive can be extremely stressful in itself. This stress can contribute to infertility, creating a vicious circle," says Alice Domar, Ph.D., director of women's health programs in the division of behavioral medicine at Harvard Medical School and author of *Healing Mind, Healthy Woman.* Women who are having difficulty conceiving need to make a point of caring for themselves mentally and physically. Proper nutrition, rest, and exercise are important. But they may also need to give themselves a much-needed day off or to seek the support of other women, she says.

Prescriptions
TO HELP YOUR MATE

It takes only one sperm to do the job. But nature demands that millions be deployed and that the majority be good candidates for fatherhood. "It's a team effort," Dr. Goldstein explains. "Sperm actually travel in packs and help each other create a pathway through the cervical mucus to penetrate the egg."

To determine a man's fertility, his sperm are examined under a microscope for quantity, motility (their ability to wriggle and thrash through the female reproductive tract en route to the egg), and form. Most cases of male infertility reflect a low sperm count—less than 20 million sperm per milliliter, which is about one-eighth of a teaspoon. (The average count is 66 million per milliliter or, on average, 200 million per ejaculation.) Poor-quality sperm can also cause problems, Dr. Goldstein says. For a man to be considered fertile, more than 50 percent of his sperm must be swimming vigorously, in a straight line, and have good form. They can't be sticking together, for instance, or have crooked tails.

Sometimes sperm problems are linked to a hidden infection such as chlamydia, a treatable sexually transmitted disease. (Both you and your partner need to be treated, however.) Prescription drugs and thyroid problems can also cause difficulties. Here are some things that your mate can do to boost your chances of conceiving.

❏ Have him wear boxer shorts and baggy pants as much as possible. Tight underwear and pants tuck the testicles too close to the body, causing their temperature to rise. And anything that cooks a man's testicles can lower his sperm count, says Dr. Meletis. Research has shown that sperm production drops sharply at temperatures above 96°F.

❏ Have him take 1,000 to 2,000 milligrams of vitamin C, 400 international units of vitamin E, and 100 micrograms of selenium each day. These nutrients help keep sperm from becoming misshapen, sticking together when they shouldn't, and dying, says Dr. Meletis.

Note: Some people develop diarrhea when they take more than 1,200 milligrams of vitamin C a day. If he is one of them, he should simply cut back the dose to a more tolerable level.

❏ Have him take 30 to 50 milligrams of zinc each day. Zinc is essential for male reproduction. A low level of the mineral can diminish production of the male hormone testosterone, which in turn can lead to a reduced sperm count, says Dr. Meletis.

Your partner should take this much zinc only with medical supervision. A too-high intake of the mineral can cause problems of its own.

Prescriptions
for Both of You

Rx

Here is what men and women can do to achieve optimum fertility.

❐ Give up smoking. It's just plain bad news if you or your partner continues smoking while you are trying to conceive, says Dr. Gutman. In women, smoking has been found to reduce blood levels of estrogen as well as the motion of the fallopian tubes, which encourages the union of egg and sperm. Nicotine, which is toxic to sperm, is found in the cervical mucus of female smokers.

In men, cigarette smoking in particular is associated with decreased sperm counts and sperm motility as well as an increased frequency of abnormal sperm, Dr. Meletis says.

❐ Limit alcohol consumption to three drinks per week, with a drink equaling one 12-ounce beer, one 5-ounce glass of wine, or a mixed drink made with 1½ ounces of liquor. This goes for you and your partner. Experts agree that alcohol is a reproductive-tract toxin for both men and women. The more you consume, the more you jeopardize your chances of parenthood.

A study by Harvard researchers found that women who had more than seven drinks a week were 60 percent more likely to be infertile because of ovulation problems than women who were teetotalers. Even moderate alcohol consumption (four to seven drinks a week) increased women's risk of infertility by 30 percent.

❐ Seek your most fertile weight. Body fat plays an important role in hormone levels, especially for women but also for men, experts say. "Thin women may have too little estrogen, and overweight women too much, to become pregnant," Dr. Gutman says. Thin women need to gain enough weight to ovulate regularly. "They may not need to gain a lot, just five pounds or so," she says. And overweight women don't need to become svelte, but they do need to lose enough to get within 30 percent of their ideal body weight.

Thin men, especially those on no-fat, no-cholesterol diets, may have low sperm counts. "You actually need some cholesterol every day to produce hormones, including testosterone," Dr. Goldstein says. "And extremely overweight men have high estrogen levels and, frequently, over-heated testes, which impede sperm production." Losing some weight can set things right. Staying within 30 percent of their optimum body weight is a good guideline for men to follow, too, he says.

 MONTHLY   ❐ Plan to attempt conception either two days before ovulation or the day of ovulation. These are the best times of the month to make babies, says Allen Wilcox, M.D., Ph.D., a researcher at the National Institute of Environmental Health Sciences in Research Triangle Park, North Carolina. In fact, your odds of conceiving remain decent for up to six days before ovulation, but they drop dramatically within 24 hours after ovulation. "One possibility is that changes occur in the cervical mucus after ovulation, blocking sperm from entering the uterus," he explains. "In any event, it's better not to wait until ovulation and possibly miss your chance."

To determine when you are ovulating, use a urine test that measures luteinizing hormone, advises Dr. Gutman. This test turns positive about 24 hours before ovulation occurs. Women with regular, 28-day menstrual cycles tend to ovulate 10 to 14 days prior to menstruation. Ovulation test kits are available in drugstores.

TIME IT RIGHT   ❐ If your partner has a low sperm count, abstain from sex for 48 to 72 hours before attempting to conceive. Waiting will encourage a higher concentration of sperm in the semen, and you'll have a better chance of succeeding, says Dr. Goldstein.

Medical **Alert**

If you are under age 35 and you and your partner have not been able to conceive during a year of unprotected sex, see your gynecologist, says Dr. Gutman. If you are age 35 or over, see your doctor after waiting six months.

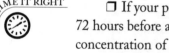

Hot Flashes

Looking back, Carol Lewis realizes that she had been having barely noticeable hot flashes for most of the summer. But in mid-October, just about the time the first cold front swept south into her eastern Pennsylvania suburb, things really started to heat up for the 44-year-old middle-school teacher.

"Our bedroom was cool. We even had a window open," Lewis recalls. "But I kept throwing off the blankets in my sleep, and my husband kept covering me back up. This went on all night long." In fact, Lewis became such a restless sleeper that her normally loyal spouse decided to sack out in the guest room until the situation settled down some—which, thankfully, it finally did after about a year.

Lewis's experience is fairly typical among women who are approaching menopause. In fact, three of four women in the United States experience hot flashes as a prelude to "the change"—sometimes beginning years before their last periods. A much smaller number of women must endure hot-flash hell, with episodes so severe that they are changing out of soaked clothes every couple of hours or waking up every night drenched in sweat.

LIFETIME

No one knows exactly what triggers hot flashes, but they seem to be linked to the hormonal changes that occur before and during menopause. "These changes somehow stimulate the part of the brain that controls body temperature, throwing off its usually fine-tuned control," explains Robert Freedman, Ph.D., director of the Behavioral Medicine Laboratory at Wayne State University in Detroit. As a result, the brain signals the body to dissipate heat—in other words, to flush and sweat.

If you took your temperature during a hot flash, you wouldn't have a fever. "But hot flashes are synchronized with your core temperature (deep inside your body), which rises and falls in a predictable pattern over a 24-hour period," notes Dr. Freedman. Things start sizzling just about the same time your body reaches its peak core temperature for the day—usually late afternoon or early evening. For women on a typical nine-to-five schedule, the prime time for hot flashes is 5:35 P.M., according to Dr. Freedman. But hot flashes can occur at any time of the day or night.

TIME IT RIGHT

During a hot flash, blood surges to the surface of the skin on your chest, neck, and head. With this increase in blood flow comes a rise in skin temperature, a slight acceleration of heart and breathing rates, and perspiration. As the hot flash dissipates heat, your body's core temperature drops (which is why you may feel cold and clammy afterward). The entire episode lasts just two to five minutes.

Hot flashes are physically harmless, according to Dr. Freedman—but they can make you flustered and self-conscious.

And if they interrupt your sleep often enough, they can leave you irritable and depressed during the day, says June LaValleur, M.D., assistant professor of obstetrics and gynecology at the University of Minnesota Medical School and director of the Mature Women's Centers at the University of Minnesota Hospital, both in Minneapolis. In fact, some of the mental symptoms attributed to hormonal changes before and during menopause—foggy thinking, for instance—more likely result from sleep deprivation, she suggests.

The good news about hot flashes is that they actually cool down once menopause finally arrives. For the women in one study, the number of incendiary episodes dropped to 20 percent of their peak frequency within four years after the onset of menopause.

Rx —— *Prescriptions*
TO COOL DOWN QUICKLY

Hot flashes may take you by surprise the first couple of times they occur. But if you are like many women, you will eventually be able to tell when one is coming on (except when you are asleep, of course). The following strategies can help you weather a hot flash and prevent it from becoming too severe.

❒ Practice deep breathing. In one study, women who had been having 20 or more hot flashes a day reduced that number by half with the help of deep breathing, says Dr. Freedman. "This technique seems to short-circuit the arousal of the central nervous system that normally occurs in the initial stages of a hot flash," he explains.

When you feel a hot flash creeping up on you, prepare for deep breathing by sitting up straight and loosening your belt or waistband if it feels tight. Begin by exhaling through your nose longer than you normally would. Then inhale through your nose slowly and deeply, filling your lungs from the bottom up while keeping your belly relaxed. When your chest is fully expanded, exhale slowly and deeply, as if sighing. Continue this pattern of inhaling and exhaling until the hot flash subsides.

❒ Combine deep breathing with visualization. Using the two techniques together may enhance their chill factor, so they stop a hot flash more quickly, says Carol Snarr, R.N., a psychophysiological therapist (one who teaches biofeedback and other mind/body skills) at the Life Sciences Institute in Topeka, Kansas.

Try this visualization when you feel a hot flash coming on, suggests Snarr. Begin by assigning your hot flash a color, such as red. As you exhale, envision the color leaving your body, releasing the heat, and sending it away from you. Then as you inhale, see your breath as blue or another cool color. Allow the color to bathe your body, soothing your chest, your neck, and your head. When you feel that the hot flash has passed, you can end your visualization by imagining yourself as you would like to feel—cool and refreshed.

❒ If you can, adjust the temperature of the room you are in to 60°F. Simplistic as it may seem, turning down the heat or cranking up the air conditioning is solid advice, according to Dr. Freedman. "Anything that raises body temperature even a tiny bit, such as being in a too-hot room, can aggravate a hot flash," he says.

❒ Wear undergarments made from polypropylene. This fabric wicks moisture away from your skin and dries quickly. You will find such clothes in outdoors and sports catalogs such as L. L. Bean (Freeport, ME 04034) and Patagonia (P.O. Box 32050, Reno, NV 89533).

❒ Dress in layers. This way, you can slip off clothes as your body temperature rises so that you stay comfortable. Instead of a bulky turtle-neck sweater, for instance, wear a cardigan or vest over a blouse.

Prescriptions   Rx
TO HEAD OFF HOT FLASHES

Depending how frequent or intense your hot flashes are, you may want to find a way to stop them altogether. Many doctors initially prescribe hormone-replacement therapy just for this purpose, says Dr. LaValleur. If you would prefer a nondrug approach, try these preventive measures instead.

❒ Try an herbal preparation specifically formulated for hot flashes or menopause, such as Remifemin or Femtrol. Such a product may include a combination of a few or many herbs, such as chasteberry, black cohosh, dong quai, panax ginseng (sometimes called Asian ginseng), and licorice root. These herbs complement and balance each other, increasing the effectiveness of the product and minimizing its side effects, says James E. Williams, O.M.D., a doctor of Oriental medicine with the Center for Women's Medicine in San Diego. He suggests consulting a doctor who is knowledgeable about herbs so that she can recommend a good product and explain how to use it effectively and safely. If you choose a product on your own, be sure to follow the dosage recommendations on the label. You will find these herbal blends in health food stores.

Note: If the product contains licorice root, limit your intake of the herb to five grams (less than one-quarter ounce) a day. Larger doses can produce side effects such as high blood pressure, headache, and lethargy. If you use dong quai, avoid exposure to the sun. Some people become photosensitive when they use dong quai and develop a rash or sunburn easily.

NIGHTTIME

❒ Before going to bed, draw a comfortably warm—not hot—bath. Then soak in it long enough for the water to cool, which should take about 20 minutes. This bedtime ritual may interrupt a pattern of night sweats (nocturnal hot flashes) so that they occur less frequently and are less severe, according to Helen Healy, N.D., a naturopathic doctor and director of the Wellspring Naturopathic Clinic in St. Paul, Minnesota.

❒ To enhance the therapeutic effects of your bath, add the following essential oils: 4 drops of chamomile, 6 drops of lemon, and 10 drops of evening primrose. Chamomile is said to relax the body, while lemon cools and destresses and evening primrose aids hormonal balance, according to Mary Muryn, an aromatherapist in Westport, Connecticut, and author of *Water Magic.* You can buy essential oils in health food stores and some specialty bath-and-beauty shops.

MORNING

❒ Apply a cream containing natural progesterone to your skin. A cream delivers the hormone directly to your bloodstream so that it takes effect more quickly, according to Marcus Laux, N.D., a naturopathic doctor in Santa Monica, California, and co-author of *Natural Woman,*

Natural Menopause. Clinical evidence suggests that the cream may help reduce hot flashes by balancing a woman's hormonal makeup, he explains. Also, your body can convert progesterone to estrogen or other sex hormones as needed, whenever it runs low on these substances.

Buy a product that contains a minimum of 400 milligrams of progesterone per ounce and apply one-half teaspoon two times per day, morning and night, until your hot flashes decrease, recommends Dr. Laux. At that point, reduce your dosage to one-quarter teaspoon two times a day. Then once your hot flashes are under control, cut your dosage again to one-quarter to one-half teaspoon per day. Rub the cream into your wrist, neck, chest, breasts, abdomen, and/or inner thighs (make sure that your skin is clean first).

While you can buy progesterone cream over the counter, Dr. Laux recommends consulting your doctor first to find out if progesterone cream is appropriate for you and to get a prescription for the proper strength. These products are not appropriate for women who have had cancer or who are at high risk for the disease, he adds.

Beware of the so-called wild yam progesterone creams, however. A laboratory analysis found that most of these products actually contain very little to none of the hormone, notes Dr. Laux. He recommends avoiding them completely.

Prescriptions ———— NUTRITION Rx
to Beat the Heat

What you eat can either ease or aggravate your hot flashes. The following dietary strategies can help you keep your cool.

❐ Consume 30 to 50 milligrams of isoflavones each day, says Dr. Laux. Isoflavones are plant substances that are found in abundance in soy foods and have a weak estrogen-like effect in the human body. These compounds may help cool hot flashes as well as ease the physical effects of menopause.

You need to eat three to five ounces of soy products like tofu, soybeans, and texturized vegetable protein to meet the recommended daily intake of isoflavones. (For top-notch food sources of isoflavones, see "Get Your Isoflavones Here" on page 270.) There are also soy-based phytoestrogenic supplements available in health food stores, like Nature's Herbs Phyto Estrogen Power, Carlson EasySoy, and Solaray Phyto Estrogen.

❐ Take 800 international units (IU) of vitamin E each day. So far, the evidence is mostly anecdotal, but some doctors say that their patients who take vitamin E have less trouble with hot flashes, according to Michael Murray, N.D., a naturopathic doctor in Bellevue, Washington, in his book *Menopause: How You Can Benefit from Diet, Vitamins, Minerals, Herbs, Exercise, and Other Natural Methods*. He suggests cutting your dose to 400 IU each day once your hot flashes are under control.

Note: Because high doses of vitamin E can cause side effects, it is a good idea to consult your doctor before taking more than 600 international units a day.

❐ Monitor your reaction to garlic, ginger, ground red pepper, onions, and highly acidic produce such as citrus fruits and tomatoes. These foods may fuel your hot-flash fire, according to Judyth Reichenberg-Ullman, N.D., a naturopathic doctor with the Northwest Center for Homeopathic Medicine in Edmonds, Washington, and co-author of *Homeopathic Self-Care*. If you tend to experience hot flashes after eating one of these foods, eliminate the food from your diet for a week or so and note if your symptoms improve.

❐ Stick with decaffeinated beverages. Researchers cannot yet explain why, but coffee, tea, and chocolate can trigger hot flashes in some women, notes Pamela Schwingl, Ph.D., senior epidemiologist at Family Health International in Research Triangle Park, North Carolina.

Rx —— *Prescriptions*
FOR A HOT FLASH–FREE LIFESTYLE

Besides good nutrition, other healthy habits can help you get rid of hot flashes for good. Here is what the experts recommend.

TIME IT RIGHT

❐ Exercise for at least 30 minutes each day. Swedish researchers found that women who worked out regularly had fewer and milder hot flashes than women who were sedentary. What's more, those who worked up a sweat for at least 3½ hours a week—or 30 minutes a day—were most likely not to have hot flashes at all. If you have been relatively inactive, you can safely start up your fitness routine with walking, advises Mona Shangold, M.D., director of the Center for Women's Health and Sports Gynecology in Philadelphia.

❏ **Avoid alcoholic beverages.** Alcohol causes you to flush even when you aren't in a state of hormonal upheaval. It can certainly fan the flame of hot flashes.

In a study at the University of North Carolina at Chapel Hill, women who had at least one alcoholic beverage a week were about 13 percent more likely to experience hot flashes than women who never drank. "Alcohol consumption proved to be one of the strongest lifestyle risk factors for hot flashes," according to Dr. Schwingl, the study's main author.

❏ **Give up smoking.** Smoking depletes your body's level of the hormone estrogen, making you more susceptible to hot flashes, notes Dr. Schwingl. In addition, some studies have shown that women who smoke go through menopause one to two years earlier than women who don't.

Medical **Alert**

See your doctor if your hot flashes become so frequent or severe that they disrupt your daily routine, advises Dr. LaValleur. Also see your doctor if night sweats continue for several weeks and you are having trouble sleeping as a result.

Labor Pain

It has been compared to running a marathon—all 26.2 miles—or to climbing a mountain. It has been referred to as the hardest work that most women will ever do in their lives. Both of these descriptions make an important point about childbirth. As with any physically demanding activity, you are better off preparing for it. If you know what to expect and you prime your body beforehand, your baby's arrival will be a positive, joyous experience.

You must make a lot of important decisions in the weeks and months leading up to your baby's birth. Do you want to be attended by an obstetrician or a midwife? Do you want to deliver in a hospital or a birthing center? Do you want to take childbirth education classes—and if so, which kind?

You also need to consider whether or not you want pain-relieving drugs during labor. Sometimes they are absolutely necessary—for example, during prolonged labor. But if you don't need them, you may want to try to go without, advises Debra Grubb, M.D., director of the Natural Choice Birth Center in Pasadena, California. An epidural—the most common means of controlling pain during childbirth—actually slows down labor and increases the likelihood of a forceps delivery or a cesarean section.

Rx

Prescriptions
TO PREPARE FOR THE BIG EVENT

Yes, labor hurts. It hurts a lot. But you can control the pain naturally, without medication. In fact, you can get started as soon as you find out that you are pregnant. Here is what you need to do.

TIME IT RIGHT

❐ Drink one to two cups of raspberry leaf tea each week during your second trimester, building up to one cup a day during your third trimester. "Raspberry leaf is considered a tonic herb," explains Lise Alschuler, N.D., a naturopathic physician and director of botanical services at Bastyr University in Seattle. "It contains an abundance of minerals and other ingredients that, over time, help tone the muscular layer of the uterus. This enables the uterus to expand more to accommodate a growing fetus and to contract more efficiently during labor." To make raspberry leaf tea, steep one teaspoon of dried herb in a cup of freshly boiled water for 10 to 15 minutes. Strain the tea and allow it to cool before drinking it. You can buy the herb in health food stores.

❐ Do exercises to strengthen and tone the muscles that you will use during childbirth. Kegels, tailor sitting, pelvic rocking, and squatting help prepare your body for labor and ease the actual delivery, says Marjorie Hathaway, co-founder and executive director of the Bradley Method, a natural childbirth organization based in Sherman Oaks, California.

Kegels work the pelvic-floor muscles, which support the pelvic organs. To do Kegels, squeeze the pelvic-floor muscles as though you were trying to stop the flow of urine. Hold for a count of 10, then release. Do

TAILOR SITTING

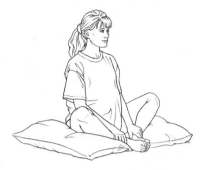

Tailor sitting is an exercise that encourages a feeling of openness in the pelvis, helps to release tension, and improves flexibility.

Sit on the floor and stretch your legs out in front. Keeping your back straight, bend your knees and grasp your ankles (not your toes). Bring the soles of your feet together, then pull them toward your groin without pushing or bouncing your knees. To avoid pain in your pubic area, place cushions under your knees or keep your feet farther away from your body. Ask your doctor or midwife if tailor, or tailbone, sitting is safe for you.

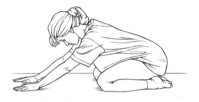

PELVIC ROCKING

Rocking helps to shift the pressure of your baby's weight away from your back to relieve back pain.

Kneel on all fours on a soft surface with your weight evenly distributed between your hands and knees. Your hands should be under your shoulders, and your knees should be under your hips. Inhale, bringing your weight forward onto your hands without arching your back. This helps you to press your hips toward the ground. Exhale, bringing your pelvis back toward your heels. Repeat this motion five times. Relax in the resting (back) position.

SQUATTING

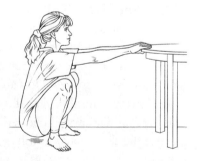

Squatting makes your pelvis more flexible, stretches your thigh and back muscles, and can relieve back pain.

Stand with your feet shoulder-width apart and your toes pointed out. Squat down as low as you can, an arm's length away from a chair, table, or low stool. When you reach the lowest position, use the chair, table, or low stool for balance. Try to keep your heels on the ground and distribute your weight evenly between your feet. Hold this position for as long as is comfortable. If no chair is available, you can also lean your back against a wall for support. Ask your doctor or midwife if it is safe for you to practice squatting.

20 repetitions, five times a day. Although these directions may seem simple, you would do best to learn proper technique from a trained health professional.

❐ Learn relaxation techniques that you can use during childbirth. You can choose from various techniques, such as progressive relaxation, which releases the tension muscle by muscle, according to Wendy Hoffman, a certified childbirth educator and labor assistant in Emmaus, Pennsylvania.

"Being able to relax fully between contractions is an important skill to learn," says Dr. Grubb. "It helps your uterus work more efficiently, and it prevents you from wearing out."

Studies have shown that it takes about three months of practice to become proficient in a particular relaxation technique, so start your training early.

To do progressive relaxation, for example, you simply tense and then release each muscle group in your body, starting with the top of your head and working your way down to your toes. The goal is to become so accustomed to relaxing your muscles that you can do them all at once, as if your body was an egg splattering on a tile floor.

A good childbirth education class should teach you a number of relaxation techniques. "You may need just one to get you through labor and delivery, or you may need to switch from one to another as the process becomes more intense," notes Hoffman.

❐ Attend childbirth education classes. "The more you know about childbirth, the less you will fear the experience," says Carrie Klima, R.N., a certified nurse-midwife and assistant professor at the Yale University School of Nursing. "Fear can make you anxious, and anxiety can make you more sensitive to pain and less able to control it."

Don't wait until the last three months of your pregnancy to enroll in a class, adds Hathaway. "The earlier you start, the more time you have to practice the skills that you will need during labor," she explains. About a half-dozen different "schools" of childbirth education operate nationwide. You may want to attend a few different types of classes to compare their philosophies and methods.

"Families need to decide what they feel will be an effective class for them," Hathaway says. "Labor is like an athletic event. Mothers need physical, mental, and emotional support throughout the process. And they need to cultivate a positive outlook toward the birth of their babies."

❒ Encourage your husband to attend classes with you. These days, every hospital allows husbands to stick around for the duration of the childbirth process. You are both better off if he has at least some knowledge of what to expect. "He may see you in pain and want to do something to stop it, which is exactly *not* what he should do," says Dr. Grubb. "You want him to say, 'I know it hurts, but you're doing wonderfully, and it'll all be over soon.'" Most childbirth education classes include husbands, but the Bradley Method is specifically geared toward them.

❒ Consider hiring a certified labor assistant, says Dr. Grubb. This person stays with you throughout your entire labor. Like a midwife, she can help you (and your husband) with all sorts of pain-relieving tactics: getting you into a comfortable position, giving you a massage, and coaching you through your relaxation techniques. Labor assistants are certified by a number of organizations. Your childbirth educator may also be a labor assistant.

One organization that certifies, trains, and makes referrals to labor assistants is the Association of Labor Assistants and Childbirth Educators. You can reach the organization by writing to P. O. Box 382724, Cambridge, MA 02238-2724.

Prescriptions
FOR AN EASY DELIVERY

You've been preparing for months. And now you're just hours away from experiencing the miracle of childbirth. The following strategies can help keep you calm and comfortable until baby makes his grand entrance.

❒ Move around rather than lying down. Take a walk, practice your squats—do whatever feels right for you at the moment. "Labor is a dynamic process," explains Dr. Grubb. "Your baby is trying to maneuver into the birth canal. By changing positions frequently, you give your baby a number of opportunities to find his way out, however he fits best." Also, research has shown that staying mobile decreases the length of labor and makes it more comfortable for the mother.

❐ Avoid lying flat on your back. It is the worst position that you can be in when you are in labor. "It shifts the weight of your uterus, impedes blood flow to the uterus and your baby, and limits your baby's ability to rotate into the proper position for delivery," according to Klima. It's better to lie on your side, sit up, or walk around.

❐ Take a warm shower or sit in a warm bath. Being surrounded with and supported by water helps relax tense muscles, explains Klima. This, in turn, lowers your perception of pain and encourages relaxation. Some birthing centers and hospitals have tubs in which you can sit during labor. And some even perform deliveries right in the water.

❐ Using your thumbs, apply pressure to the left and right sides of your sacrum (the triangular bone at the base of your spine). This acupressure technique works especially well if you are having back labor, in which pain settles into your lower back, says Ming Ming Molony, O.M.D., a licensed acupuncturist and doctor of Oriental medicine in private practice in Catasauqua, Pennsylvania. You will know when you have hit the right points. They will feel tender at first, but as you press them, the pain will ease up. You can apply pressure as long as it feels good or helps the pain. If you have difficulty reaching your back, ask your husband or labor assistant to lend a hand.

❐ Focus on relaxation, and natural breathing will follow. "Your breathing pattern adjusts automatically, according to your body's needs," says Hathaway. "You don't have to hold your breath or count it or alter it in any way. It takes care of itself."

"You instinctively know how to breathe during labor, and you are going to do it right no matter how you are trained," adds Dr. Grubb. "Just be aware that your breathing pattern is going to change and that you shouldn't try to fight it."

❐ Practice guided imagery. This mind/body exercise supports childbirth by helping you to relax, relieving pain, and creating a positive emotional environment, explains Carl Jones, a certified childbirth educator in Jefferson, New Hampshire, and author of *Mind over Labor* and *Childbirth Choices Today*. Like other relaxation techniques, guided imagery works best if you learn and practice it before you go into labor.

One exercise, called opening flower, can help you relax as your cervix dilates during the early stages of labor. To try it, simply create a mental picture of a flower bud slowly opening into full bloom, coaxed along by the sun's rays.

Another exercise, called radiant breath, is especially helpful during the final stages of labor, when contractions are coming fast and furious. As the name suggests, you "see" your breath as soft, radiant, and golden. With each inhalation, imagine your breath filling your womb with energy.

If you have difficulty conjuring either of these images, you may do better to visualize what is really happening, says Jones. "See your baby's head pushing through and widening the cervix, as though he were slipping on a turtleneck sweater," he suggests.

❐ Listen to music. Any soft, harmonious composition can help you relax. And if you have played it for your baby in utero, the baby may respond to it, too, says David Chamberlain, Ph.D., president of the Association for Pre- and Perinatal Psychology and Health in San Diego. Keep in mind, though, that loud music with a strong beat seems to make babies move and kick a lot—not what you want during childbirth. In one study, babies preferred Mozart to rock 'n' roll. Lullabies are always safe.

You can buy recordings of music created specifically to soothe you and your baby during labor. For information, write to Transitions Music at P.O. Box 8532, Atlanta, GA 30306.

❐ Accept pain as part of childbirth. "Pain is totally subjective," notes Dr. Grubb. "A woman who views labor as hurtful or even life-threatening will experience a lot more pain than a woman who welcomes labor as the final step toward having the baby that she has waited so long for. It really comes down to trusting the process. Childbirth has evolved over millions of generations, and it works."

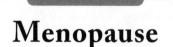

Menopause

No, menopause isn't a disease, although it is sometimes treated as such. Like puberty, it is a time of transition that all women go through sooner or later, like it or not. Most women actually reach menopause (officially defined as one year without periods) somewhere between the ages of 48 and 52. Many women, though, have at least a few years of so-called perimenopausal symptoms before this, as hormonal fluctuations cause symptoms such as hot flashes, irregular periods sometimes accompanied by heavy bleeding, and mood swings.

Surveys show that some women have a particularly tough time during menopause, while others breeze right through it. The majority are somewhere in between, with bothersome but tolerable symptoms. "Women who have had their ovaries surgically removed or who have gone through early menopause (before age 50) are especially likely to have more severe symptoms," says June LaValleur, M.D., assistant professor of obstetrics and gynecology at the University of Minnesota Medical School and director of the Mature Women's Centers at the University of Minnesota Hospital, both in Minneapolis.

There is no preventing menopause. Even replacement hormones can't fully mimic your body's natural cycle. But whether you decide on hormone-replacement therapy or choose to sweat it out, you have plenty of ways to minimize menopause's impact on your mind and body.

Rx

Prescriptions
TO MASTER MENOPAUSE

Dietary and lifestyle changes, along with certain herbs, can protect your health as you go through menopause. Here is what the experts recommend.

❐ Consume 30 to 50 milligrams of isoflavones each day. Isoflavones are weak, plant-derived forms of the hormone estrogen that are found in soy foods such as tofu, tempeh, and soy milk. Studies have shown that women who eat about four ounces of soy foods a day—which supplies 30 to 50 milligrams of isoflavones—are less likely to have bothersome menopausal symptoms such as hot flashes and vaginal dryness, says James E. Williams, O.M.D., a doctor of Oriental medicine with the Center for Women's Medicine in San Diego.

❐ Consume about one tablespoon ground flaxseed each day. "Flaxseed contains lignans, plant compounds that, like isoflavones, have some weak estrogen-like activity in the body," notes Dr. Williams. In

Hate Tofu? Try This

If tofu-phobia prevents you from trying this spongy white food, try Tofu Teriyaki, suggests Elaine Moquette-Magee, R.D., author of *Eat Well for a Healthy Menopause*. "Even women who claim that they don't like tofu like this dish," she says.

Begin by vertically cutting a 14-ounce block of firm tofu into about 10 rectangular slices. Then in a large measuring cup, blend 6 tablespoons light soy sauce; 1 teaspoon sesame oil; 1 teaspoon sesame seeds; 2 tablespoons sugar; ½ cup plus 2 tablespoons apple juice; 1 clove garlic, crushed; and 1 teaspoon finely minced fresh ginger (or ¼ teaspoon ground ginger).

Pour this sauce into a 9- by 9-inch baking pan. Arrange the tofu slices in the pan, turning them over to coat them with the sauce. Broil the slices for 10 to 15 minutes, then flip them over and broil them for 8 to 10 minutes.

This recipe makes about four servings. You can ladle the Tofu Teriyaki over noodles or rice, stuff it into pita bread, or eat it plain or with crackers.

---

studies, lignans also seem to confer some protection against breast cancer and other hormone-dependent cancers, adds Dr. Williams. In addition to baking with it, try sprinkling flaxseed on cooked foods, cereals, and salads.

You would do best to buy fresh flaxseed and grind it yourself (you can find it at health food stores). And keep it refrigerated when you are not using it, since it tends to go rancid rapidly.

❒ Eat at least one serving (about a half-cup) of *Umbelliferae* each day. This group of plants—which includes fennel, parsley, and celery—contains compounds with estrogen-like activity. "Fennel is particularly

Get Your Isoflavones Here

The following foods provide the most hot-flash-cooling isoflavones per serving. All isoflavone values are approximate.

FOOD	SERVING SIZE	ISOFLAVONES (mg.)	FAT (g.)
Nutlettes breakfast cereal	½ cup	122	1.5
Beef(Not) textured soy protein granules	¼ cup, dry	62	1
Roasted soy nuts	¼ cup	60	9.5
Low-fat tofu	½ cup	35	1.5–2.5
Regular tofu	½ cup	35	5.5–6.5
Tempeh	½ cup	35	6
Regular soy milk	1 cup	30	4
Low-fat soy milk	1 cup	20	2
Roasted soy butter	2 Tbsp.	17	11

NOTE: You can order Nutlettes and Beef(Not) from Dixie USA by writing to P.O. Box 55549, Houston, TX 77255.

rich in phytoestrogens," says Michael Murray, N.D., a naturopathic doctor in Bellevue, Washington, and author of *Menopause: How You Can Benefit from Diet, Vitamins, Minerals, Herbs, Exercise, and Other Natural Methods.* Fennel root is a large bulb that has a delicate, licorice-like flavor and that can be sliced into a salad or stir-fry or used to season soups.

MORNING ❏ Take 1,000 milligrams of vitamin C and 50 milligrams of B-complex vitamins twice each day. (Make sure that your B-complex supplement contains pantothenic acid.) These vitamins support your adrenal glands, tiny powerhouses on top of your kidneys that continue to produce small amounts of estrogen, says Helen Healy, N.D., a naturopathic doctor and director of the Wellspring Naturopathic Clinic in St. Paul, Minnesota. "I especially recommend this to women who are leading stressful lives or who, in the past, tended to burn the candle at both ends," she says. "Their adrenals have less reserve power."

Note: Some people experience diarrhea when they take more than 1,200 milligrams of vitamin C a day. If this happens to you, simply reduce your intake of the vitamin until the diarrhea subsides.

❐ Take 400 international units of vitamin E each day. Scientists have yet to determine exactly how vitamin E helps to ease menopausal symptoms. But the nutrient seems to alleviate hot flashes and vaginal dryness for some women, says Dr. Murray.

Many experts believe that you can take this much vitamin E without side effects. But if you have had a bleeding disorder or a stroke, if you are taking anticoagulants, or if your family has a history of stroke, you should use vitamin E supplements only under medical supervision. It is possible that large amounts of vitamin E interfere with the absorption and action of vitamin K, which is involved in blood coagulation.

❐ Eat small meals two to three hours apart. To make this easy, you TIME IT RIGHT can divide your breakfast and lunch in half, then make your dinner roughly the same size. All-day-long grazing maintains a normal blood sugar level and may even help you eat less because you never become ravenously hungry, explains Elaine Moquette-Magee, R.D., author of *Eat Well for a Healthy Menopause.* Both of these factors may help you avoid menopausal weight gain.

❐ Try an herbal product specifically formulated for menopause. Such a product usually contains some combination of the following herbs: chasteberry, black cohosh, dong quai, panax ginseng (sometimes called Asian ginseng), and licorice root. The herbs balance and complement each other, which enhances their effectiveness and reduces side effects, explains Dr. Williams.

You will find these herbal blends in health food stores. Dr. Williams suggests looking for a product that contains standardized extracts. A standardized extract is guaranteed to contain a specific amount of an herb's active ingredient.

Note: Dong quai causes some people to become more sensitive to the sun. So if you choose a product containing this herb, be especially cautious when you head outdoors. Also, if you choose a product containing licorice root, keep in mind that you should limit your consumption of the herb to five grams a day.

TIME IT RIGHT

❐ Regularly engage in aerobic activity. How long and how often you get a move on depends on your current level of fitness. If you have been inactive, for instance, start by walking at a comfortable pace for 15 minutes, three days a week. Gradually increase your time, frequency, and intensity until you are going for 20 to 60 minutes every day. If you like, you can switch from walking to bicycling, swimming, rowing, or aerobic dance—any activity that elevates your heart rate.

Research has proved that regular exercise helps combat weight gain, heart disease, and osteoporosis—conditions for which a woman's risk increases following menopause, says Mona Shangold, M.D., director of the Center for Women's Health and Sports Gynecology in Philadelphia. It may also improve your mood and the quality of your sleep.

❐ Lift weights two or three times a week. Strength training helps to prevent the muscle loss and weakness that is inevitable in older, sedentary women after menopause, explains Dr. Shangold. You can use dumbbells, a barbell, or strength-training machines—whichever you are most comfortable with.

If you haven't tried lifting weights before, contact your YWCA or local health club for a reference to an experienced, knowledgeable instructor. An instructor can show you proper form and technique, then supervise you until you have it down pat.

Medical Alert

Many women have irregular periods as they approach menopause. In most cases, there is no need for concern, Dr. LaValleur says. Do see a doctor, though, if your periods are less than 21 days apart, if you bleed between periods, or if your periods become much heavier. See a doctor, too, if you become unusually tired. Thyroid problems are more common at this stage of life.

Even if your menopausal years go smoothly, you should see your gynecologist for preventive care, advises Dr. LaValleur. This includes regular Pap tests, mammograms, and cholesterol, blood pressure, and bone-density screenings.

Menstrual Discomforts

Figure one or two days a month, 12 months a year, from age 14 to age 50 or so. Subtract some time off for pregnancy, and that's about two years' worth of menstrual cramps by the time a woman reaches the end of her reproductive years. Add in tag-along symptoms—backaches, bloating, nausea, diarrhea, fatigue, and headaches—and that's a heck of a lot of time spent feeling not-so-great.

Most women have some menstrual discomfort at some point in their lives. Older teenagers and women in their thirties typically experience the most pain.

MONTHLY

Cramps, headaches, diarrhea, and fatigue are caused by chemicals called prostaglandins that are released into the body during menstruation. Certain prostaglandins cause blood vessels in the uterus to constrict, for example, decreasing blood flow to the area. The uterine muscle then goes into spasm, tensing up like a tight fist. Older women sometimes have so-called congestive menstrual pain, thought to be due to poor fluid flow in the pelvis and usually preceded by premenstrual bloating, headaches, and breast pain, explains Mary Bove, N.D., a naturopathic doctor and director of the Brattleboro Naturopathic Clinic in Brattleboro, Vermont.

Ibuprofen—the standard drug approach for relieving menstrual discomfort—targets prostaglandins. Some women swear by ibuprofen, and, apparently, for good reason. In several studies, ibuprofen beat out aspirin and acetaminophen in relieving menstrual cramps, backache, and headache. Some women also report that it helps reduce the diarrhea and nausea that they have during the first day or two of their periods.

"This drug inhibits the body's production of cramp-causing prostaglandins, and it works best if you start taking it before the specific prostaglandin that causes the uterine spasms is released into the bloodstream," says Robin Phillips, M.D., a doctor in the department of gynecology at Mount Sinai Medical Center in New York City. If you go this route, she suggests taking 400 milligrams of ibuprofen just prior to or at the onset of pain and then every six to eight hours, with food, for the first day or two of your period. *(Note:* If you have a history of ulcers, Dr. Phillips cautions against using ibuprofen.)

TIME IT RIGHT

Nondrug strategies—offered below—may cut down (or eliminate) reliance on ibuprofen.

Rx

Prescriptions
FOR STOPPING CRAMPS

Some natural prescriptions for menstrual discomfort work by fighting prostaglandins. Others simply relax muscles or stimulate blood flow to the pelvis. You have probably already discovered some remedies by trial and error: curling up in a fetal position, holding a heating pad against your abdomen, or taking a hot bath. Here is what experts recommend for relief.

❐ Try cramp-easing herbs. Two in particular, black haw and cramp bark (both members of the viburnum family), have a long history of use to relax the muscles of the uterus and relieve menstrual cramps, says Dr. Bove. In fact, black haw works so well that it is sometimes used to help prevent miscarriage. "I tend to use both, interchangeably or in combination," she says.

TIME IT RIGHT

If your cramps are mild, make a tea: Add two teaspoons dried black haw or cramp bark per cup of water. Boil 10 minutes, cool, strain, and drink up to three cups a day. Severe cramps may require stronger medicine: a teaspoon dose of herbal tincture every half-hour for two to three hours, Dr. Bove says. It is best not to wait until your pain peaks to start dosing, she adds. "Women who regularly have cramps may want to start taking this a few days before they expect their periods." Since these herbs (which can be purchased at health food stores) contain an aspirin-like compound, they should not be used by women sensitive to aspirin.

❐ Sip ginger tea. This pungent spice has several properties that make it a good choice for menstrual cramps: It reduces inflammation and muscle spasms, it dilates blood vessels and so increases blood flow, and it has warming, energizing character that helps dispel sluggishness, Dr. Bove says. Add six to eight thin slices or a couple of teaspoons grated fresh or ground ginger to two cups freshly boiled water and simmer 15 to 20 minutes. Strain before drinking. "You can add ginger to cramp bark tea to augment the effects of cramp bark," she adds.

❒ Head for the tub. Fill your tub with comfortably warm water, then add 5 drops each of bergamot, chamomile, and rosemary essential oils, along with 10 drops of evening primrose oil. Then soak in the tub, adding hot water as necessary to keep the water warm, suggests Dr. Bove. "These essential oils have tension-relieving and muscle-relaxing qualities."

❒ Press the traditional Chinese acupressure points for relieving menstrual cramps—in the middle of the crease where the leg joins the trunk of the body, explains Michael Reed Gach, Ph.D., director and founder of the Acupressure Institute in Berkeley, California, and author of *Acupressure's Potent Points*. You can press here with your fingertips, or you can stimulate these points one at a time by positioning your left fist over the points on your left side and your right fist over the right side, then, lying on your stomach with your fists in place, using the weight of your body to apply pressure. Find a comfortable position to relax in for at least two minutes, Dr. Gach says.

❒ Rub to relax. Add five drops each of warming, muscle-relaxing essential oils of wintergreen and lavender to a half-ounce base of olive or almond oil. Rub it over your abdomen or lower back, then apply a heating pad—for no more than 20 minutes at a time—covered in a thin towel and set on low, for quick relief, Dr. Bove suggests.

❒ Take a hip-swinging stroll. Walking stimulates the pelvic region TIME IT RIGHT and gets fluids moving through the area, so it reduces pelvic congestion, says Dr. Bove. "I tell women to work on opening their pelvis, letting their hips lead their stroke as they walk, letting their hips and arms swing freely so that their whole body has a chance to stretch out." A daily 20-minute-or-so walk will decrease the likelihood of cramps, reduce them if you have them, and brighten your mood, she says.

❒ Drink lots of water. No one knows why, but "it's been shown sci- SUMMERTIME entifically that increased hydration relieves menstrual cramps," says Dr. Phillips. "If a woman happens to be in the hospital when she has her period and the flow of fluid through her IV is increased, the cramps get better. I tell women with cramps to drink as much water as they can until their cramps go away, then cut back. They tell me it works." This is particularly helpful during the summer, she says, when women are more likely to be slightly dehydrated.

Take a Yoga Break

Yoga can work wonders to relieve abdominal muscle tension and fluid congestion associated with menstruation, says Aadil Palkhivala, senior Iyengar yoga instructor and director of Yoga Centers in Bellevue, Washington. Try these two poses for quick relief. (You will need several thick towels or blankets to perform these poses comfortably.)

MODIFIED HEAD-TO-KNEE STRETCH

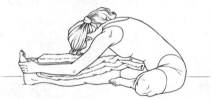

To prepare for the stretch, sit up straight with both legs touching and stretched out in front of you. Bend your left leg, bringing the foot to your right inner thigh, as shown. Lay a stack of folded towels or firm blankets on top of the thigh and calf of your extended leg. The stack should be high enough to fully support your chest and the weight of your head so that there is no strain in your back. Inhale as you lift your chest and lengthen your spine upward.

Keep your spine long and exhale as you lean forward from your hips, rotating your torso slightly and stretching your breastbone area over your extended leg, toward your toes, as shown. Catch hold of your extended foot, using a belt instead of your hands, if necessary. Rest your forehead on a towel, to keep your neck relaxed. Keep your toes pointed up. Hold the pose for two to three minutes, breathing gently and surrendering your weight on the exhales. Then repeat the pose with the opposite leg extended.

MODIFIED BUTTERFLY STRETCH

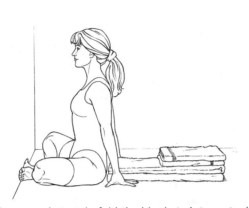

To prepare for the second stretch, fold the blankets into a stack about four to six inches high, as wide as your chest and the length from your waist to your head. Sit down facing a wall and place the stack of blankets behind you lengthwise, just touching your buttocks, as shown. Bring the bottom of your feet together and rest your toes against the wall, getting as close to the wall as you can.

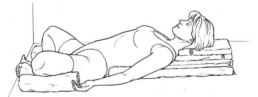

Use your arms to help you recline backward until your waist, spine, and head are comfortably supported on the towels, as shown. Shut your eyes and concentrate on your breath, inhaling and exhaling gently. Feel your chest and abdomen expand and release constriction. Also, feel your belly and pelvis expand and relax, releasing tightness in the groin and uterine walls. Hold this pose for 5 to 10 minutes. You should be absolutely comfortable, with no strain at all. Remove any strain in your inner thighs by putting towels under your thighs, as shown, and/or by moving away from the wall.

    To release the pose, use your hands to bring your knees together and roll to the right off the blankets. Rest in the fetal position before slowly pushing yourself up with your hands, letting your head dangle and come up last.

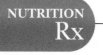

Prescriptions
FOR PAINFUL PERIODS

The natural prescription for long-term prevention of menstrual discomfort rests on dietary changes. Doctors offer these recommendations.

❐ Reduce meats; dairy products such as butter, full-fat cheese, and whole milk; and egg yolks. The saturated fat in these foods contains a type of prostaglandins that triggers muscle contractions. So you will want to cut back on fat from these sources.

❐ Eat more fish and raw nuts and seeds. Flax, sunflower, sesame, and pumpkin seeds and certain fish, such as trout, mackerel, and salmon, contain two kinds of fatty acids—linoleic and linolenic. These fatty acids help relax muscles, says Dr. Bove.

❐ Consider capsule supplements of evening primrose or black currant oil, which also contain linoleic and linolenic acids, says Dr. Bove. She prescribes 1,000 to 3,000 milligrams a day, depending on the severity of the symptoms. Make sure to take the supplements daily with meals for about three to six months. Both supplements can be purchased at health food stores.

❐ Add 500 to 600 milligrams each of magnesium and calcium a day. Both minerals play an important role in maintaining normal muscle tone. Getting enough of both can help your muscles relax and so reduce the severity of menstrual cramps, says Dr. Bove. (In fact, intravenous magnesium sulfate is used to stop the contractions of premature labor.) "I like to use equal amounts of both, as liquid or buffered supplements, which seem to get into the muscles faster than tablets," she says. Some women report relief within a few hours of taking this mix; for others, it may take a few menstrual cycles. "I tell women to try these daily supplements and other dietary changes for at least three months because it often takes some time to see an improvement."

Taking magnesium and calcium only when you have cramps isn't likely to be helpful, adds Adriane Fugh-Berman, M.D., chairman of the National Women's Health Network and author of *Alternative Medicine*. "You need to take them during the entire month."

Note: If you have heart or kidney problems, you should talk to your doctor before taking supplemental magnesium. Also, if you experience diarrhea when taking these supplements, cut back your dosage until your symptoms subside.

❏ **Balance out with the B vitamins.** These are important—especially vitamin B$_6$—because they help your body metabolize hormones. Dr. Fugh-Berman recommends a daily 50-milligram supplement of a B-complex vitamin formula. "I tell women to take this all month long."

❏ **Add vitamin E.** In clinical studies, 150 international units (IU) of vitamin E—administered daily for 10 days premenstrually and during the first four days of the menstrual cycle—helped relieve menstrual discomfort within two menstrual cycles in approximately 70 percent of the women who tried it.

Vitamin E also seems to relieve heavy bleeding, Dr. Bove says. "I'll start someone on 800 IU daily, and then increase to 1,200 IU in the days before menses begins. I might have them use 1,200 to 1,600 IU during days of heavy bleeding, and then, as their bleeding decreases, decrease the dosage." Usually, she says, "by the second or third cycle, they no longer have heavy days."

Vitamin E was initially identified as a fertility-protecting nutrient. (Its scientific name, *tocopherol*, means "child-bearing.") But no one really knows exactly how it might influence hormone production, Dr. Bove admits. Before taking amounts above 600 IU, you should check with your doctor, she adds.

❏ **Check your iron status.** If you have been having heavy periods, you may be low on iron, since blood is rich in iron. And iron deficiency can cause heavier bleeding as well, creating a vicious cycle that isn't stopped unless you replace the iron you have lost, says Dr. Phillips. "If you think that you may be low on iron, ask your doctor about blood tests that measure iron status." Don't take more than 18 milligrams (the Daily Value) of iron without medical supervision, however. Too much iron can cause problems of its own.

❏ **Consider vitamin A.** Some doctors have women with heavy menstrual bleeding take extra vitamin A for several months to see if it lightens their bleeding. "I wouldn't recommend vitamin A alone but might give an amount higher than the Daily Value of 5,000 IU in a good multivitamin or even a prenatal vitamin," Dr. Bove says. In one study, 71 women with heavy bleeding had significantly lower blood levels of vitamin A than women with normal periods. And when these women were given 25,000 international units of vitamin A twice a day for 15 days, blood loss returned to normal or was reduced in more than 90 percent of the women. "I'd stick with no more than 25,000 international units a day," she adds.

Note: Any vitamin A supplement of more than 15,000 IU a day should be taken only with medical supervision. Women who are pregnant should rely on their doctor-prescribed prenatal vitamins and avoid taking vitamin A supplements altogether.

ALTERNATIVE Rx — *Prescriptions* for Menstrual Complaints

Practitioners of alternative medicine offer these additional nondrug tactics against painful periods.

❏ Take a standard capsule or dropperful of the tincture dong quai a day. This herb, also called Chinese angelica or dang-quai, has long been used in Oriental medicine to tone the uterus and balance female hormones, says Andrew Weil, M.D., director of the integrative medicine program at the University of Arizona College of Medicine in Tucson and best-selling health book author. Dong quai helps to regulate the menstrual cycle and ease painful menstruation and heavy flow. It has smooth-muscle-relaxing and pain-relieving properties. "You can take one standard capsule of the herb or one dropperful of the herbal tincture twice a day as a preventive measure to even out irregular menstrual cycles," he says.

Note: If you use this herb, avoid exposure to the sun. Some people become photosensitive when they use dong quai and develop a rash or sunburn easily.

❏ Give homeopathy a chance. This branch of medicine uses extremely dilute solutions of substances to help your body shake off whatever is ailing it, explains Judyth Reichenberg-Ullman, N.D., a naturopathic doctor with the Northwest Center for Homeopathic Medicine in Edmonds, Washington, and co-author of *Homeopathic Self-Care*. Selecting a particular homeopathic remedy takes into consideration physical and psychological symptoms, she says.

Some of the remedies that she might use for menstrual cramps are as follows. They are available in tablet form in health food stores.

Pulsatilla. Try this for symptoms that include changeable menstrual flow from month to month, occasional nausea, tendency to feel worse when exposed to heat, and weepiness.

Belladonna. This works best for symptoms that include intense bearing-down pains or cramps that come and go away suddenly or are aggravated by motion, occasional headaches, and fitful sleep with wild dreams.

Magnesia phosphate. Take this remedy for cramps that are relieved by bending over, by firm abdominal massage while bending forward, or by warm applications and for cramps aggravated by cold.

Selecting the correct homeopathic remedy takes some expertise and training. If these remedies don't help after taking several doses according to the directions on the label, discontinue and consult a homeopathic doctor.

Medical **Alert**

If you have severe cramps and heavy bleeding (defined as bleeding through a pad and or tampon every hour), try lying down, suggests Mary Lake Polan, M.D., Ph.D., professor and chairman of the department of gynecology and obstetrics at Stanford University School of Medicine. If the bleeding continues at that rate for 12 to 24 hours, call your doctor.

You should also call your doctor in the following circumstances, says Dr. Polan: if you have heavy bleeding and lower abdominal pain and cramping and believe that you could be pregnant; if you have heavy bleeding and feel weak and light-headed; if you have severe menstrual cramps for the first time or start passing clots for the first time; if you are on birth control pills and have severe cramps; if you have nausea, headaches, fever, diarrhea, and vomiting as well as cramps; or if your cramps interfere with normal activity and aren't relieved by self-care, including normal doses of aspirin or ibuprofen.

Morning Sickness

It may be one of the first signs that a woman is really, truly pregnant. The wave of nausea, the dash to the bathroom, the old heave-ho. A couple of days of this, and a pregnancy test simply confirms what she already knows.

LIFETIME

Morning sickness got its name because it is most likely to occur between 6:00 A.M. and noon. "Some women wake up with it; for others, it begins when they get up and start moving around," says Lise Alschuler, N.D., a naturopathic physician and director of botanical services at Bastyr University in Seattle. But truth is, pregnant women can have episodes of nausea and vomiting at any time throughout the day. Symptoms start during the 4th to 6th week of pregnancy, end by about the 14th week, and usually hit their stay-near-a-bathroom worst during the 9th week.

Surging hormones, including what's called the pregnancy hormone, human chorionic gonadotrophin, all contribute to queasiness, although exactly how—or why—is a matter of speculation, says Jerome Yankowitz, M.D., a perinatalogist and assistant professor of obstetrics and gynecology at the University of Iowa School of Medicine in Iowa City. "We know that 50 percent or more of pregnant women get it, and that before intravenous fluids were available, women sometimes died from it. But a lot of the things that we recommend to make things easier are simply common sense."

Rx

Prescriptions
FOR QUEASINESS

"Nothing works for everybody, so you have to experiment and sometimes combine things," says Miriam Erick, R.D., a senior perinatal dietitian in the department of nutrition at Brigham and Women's Hospital in Boston and author of *No More Morning Sickness.* Here's what experts suggest.

❏ **Wear the Sea-Band.** The same wrist bands that are used to prevent seasickness can help to reduce nausea in some women, Dr. Alschuler says. Worn snugly, these bands stimulate an antinausea acupuncture point just above the wrist. "It is something I would definitely recommend because it is completely safe. It doesn't seem to be enough by itself, but along with other measures, it is definitely helpful."

One way to increase the band's effectiveness, apparently, is to wear it all the time, Dr. Yankowitz says. "I've had women who swear by them, but they wear them even in the shower," he says. "They tell me that if they take them off to shower, within an hour they are throwing up." Look for Sea-Bands at drugstores.

❐ Eat or drink some ginger. This spice has an age-old reputation for soothing out-of-sorts stomachs. In one study, women with the worst form of morning sickness, hyperemesis gravidarum, who took 250 milligrams of powdered ginger four times a day had a significant reduction in the number of attacks.

"For some women, ginger seems to be the perfect thing," Dr. Alschuler says. She recommends fresh ginger, which contains more of ginger's active ingredients than powdered ginger. Chop about one-quarter inch fresh ginger into small cubes, place in a non-aluminum pot, add one cup water, cover the pot, and simmer for 15 to 20 minutes. "It's really important to keep the pot covered so that you don't boil away the volatile oils that are the active ingredients in the ginger," she points out. Ginger is considered relatively safe both at the time morning sickness occurs and to help prevent future bouts. Two or three cups daily is usually recommended.

Erick prefers that women get their ginger from foods. "We use a ginger ale or ginger beer, a nonalcoholic soda that has a lot of kick," she says.

Time it right

❐ Supplement with B$_6$. In one study of 59 pregnant women with nausea and vomiting problems, half the women took 25 milligrams of vitamin B$_6$ every eight hours for three days. (They were given instructions to take the medication between 6:00 and 8:00 A.M., between 2:00 and 4:00 P.M., and then between 10:00 P.M. and midnight.) The other half took placebos—pills that looked like the real thing but did nothing. At the end of the study, only 8 of the women in the vitamin B$_6$ group were still vomiting, compared to 15 in the placebo group. Vitamin B$_6$ worked best for those women having the worst problems—vomiting more than seven times a day.

"B$_6$ can be helpful for some people, but it doesn't help every woman," Dr. Alschuler notes. She recommends that women take a prenatal multivitamin that contains vitamin B$_6$. "I'll give that, and if the problem continues, I might add 25 milligrams twice a day, for a total of no more than 100 milligrams of B$_6$ per day."

LONG-TERM Rx
Prescriptions
FOR FEEDING AN UNSETTLED STOMACH

When you are having a bout of morning sickness, food may be the last thing on your mind. Still, you have to eat. Here is what to do when you think you can try to eat.

❐ Eat a little a lot. The advice about crackers, dry toast, and rice cakes has evolved into a broader notion—frequent mini-meals. "Volume is a big deal," Erick says. "We feed women bite by bite, because the more you try to put in at any one time, the faster it is going to come back out."

❐ Honor your cravings. The foods that you desire most are the least likely to upset your stomach, Erick says. "Women say that they want spaghetti, pizza, spicy things, and foods that appear to be unusual to other people, like pickles. We don't know why, but women are particular about what foods they think are going to make them feel better, and the foods they say they think will make them feel better usually do."

❐ Get your quarter-cup quota. The average pregnant woman needs about 10 cups of fluids a day, but women with severe morning sickness might not be able to stomach more than one-quarter cup of fluid at a time, Erick says. So they need to figure out how much they can handle at one time, and drink that amount frequently, she says.

❐ Have a "solid liquid." Fruits such as watermelon or grapes are mostly fluid, and they seem to stay down better than juices for some people, Erick says.

❐ Don't limit salt. Salt is important during this time for two reasons, says Dr. Alschuler. First, salt is lost in body fluids, so you need to replace it. And second, salt makes you thirsty, driving you to drink the fluids you need. She recommends simply eating salt to taste, but not putting extra salt on already salty food. In her experience, this keeps women hydrated, and women are less likely to experience nausea if they are adequately hydrated.

❑ Smell some lemons. Lemon is one smell that seems to settle the stomach, Erick says. "We use a lot of lemons around here." Lemonade and lemon water are popular beverages. And lemon water is used to swish and spit to get rid of the bad mouth taste pregnant women often develop. "That taste can be bad enough to cause nausea," she says.

❑ Suck on red-hot fireball candy. They, too, seem to quell queasiness, but here again, no one knows why, Erick says.

❑ Watch out for iron supplements. They are associated with a high incidence of nausea as a side effect and can make morning sickness worse, Dr. Yankowitz says. "Unless a woman is anemic, I might tell her to back off the iron during this time."

❑ Stay upright or even active for at least half an hour or so after you have eaten a meal, Dr. Yankowitz recommends. "Otherwise, you can get this acidy taste in your mouth and a burning sensation in your throat as stomach acid backs up, and that can set off the whole reflex of nausea and vomiting."

Mealtime

Medical **Alert**

If you are losing weight or feeling weak or light-headed, if your skin stays raised after you pinch it (a sign of dehydration), or if your symptoms persist after the third month of pregnancy, see your doctor, says Dr. Yankowitz.

And make sure that your doctor takes your symptoms seriously, Erick says. "In my opinion, morning sickness has not been taken seriously for a billion years; doctors simply assume that it is a part of pregnancy, and by the time women end up in the hospital, they are a real disaster emotionally and physically."

A simple urine test to check for ketones, "the poor man's test for starvation," can help a doctor determine whether a woman is sick enough to require hospitalization and intravenous fluids, Dr. Yankowitz says.

Postpartum Depression

New moms can't be blamed for getting a certain, shall we say, skewed view of motherhood. Television, magazines, and most books portray this time as one of unabashed bliss—with nary a single dirty diaper, screaming baby, or overbearing mother-in-law to deal with.

Reality is seldom so rosy. In fact, up to 70 percent of new moms experience the "baby blues." These women become teary, anxious, irritable, restless, and super-sensitive within three or four days after baby arrives. "You are weepy and irritable," says one former baby-bluer. "You can't sleep, and you don't know why—but you could just as soon cry as look at the clock." These symptoms tend to peak between 7 to 10 days after delivery, then subside around day 14.

In a much smaller number of women—no more than 1 in 10—the blues don't spontaneously disappear. They persist, and they may even intensify. This condition is called postpartum depression. "The difference between baby blues and postpartum depression may not always be clear at first to a woman or her family or her doctor," says Ann Dunnewold, Ph.D., president of Postpartum Support International and co-author of *Postpartum Survival Guide*. "So the point I always make is this: When the balance shifts, when there is more negative than positive, then you need some outside help—whether it is a support group or counseling or therapy or medication."

Two things conspire to make mom blue, Dr. Dunnewold explains. One is unrealistic expectations. "Simply realizing that what she is going through is normal, that being a mother really is demanding, may be enough to lift the guilt and self-blame that only make things worse," she says. "New mothers are sleep-deprived, exhausted, and typically overwhelmed. They are thrown into a new job for which there is no adequate training available and are given sole responsibility for a completely vulnerable and complex human being that arrives in the world without an instruction manual."

LIFETIME

The other is biology. The soaring hormones that can make a pregnant woman glow drop sharply after delivery and take time to return to normal, says George Chrousos, M.D., a researcher in the developmental endocrinology branch of the National Institute of Child Health and Human Development in Bethesda, Maryland. And it is not just female hormones such as estrogen and progesterone that are low, he says. He has found that a hormone that offers protection from stress, called corticotropin-releasing hormone, remains abnormally low in women for about three months after delivery.

For some women, taking care of themselves during this time may prevent the baby blues from slipping into postpartum depression, says Lisa Weinstock, M.D., a psychiatrist at the Westchester division of the New York Hospital/Cornell University Medical Center in White Plains, New York. But women who are at the highest risk—including those who have been depressed before, and especially those who have had postpartum depression previously—need to have a plan of action in place before they have their babies to make sure that they get the professional help they may need, she adds.

Prescriptions
TO CHASE AWAY THE BLUES

Rx

Two things need to happen for you to start feeling better, Dr. Dunnewold says. First, you need to stop blaming yourself for what is happening. Second, you need to figure out your real needs. Here is how you can make those things happen.

❐ Look on the brighter side. Know that you are not alone, that you are not to blame, and that you can feel better, Dr. Dunnewold says.

❐ Replace negative self-talk with positive messages. You may find yourself being extremely self-critical, telling yourself things like "You are so stupid. What's wrong with you that you can't even take care of your baby? You wanted this baby so badly, and now all you can do is cry." When such a thought enters your mind, pause to acknowledge it, suggests Dr. Dunnewold. Then imagine that you are talking to a child or a close friend who is tormenting herself in this way. What would you tell her to make her feel better? Close your eyes, take four deep breaths, and say to yourself, "You are strong and competent, and this is really hard work. Just hang in there. Everything's going to be all right. Things will get easier soon."

❐ Once you recognize and set aside your self-blame, focus on what would make you feel better. Whether it is time away from the baby, help around the house, home-cooked meals, or a sympathetic ear, you can develop a plan to get the support you need, Dr. Dunnewold says.

❐ Create a social support network for yourself. In countries like Japan, where the new mother and her infant are cared for by others, the rate of postpartum depression is lower, Dr. Weinstock says. "But in this country, we expect women to have their babies, then get right back into the swing of things within two months. This is very unrealistic. You need to put other goals aside and focus on recovering from this huge change in your life."

"Just getting together with other parents who have similar concerns and needs has been shown to prevent postpartum depression," adds Dr. Dunnewold. "Seeing other moms struggling with the same problems that you're grappling with can be validating."

MEALTIME

❐ Keep eating nutritious meals. Even if you feel fat and flabby, now is not the time to go on that 800-calorie diet. You should eat at least as well as you did while you were pregnant but reduce your intake of fatty foods a bit and increase your level of exercise, says Judith Roepke, R.D., Ph.D., a perinatal nutritionist at Ball State University in Muncie, Indiana.

❐ Continue taking your prenatal supplements. Symptoms of depression can result from shortages of certain vitamins, including folic acid, B_6, and B_{12}, says Melvyn Werbach, M.D., a psychiatrist and author of *Nutritional Influences on Mental Illness*.

"It's not unreasonable to take similar supplements for up to three months after childbirth, or for as long as you breastfeed your baby," adds Dr. Roepke.

❐ Catch up on your sleep whenever you can. "Sleep deprivation is a tried-and-true method for torturing prisoners," notes Dr. Dunnewold. It can lead to exhaustion, irritability, and irrationality.

Try to sleep when your baby sleeps. If you have trouble getting in sync with baby's odd hours, take a hot shower, retire to a darkened room or cover your eyes, and pull a blanket over you to get cozy. "If you still can't sleep, at least rest," advises Dr. Dunnewold. "Put your feet up and sip a soothing beverage, listen to soft music, watch a soap opera—do whatever you must to have some sense of getting a break from your duties."

❒ Engage in exercise for at least 10 minutes each day. You don't need a heavy-duty aerobic workout either. Even walking or practicing yoga can lift your mood, dissipate anxiety, and boost your energy, according to Dr. Dunnewold. If you want, you can put your baby in a sling in front of you while you vacuum or do another physically active chore. You may also want to check around for a postpartum exercise class where new moms and babies are welcome. (Your local YWCA or health club is a good place to start.)

❒ Schedule your workout before 2:00 in the afternoon. Exercising 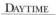 early in the day can help you sleep better at night, explains Dr. Dunnewold.

❒ Keep track of the time you spend on baby-related duties: diaper changes, feedings, burpings, walks. This can help you realize how demanding caring for a baby really is. "Women say, 'I didn't get the bills paid' or 'I didn't get the dishes washed,'" observes Dr. Dunnewold. "But maybe they changed 14 diapers. So they really did accomplish something."

❒ Plan your day the night before. "It helps to have at least one ac- tivity to look forward to each day," says Dr. Dunnewold. You could take a walk or do a crossword puzzle or call a friend. "Try to schedule at least one event involving adult contact, beyond your partner's return in the evening."

Medical **Alert**

Postpartum depression should not be taken lightly. If your symptoms haven't cleared up in two weeks, experts recommend seeing a doctor. "It's normal to feel low on energy and even kind of 'nutsy' for a time after having a baby," Dr. Weinstock says. "But if you have an array of symptoms, including an inability to enjoy things, changes in your sleep and eating habits, a lack of concentration, and feelings of guilt, that's depression." And if you have had thoughts of harming yourself or your baby, seek professional help without delay.

Premenstrual Syndrome

Virtually all women—more than 90 percent—experience some sort of premenstrual misery. They may feel tired or bloated or crabby. And it is all absolutely normal.

Premenstrual *syndrome*, on the other hand, is not normal. In fact, it has been recognized as an official psychiatric disorder (called late luteal phase dysphoric disorder) since 1987. True premenstrual syndrome, or PMS, affects a minority of women—only 3 to 10 percent of the female population.

These women experience various combinations of the more than 150 symptoms associated with PMS, including mood swings, food cravings, bloating, and fatigue. What distinguishes their symptoms from garden-variety premenstrual discomfort? In PMS, the symptoms show up in at least two of every three menstrual cycles. They get worse just prior to your period, then subside—sometimes dramatically—once your period begins.

Just what causes PMS is still a mystery, says Mary Lake Polan, M.D., Ph.D., professor and chairman of the department of gynecology and obstetrics at Stanford University School of Medicine. One theory that is getting a lot of scientific scrutiny has to do with serotonin, a brain chemical that influences your mood. Studies have shown that some women with PMS have lower-than-normal levels of serotonin. Another theory that is making the rounds links PMS to changes in the ratio of estrogen to progesterone, both female hormones.

Because PMS causes such a wide variety of symptoms, no one treatment usually handles all of them. Instead, doctors often prescribe a combination of dietary and lifestyle changes to manage the condition, says Marcus Laux, N.D., a naturopathic doctor in Santa Monica, California, and co-author of *Natural Woman, Natural Menopause*. In severe cases, doctors may prescribe antidepressants or tranquilizers—which, unfortunately, often cause side effects of their own.

Rx

Prescriptions
TO PACIFY PMS

Regardless of whether you meet the clinical definition of PMS, you can use self-care measures to ease your premenstrual symptoms. Try the following remedies for on-the-spot relief.

❐ Take time for yourself. Responsibilities and demands may seem especially burdensome when PMS is in full swing. You should find a way to give yourself a break—to indulge in something that you find pleasurable or relaxing.

❐ Practice deep breathing for 5 to 10 minutes at least twice a day. Deep breathing offers more than a pleasant time-out. "It helps the nervous system and endocrine system to balance and calm down," says Carol Snarr, R.N., a psychophysiological therapist (one who teaches biofeedback and other mind/body skills) at the Life Sciences Institute in Topeka, Kansas. "It produces a physical response that can ease the emotional upheaval associated with PMS."

To try deep breathing, sit up straight or lie on your back. Exhale through your nose, then inhale, focusing on your breath. Keep your exhalations and inhalations of equal length. "The idea is to breathe deeply, slowly, and calmly, letting your belly expand with each inhalation," explains Snarr. "As you become accustomed to the technique, you will want to increase the depth and length of your breaths."

Ideally, you should rehearse deep breathing while your PMS isn't in full swing. Snarr suggests twice-a-day training sessions—one in the morning, one at bedtime. That way, when PMS sets in, you will know exactly what to do.

❐ If you feel stressed at any time during the day, stop what you are doing and take a couple of deep breaths. This helps relieve premenstrual tension and anxiety, according to Snarr.

❐ Engage in some type of physical activity. Exercise burns up the anxiety-producing hormone adrenaline and stimulates the release of feel-good brain chemicals called endorphins. "In my experience, what works best is an activity where you get to hit something or you have an opponent to defeat," says John Lee, M.D., co-author of *What Your Doctor May Not Tell You about Menopause*, with Virginia Hopkins, M.D. "I'd recommend racquetball, which is easy to learn. Ignoring or trying to suppress PMS-related aggression just doesn't work over the long run."

❐ Take 5 to 15 drops of chasteberry tincture, mixed with a few ounces of water, three times a day. Chasteberry, also called vitex, is commonly prescribed in European countries for PMS. The herb appears to work through the pituitary, your body's master gland, to help reestablish hormonal balance, says Daniel Mowrey, Ph.D., in his book *Herbal Tonic Therapies*.

You can buy chasteberry tincture in health food stores, or you can make your own supply. Fill any size jar one-third of the way with dried chasteberries (also available in health food stores), then fill it the rest of the way with 100-proof vodka. Put on the lid and note the contents and date on the label. Allow the tincture to sit at room temperature for six weeks. During this time, the active ingredients in the berries will infuse into the alcohol. At the end of six weeks, the tincture is ready for use. If you store it in a cool place, it should be good for decades, according to Susun S. Weed, director of the Wise Woman Center in Woodstock, New York, and author of the *Wise Woman Herbal* series.

❐ Use aromatherapy. Certain essential oils have therapeutic properties that can ease PMS symptoms, according to Judith Jackson, an aromatherapist in Greenwich, Connecticut, and author of *The Magic of Well-Being*. She suggests the following remedies. (You can buy essential oils in health food stores or through mail-order catalogs.)

✔ To dispel anger, dab two drops of rose and three drops of sandalwood essential oils onto your wrists.

✔ To relieve anxiety, sniff the scent of sandalwood, ylang-ylang, or neroli (orange blossom) essential oil.

✔ To reduce fluid retention, add six drops of juniper and four drops of geranium essential oils to one-half ounce sesame oil. Rub the oil onto your abdomen, your breasts, and wherever else you feel bloated.

NUTRITION Rx

Prescriptions
to Stave Off Symptoms

Once you have addressed your immediate symptoms, you may want to find a way to manage PMS over the long term. You can start by taking a good, hard look at your eating habits. "I recommend major nutritional overhauls for most of my PMS patients," says David Edelberg, M.D., clinical instructor at Northwestern University in Evanston, Illinois, and founder of the American Whole Health Centers in Chicago, Denver, and Bethesda, Maryland. "In my opinion, dietary changes offer the most benefit for the least expense."

Which dietary changes you make really depends on the nature of your PMS. That said, many women have succeeded at controlling their premenstrual symptoms with the following strategies.

Hormonal Help for PMS

The theory that out-of-balance hormones—too much estrogen and too little progesterone—cause premenstrual syndrome (PMS) has led some doctors to recommend supplemental progesterone to women from midcycle to the time menstruation begins. This treatment remains controversial, though, since the few well-controlled scientific studies that have been done have found progesterone no more effective at relieving symptoms of PMS than placebos (pills that look like the real thing but do nothing). In both cases, about one-third of the women responded well.

Still, doctors who prescribe it say that many of their patients benefit from progesterone. "Women have to take more of the hormone for the first month that they are on it," says Marcus Laux, N.D., a naturopathic doctor in Santa Monica, California, and co-author of *Natural Woman, Natural Menopause.* "But within six months, they usually report significant relief from their PMS symptoms." Bloating, cramping, back pain, breast tenderness, and skin and bowel problems all seem less severe.

If you think progesterone therapy might benefit you, talk to your doctor about taking a natural form of the hormone. According to Dr. Laux, the natural form is nearly biochemically identical to a woman's own hormone. When used correctly, it is very safe, without the side effects of synthetics.

A product called Pro-gest Body Cream, which is available in some drugstores, is recommended by Dr. Laux. He suggests that you consult your doctor first to see if this is right for you before purchasing any products. As an alternative, a compounding pharmacist—one who makes medications by hand—can provide you with tablets or a cream made from natural progesterone.

❏ Eat a well-balanced diet that consists of 40 to 50 percent complex carbohydrates, 30 percent protein, and 20 to 30 percent fat. This mix of nutrients stabilizes levels of blood sugar and the brain chemical serotonin, both of which influence your mood, according to Mary Bove, N.D., a

Healing Meals

Good nutrition is a central component of nondrug treatment for premenstrual syndrome (PMS). "What you eat has a direct impact on the amounts of hormones and brain chemicals, or neurotransmitters, in your system," explains David Edelberg, M.D., clinical instructor at Northwestern University in Evanston, Illinois, and founder of the American Whole Health Centers in Chicago, Denver, and Bethesda, Maryland. "These compounds help determine whether or not you experience PMS symptoms."

What's more, when you don't feed your body properly, it doesn't function properly, notes Mary Bove, N.D., a naturopathic doctor and director of the Brattleboro Naturopathic Clinic in Brattleboro, Vermont. PMS can be a symptom of poor nutrition.

The following one-day menu plan, which is based on guidelines provided by Dr. Bove, shows you what a day's worth of eating might be like for a woman who is trying to ease her PMS symptoms. The five small meals supply a total of 2,200 calories—40 to 50 percent from complex carbohydrates, 30 percent from protein, and 20 percent from unsaturated fats. Red meat, caffeine, and fatty, sugary, and salty foods have all been eliminated.

This menu plan does come up short on certain nutrients, particularly calcium and iron. So if you decide to try it, you should take a multivitamin as well, says Dr. Bove. Try following a menu plan similar to this consistently for a few months to see if it helps reduce your symptoms.

naturopathic doctor and director of the Brattleboro Naturopathic Clinic in Brattleboro, Vermont. To get your nutrients in roughly the right proportions, visualize one of those compartmentalized dinner plates. The largest of the three compartments is for complex carbohydrates (whole

BREAKFAST
>   Three-quarters cup whole-grain cereal (choose one that supplies three to five grams of fiber per serving)
>   Four ounces skim milk
>   Fruit shake (blend two ounces tofu, one-half cup orange juice, one-half cup pineapple juice, one-half small banana, and one-half cup fresh papaya)

MIDMORNING SNACK
>   One cup fresh strawberries with nonfat yogurt and raw nuts; or one-half cup serving of steel-cut oatmeal

LUNCH
>   One cup pasta with one cup grilled or steamed mixed vegetables, one-half cup tofu, and one-half cup low-fat spaghetti sauce
>   One cup green vegetables (such as broccoli) or one cup salad with balsamic vinegar

AFTERNOON SNACK
>   One cup vegetarian lentil soup
>   Two ounces whole-grain roll or about two slices bread

DINNER
>   Eight ounces baked monkfish or other white fish with garlic, lemon juice, and a drizzle of olive oil
>   One cup whole-wheat couscous
>   Six ounces steamed green beans and red peppers
>   One-half cup nonfat sorbet

grains, rice, and pasta). The two smaller compartments are for protein (lean meats, poultry, fish, and soy products) and unsaturated fat (nuts, seeds, and vegetable oils).

TIME IT RIGHT

❒ Eat small meals at three- to four-hour intervals over the course of a day. So-called mini-meals have a distinct advantage over the standard three squares. They prevent the dips in blood sugar and serotonin that precipitate the mood swings of PMS, explains Dr. Bove.

❒ Take 300 milligrams of magnesium every day. Magnesium plays an important part in the treatment of PMS, according to some studies. Supplementation of the mineral is associated with fewer cramps, less water retention, and an overall improvement in premenstrual symptoms. The best dietary sources of magnesium are nuts, legumes, whole grains, and green vegetables.

❒ Take B-complex vitamin supplements every day. Choose supplements that supply 150 to 250 milligrams of vitamin B_6 and 75 to 100 milligrams of the other B vitamins, suggests Dr. Bove. The B vitamins help your body metabolize hormones, including estrogen. While B_6 seems to capture most of the attention, all of the B vitamins are important. "After a few months of supplementation, you should notice significant improvement in your PMS symptoms," according to Dr. Bove.

Note: Consult your doctor before taking more than 100 milligrams of vitamin B_6 a day. Such a high dosage, taken for a long period of time, can cause numb feet and an unstable gait in some people.

❒ Take one tablespoon ground flaxseed every day. Flaxseed contains essential fatty acids that help reduce premenstrual bloating and inflammation, says Dr. Bove. You can buy flaxseed in your local health food store already ground, or you can grind it yourself with a coffee grinder and store it in the refrigerator. Try mixing it into recipes for baked goods or sprinkling it on cereal or yogurt.

❒ Avoid drinking alcoholic beverages during the last two weeks of your menstrual cycle, suggests Dr. Bove. Alcohol steps up your body's excretion of magnesium and B vitamins, nutrients that help protect against PMS symptoms. Loss of these nutrients can lead to a craving for sweets.

Medical **Alert**
If self-care measures fail to ease your PMS symptoms, or if PMS-related mood changes are affecting your family or your job, you should see your doctor, says Dr. Polan. You may have an undiagnosed health problem whose symptoms worsen just prior to menstruation.

Urinary Incontinence

Forget what those TV commercials for adult diapers make you think. Urinary incontinence isn't an unavoidable consequence of childbirth. Nor is it an inevitable part of aging. Even if your bladder seems to have sprung a slow leak, you probably won't have to trade in your fashionable unmentionables for the latest in bulky absorbent-wear.

Doctors have identified several types of urinary incontinence, all with slight variations in symptoms and severity. Among women ages 55 and younger, stress incontinence is most common. Women who have stress incontinence may dribble urine when they cough, laugh, lift heavy objects, exert themselves suddenly, change positions quickly—any action that increases pressure on the bladder. "For example, a woman playing tennis may leak when she serves the ball," says Stephen B. Young, M.D., director of urogynecology and pelvic reconstructive surgery at the University of Massachusetts Medical Center in Worcester.

Stress incontinence results from stretched and weakened pelvic-floor muscles. These muscles extend from the pubic bone to the tailbone, providing hammock-like support for the bladder and uterus. Both the vagina and the urethra (the one-inch-long tube that carries urine from the bladder) pass through this muscular sling. When you contract the pelvic-floor muscles, you squeeze your vagina and urethra shut.

New moms are prime candidates for stress incontinence because vaginal childbirth may damage the pelvic-floor muscles and nerves. Menopausal changes and abdominal surgery can also affect the strength and tone of these muscles.

While stress incontinence gives you no advance warning of a urine leak, urge incontinence sends the signal that you have to go. Unfortunately,

LIFETIME

it leaves you no time to get to a bathroom. "The bladder may release just a bit of urine, or it may spill its whole load," according to Dr. Young.

LIFETIME

In urge incontinence, some factor disrupts communication between your brain and your bladder. As a result, your brain gets the message that your bladder is full, but your bladder doesn't receive its instructions to wait until you find a toilet. Weak pelvic-floor muscles may contribute to urge incontinence, but other factors—such as menopausal changes, urinary tract infections, and even food irritants—likely play roles as well.

Both stress incontinence and urge incontinence can be controlled, even cured. And the earlier you begin treatment, the better off you will be, says Dr. Young.

Rx

Prescriptions
TO STEM THE FLOW

Even if you have urinary incontinence, you don't have to suffer through embarrassing accidents. The following strategies can keep spills to a minimum.

❒ **Cross your legs.** In a study at the University of Utah School of Medicine in Salt Lake City, women with stress incontinence lost urine 9½ times less often if they simply crossed their legs before they sneezed or laughed. This maneuver boosts the holding-in power of your pelvic-floor muscles, explains Dr. Young. It could mean the difference between a slightly wet pad and a change of clothes.

TIME IT RIGHT

❒ **Go to the bathroom before you exercise.** This may help prevent an accident while you work out, especially if you have only mild stress incontinence, says Linda Brubaker, M.D., director of the urogynecology and pelvic surgery section at Rush Medical College in Chicago.

❒ **Wear a tampon or diaphragm for high-impact activities** such as aerobic dance, horseback riding, karate, tennis, and volleyball. When inserted into the vagina, either device puts some pressure on the urethra, according to Dr. Young. This counteracts the pressure on the bladder when you bounce and jostle your body. Neither a tampon nor a diaphragm is made to be worn continuously, so remove it following the activity.

For an alternative to a tampon or diaphragm, you may want to ask your doctor about a prescription device called Introl. It fits into the vagina somewhat like a diaphragm, but it has two prongs designed specifically to support the bladder, explains Dr. Young.

Prescriptions
TO BENEFIT YOUR BLADDER

NUTRITION
Rx

For long-term protection against urine leaks, you may want to make some dietary changes. Here is what some experts recommend.

❏ **Drink cranberry juice.** Research suggests that cranberry juice helps prevent unhealthy bacteria from clinging to cells in the urinary tract, reducing your risk of a urinary tract infection. This is important, since a urinary tract infection can aggravate incontinence, according to Kristene E. Whitmore, M.D., chief of urology and director of the Incontinence Center at Graduate Hospital in Philadelphia and co-author of *Overcoming Bladder Disorders*. About three glasses a day should do it.

❏ **Eat eight ounces of yogurt containing live cultures each day.** The *Lactobacillus acidophilus* bacteria in the yogurt restores and maintains a healthy bacterial environment in the vagina. This helps ward off a yeast infection—which, like a urinary tract infection, can worsen incontinence, notes Dr. Whitmore. To find out whether a yogurt contains *Lactobacillus acidophilus*, just check for it in the list of ingredients or see if the label mentions live and active cultures.

❏ **Consume enough high-fiber foods each day to meet or exceed the** Daily Value of 25 grams. Fiber helps keep your bowel movements regular. Without it, you may become constipated, and constipation contributes to incontinence, says Dr. Whitmore. Among your best fiber sources are whole grains, beans, fruits, and vegetables. A cup of whole-wheat spaghetti contains more than 6 grams of fiber; a half-cup of canned refried beans, almost 7 grams; and the kernels from one ear of corn, more than 2 grams.

MEALTIME

❏ **Drink enough fluids each day.** Restricting your fluid intake won't prevent leaks. "In fact, it can actually aggravate incontinence by producing concentrated urine, which is highly irritating to your bladder," notes Dr. Brubaker. So in addition to cranberry juice, drink lots of water. How do you know that you are well-hydrated? Your urine should appear clear or pale yellow.

❐ Limit your consumption of caffeinated foods and beverages such as chocolate, coffee, tea, and cola. Caffeine can irritate your bladder and can contribute to urge incontinence, says Dr. Young.

❐ Cut back on spicy foods, citrus fruits and their juices, strawberries, pineapple, tomatoes, and aged cheeses. "Any of these foods may break down into acidic components, which irritate the bladder," says Dr. Whitmore.

The Kegel Cure

Many doctors consider Kegels the first-choice treatment for urinary incontinence. These exercises strengthen the pelvic-floor muscles—the ones that you use to squeeze off the flow of urine.

For Kegels to be effective, you need to make sure that you are contracting the correct muscles, notes Stephen B. Young, M.D., director of urogynecology and pelvic reconstructive surgery at the University of Massachusetts Medical Center in Worcester. To feel those muscles, try slowing or stopping the flow of urine or try squeezing a finger or two inserted in your vagina.

While you are working your pelvic-floor muscles, you want to relax your other muscles—especially those in your stomach, buttocks, and thighs. You shouldn't see anything moving when you are doing Kegels.

Women who have extremely weak pelvic-floor muscles may need to lie down to do Kegels, at least to start. "Lying down with your knees bent, perhaps with a pillow under your hips, takes the weight of your internal organs off the muscles," says Linda Brubaker, M.D., director of the urogynecology and pelvic surgery

❏ Eliminate artificial sweeteners such as aspartame (NutraSweet). These sugar substitutes break down into compounds that can irritate the bladder, according to Dr. Whitmore.

❏ If you take vitamin C supplements, switch to a buffered form. Buffering ingredients like calcium ascorbate neutralize the acidity of the vitamin C so that the supplements are gentler on your bladder, explains Dr. Whitmore.

❏ Keep a detailed diary of your dietary and voiding (urinating) habits. Dr. Whitmore has her patients write down what and when they

section at Rush Medical College in Chicago. "This can be especially helpful after childbirth."

As for how many Kegels you need to do, doctors' prescriptions vary. "It's kind of like any other kind of strength training," observes Dr. Brubaker. "You need to determine an appropriate starting point and progress in a logical fashion."

One common recommendation is to begin with three sets of 10 Kegels each day, holding each contraction for a count of five. Then gradually work your way up to three sets of 20 Kegels each day, holding each contraction for a count of 10, suggests Dr. Brubaker.

Kegels take time to work. Some women see results in six to eight weeks. But Dr. Young suggests giving yourself at least six months before considering other treatment options, such as surgery.

For more detailed instruction on proper Kegel technique, you may want to invest in an audiotape. The National Association for Continence offers one of the best. To order your copy, write to the organization at P.O. Box 8310, Spartanburg, SC 29305.

eat and drink, along with how often and how much they urinate (including accidents). Based on their notes, she asks her patients to give up the offending foods and beverages for one to three months. Then folks add the suspected triggers back into their diets, one at a time. All the while, they continue to track their voiding habits. "This exercise gives us a complete picture," she says. "We can be fairly certain which foods and beverages cause problems and whether eliminating those items leads to an improvement in symptoms."

Rx ——— *Prescriptions*
TO CONTROL NATURE'S CALL

To get your bladder back on track, you need to look at other lifestyle factors besides diet. Be sure to include the following self-care measures in your treatment regimen.

TIME IT RIGHT ❏ Retrain your bladder to void on schedule. This works especially well for women with urge incontinence, notes Dr. Young. Begin by allowing yourself one bathroom trip per hour every day for a week or two. Then extend the time between trips by a half-hour for another week or two. Continue this pattern of adding half-hour increments every couple of weeks until you are able to hold your urine for three to four hours at a time. "This exercise teaches your bladder to hold more urine and to become less spastic when it's full," he explains. And because your bladder becomes accustomed to postponed voiding during the day, you are less likely to be awakened at night by the sudden urge to go.

❏ Ask your doctor whether any medicine that you are taking—prescription or over-the-counter—could cause bladder leakage. "If symptoms set in when you start a new medication and disappear when you stop the medication, then the source of the problem is fairly obvious," says Dr. Brubaker. "Your doctor should switch you to a different drug or at least reduce your dosage."

Among the medicines linked to incontinence are diuretics, which increase urine flow and may overwhelm the bladder; certain blood pressure medications, including alpha blockers and calcium channel blockers; antidepressants; sedatives; and over-the-counter sleep and cold medications.

❒ **Quit smoking.** Women who smoke cigarettes are more than twice as likely to develop stress incontinence as women who have never smoked, according to a study performed at the Medical College of Virginia at Virginia Commonwealth University in Richmond. Cigarettes deliver a double whammy to your bladder: Nicotine irritates it, and coughing (as most smokers do) puts pressure on it, explains Dr. Young.

Medical **Alert**

See your doctor if you leak more than an occasional drop or two of urine, advises Dr. Young. Incontinence can be a symptom of an underlying health problem such as diabetes, chronic bladder infection, or prolapse of the uterus or bladder (the organ slips out of its normal position, often after a hysterectomy).

Vaginal Dryness

Sex seemed like a good idea at the time. The mind was certainly willing, but the body—or rather, a very specific part of the body—said, "Nothing doing." Instead of being its usual moist, receptive self, the vagina felt painfully dry—inhospitable, even.

"I didn't used to have to worry about vaginal dryness. It was never anything a little spit couldn't fix," says one newly remarried 44-year-old woman. "But now I won't even begin to fool around without having a tube of lube handy." Neither she nor her husband considers the need for additional lubrication a terrible inconvenience. "We just make it part of the fun," she says.

Many women develop vaginal dryness as they get older, thanks to dwindling supplies of the hormone estrogen. Estrogen helps keep vaginal tissue moist and healthy. Levels of the hormone begin to drop off when women reach their late thirties.

But at that age, well before menopause, a woman seldom makes the

Lifetime

connection between hormonal decline and vaginal dryness. "She thinks the irritation is from a yeast infection or her panties—anything except less estrogen," says Georgia Witkin, Ph.D., a supervisor of the human sexuality program and director of the stress program at Mount Sinai School of Medicine of the City University of New York in New York City. "She may not find out the real cause for years. In the meantime, she lives with enormous discomfort."

When menopause does finally arrive, it brings significant changes to the vaginal environment. Within a few years, a woman's vagina shrinks and loses muscle tone. Its normally thick walls become thin and delicate. And its secretions become less acidic, which sets the stage for infection.

Hormonal fluctuations can affect a woman's vaginal health at other times of life, too. For instance, many new moms experience vaginal dryness while they are nursing their babies. The reason is that prolactin, the hormone that stimulates the breasts to make milk, also suppresses the production of estrogen, explains Larry Grunfeld, M.D., clinical associate professor of obstetrics and gynecology at Mount Sinai Medical Center in New York City. The lack of estrogen can suppress ovulation. This is why breastfeeding acts as something of a contraceptive.

Other, nonhormonal factors can cause vaginal dryness, too. Stress can take its toll, as can certain medications (such as fluid-depleting diuretics and mucous membrane–drying decongestants and antihistamines).

While vaginal dryness poses no serious threat to your health, it does make sex uncomfortable—even impossible. "If you let it go for too long, it can change your entire attitude toward sex," says Lonnie Barbach, Ph.D., assistant clinical professor of medical psychology at the University of California, San Francisco, School of Medicine, and author of *The Pause: Positive Approaches to Menopause.* "You may start avoiding intercourse and intimacy. In that way, vaginal dryness affects not only your relationship with your mate but also your sense of self."

Rx ——— *Prescriptions*
FOR ON-THE-SPOT RELIEF

For women who have menopause-related vaginal dryness, many doctors recommend hormone-replacement therapy (HRT). HRT restores moisture to vaginal tissue and thickness to vaginal walls, explains Dr. Grunfeld. Vaginal creams that contain estrogen do pretty much the same thing.

If you want to try self-care before bringing in the heavy artillery, here is what you can do.

❏ **Use a lubricant each time you have intercourse.** Dr. Grunfeld suggests choosing a product that is water-soluble (such as K-Y jelly or Astroglide). The advantage of Astroglide is its staying power: It doesn't dry out or become tacky as quickly when exposed to air.

If you are trying to conceive, however, you are better off using either pure mineral oil or egg whites. "Neither one kills sperm," notes Dr. Grunfeld. In fact, mineral oil plays a role in the in vitro fertilization process. If you prefer to use egg whites, just separate them from the yolks and let them warm to room temperature. You don't need to whip the whites—just apply them with a finger as needed. Dispose of any leftover egg whites after one day.

One lubricant that all women should avoid is petroleum jelly. It remains in the vagina and harbors yeast and other infection-producing microbes.

❏ **For vaginal itching and irritation, apply a lubricant.** You can choose a product that is designed for use during sexual intercourse, such as those mentioned above. Or you can try a vaginal moisturizer that contains polycarbophil, such as Replens. This lubricant lasts longer and balances vaginal pH, helping to restore it to a more normal state. And since one application works for several days, you don't need to reapply as often.

"You can use any of these lubricants as much as you like to stay comfortable. If they don't give you the results that you want, though, you should consult your family doctor," says Leslie Shimp, D.Pharm., associate professor of pharmacy at the University of Michigan in Ann Arbor.

❏ **For menopause-related vaginal dryness, try a vaginal suppository** containing vitamin E and a beeswax base. Begin by using one suppository every night for six weeks, then cut back to one suppository one night a week for as long as needed. "I've recommended this regimen to countless women, and the great majority find the suppositories to be very helpful in relieving vaginal dryness and irritation," reports Judyth Reichenberg-Ullman, N.D., a naturopathic doctor with the Northwest Center for Homeopathic Medicine in Edmonds, Washington, and co-author of *Homeopathic Self-Care*. You can either buy vitamin E suppositories in health food stores or get them from a naturopathic doctor.

HERBAL Rx

Prescriptions
FOR RESTORING MOISTURE

Certain herbs are effective in treating vaginal dryness. Two of the best are licorice root and ginseng. To make the most of their therapeutic properties, follow this advice from the experts.

TIME IT RIGHT

❐ Chew two tablets (a total of 380 milligrams) of deglycyrrhizinated licorice root about 30 minutes before each meal. Licorice root targets vaginal dryness in two ways, according to Helen Healy, N.D., a naturopathic doctor and director of the Wellspring Naturopathic Clinic in St. Paul, Minnesota. For starters, the herb stimulates mucous production in your body, even increasing the number of goblet cells (cells that manufacture mucus). Plus, licorice root contains compounds that act as weak forms of estrogen.

You can buy chewable tablets of deglycyrrhizinated licorice root in health food stores. (Deglycyrrhizinated means the compounds that elevate blood pressure have been removed.) The tablets work so well, says Dr. Healy, that you may find yourself having to blow your nose as you chew them. Forget about munching on licorice candy, though—it doesn't even contain real licorice.

❐ Take 100 milligrams of panax ginseng (sometimes called Asian ginseng) in the form of a standardized extract, once or twice a day. Ginseng is useful for all typical menopausal symptoms, including vaginal dryness, hot flashes, insomnia, and energy loss, says James E. Williams, O.M.D., a doctor of Oriental medicine affiliated with the Center for Women's Medicine in San Diego. The active compounds in ginseng apparently have an estrogen-like effect on vaginal tissue, helping the tissue stay moist and supple. "In traditional Chinese medicine, ginseng is often prescribed to women in their menopausal and postmenopausal years as a general tonic," he explains.

A standardized extract ensures that you are getting a consistent amount of the active compounds in ginseng—unlike most teas and herbal formulas, which contain very little of the stuff. Ask a medical professional who is knowledgeable about herbs to recommend a product to you, Dr. Williams suggests. You can buy the extracts in health food stores. Just look for the words *standardized extract* on the label.

Prescriptions
FOR VAGINAL HEALTH

NUTRITION
Rx

To get rid of vaginal dryness for good, some lifestyle changes may be in order. For instance, consider your dietary habits. If you are not already doing the following, why not start now?

❐ Take 400 international units of vitamin E each day. Recent research has paid little attention to the effects of vitamin E on vaginal dryness. But two studies done in the 1940s indicated that vitamin E supplements can improve symptoms of vaginal atrophy, says Michael T. Murray, N.D., a naturopathic doctor in Bellevue, Washington, and author of *Menopause: How You Can Benefit from Diet, Vitamins, Minerals, Herbs, Exercise, and Other Natural Methods.* These days, many doctors recommend vitamin E for vaginal dryness and other physical changes associated with menopause. If you decide to try vitamin E, give yourself at least four weeks to see results, he advises.

❐ Consume up to 200 milligrams of isoflavones each day. Isoflavones are compounds found in soy foods such as tofu and soy flour. In studies, these compounds appear to have a mild, estrogen-like effect. One study found that postmenopausal women who ate enough soy foods to get about 200 milligrams of isoflavones each day (a little more than one-half cup soybeans) experienced an increase in the number of cells lining the vagina. This increase helped to offset vaginal dryness and irritation. (For top-notch sources of isoflavones, see "Get Your Isoflavones Here" on page 270.)

❏ Drink at least eight eight-ounce glasses of water or fresh juice each day. Even mild dehydration—the kind that is barely noticeable to most people—can dry out mucous membranes, including those in the vagina, says Dr. Healy. You may notice that your eyes and mouth feel parched.

MORNING

❏ Cut back on caffeinated beverages such as coffee, tea, and cola. Caffeine depletes your body of fluid, notes Dr. Healy.

Rx — *Prescriptions*
FOR BETTER, WETTER DAYS

Once you have your dietary habits on track, add these lifestyle strategies for optimum vaginal health.

❏ Do Kegels. These exercises strengthen your pelvic-floor muscles, which extend from your pubic bone to your tailbone and support the organs in your pelvic region. Kegels have traditionally been prescribed to treat urinary incontinence, but they help keep the vaginal area healthy as well. "Kegels counteract the loss of muscle tone that leads to vaginal atrophy," explains Dr. Barbach. (To learn how to do Kegels, see "The Kegel Cure" on page 300.)

❏ Refrain from douching. Commercial douche solutions contain astringent ingredients that dry out vaginal tissue. "If you already have vaginal dryness, a douche is likely to make your problem even worse," says Dr. Shimp. "I don't ever recommend douching to my patients."

❏ Stay sexually active. Research has shown that women who are sexually active have less vaginal atrophy than women of the same age who are celibate. One theory is that sexual arousal improves blood circulation to vaginal tissues, helping them stay healthy.

Most women don't want to abandon their sexual selves as they grow older, notes Dr. Barbach. But they may need to find new ways to comfortably express their sexuality.

❏ Pay attention to what your body is telling you. If you are a healthy young woman who normally has no problem with vaginal dryness, experiencing vaginal dryness may indicate the presence of an underlying emotional issue that is inhibiting your arousal. It could be stress or anger or fear. "Instead of trying to work like a machine, pull back and think about what is going on," suggests Dr. Barbach. "Know that your body holds the larger truth and that you could benefit from listening to it." Working through the problem with your partner may ease your vaginal symptoms.

Medical **Alert**

If self-care measures fail to stop vaginal dryness from putting a crimp in your quality of life—and your sex life—see your gynecologist. "Even women who have had breast cancer or another hormone-dependent cancer, who may think that vaginal dryness is something they have to live with, can get help," says Dr. Grunfeld. You should also see your gynecologist if you experience vaginal soreness that doesn't go away in one week or bleeding (other than menstruation).

Chapter 4

Prescriptions
for Looking Your Best

Age has a way of putting things in perspective, especially when it comes to appearance. As teenagers, we thought a mere pimple was the end of the world. Now we know better. Oh, we may still get the occasional pimple. But we must also contend with graying hair, fine facial lines, and cellulite-dimpled thighs.

Living in a society that prizes youth, we don't exactly roll out the welcome mat for these physical changes. Sure, we could do without them. But this doesn't necessarily mean that we long for the face and physique of a twenty-something supermodel. On the contrary, many of us simply want to wear our age well—to look and feel vibrant, whether we are 35, 55, or somewhere in between.

What's responsible for this new, healthy attitude toward beauty? Well, we would like to think that today's woman feels comfortable with and confident about who she is. Just as likely, though, she simply doesn't have the time to primp and preen in front of a mirror. Heck, some mornings she can barely squeeze in a shower.

This section is especially designed for women who want to look sensational without a lot of fuss. You will find hair- and skin-care strategies that you can easily adapt to your own daily grooming regimen. "Recipes" for homemade bath and beauty products. Tips from the pros on styling hair and applying makeup. Plus suggestions for dietary and lifestyle changes that can make a world of difference in hair and skin health.

And if you are bothered by undesirable body fat on your upper arms, hips, buttocks, or thighs, try the simple workout on page 366. In combination with regular aerobic exercise, this resistance-training routine can shape up even the toughest trouble zones.

Hey, you know that you feel young. So why not let it show? With the natural prescriptions in this section, you can put your best face (and body) forward.

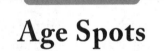

Age Spots

Allison T. Vidimos, M.D., a staff dermatologist at the Cleveland Clinic Foundation in Cleveland, usually can tell if women she sees in her office play golf just by looking at them.

How does she know? It's easy: They have age spots on only one hand as well as on the face, neck, chest, and forearms. Since male and female golfers alike typically wear just one glove to aid in grasping the club, the other hand gets all the sun. With time, age spots appear on the unprotected skin.

Despite their name, age spots—also known as liver spots and solar lentigines—may have little to do with age, says Dr. Vidimos. These small, brown, flat patches of increased pigmentation appear mostly on the face, neck, upper chest, and back of the hands. They are caused by overexposure to the sun. "Calling them 'age spots' is misleading because they are not due to aging alone," she explains. "They are due to the cumulative effect of sun exposure over the years. A 30-year-old can develop age spots as well as an 80-year-old."

Heredity also plays a role in who will develop age spots, according to Edward Bondi, M.D., professor of dermatology at the University of Pennsylvania Medical Center in Philadelphia. "Some people get lots of sun and never get age spots," he says. "And for other people, they appear after very little exposure."

At first, age spots resemble a freckle or small mole. But with time, they take on their own size, shape, and color characteristics. So what is the difference between an age spot, a freckle, and a mole?

Early on, the three look very similar, according to Dr. Bondi. But moles tend to darken over time and often raise above the skin, whereas freckles and age spots stay flat. Freckles generally stay small and fade away during the winter, but age spots never disappear on their own without treatment and grow larger and darker as you spend more time in the sun.

Rx ——— *Prescriptions*
FOR PREVENTING AGE SPOTS

Age spots are preventable, says Marianne O'Donoghue, M.D., associate professor of dermatology at Rush–Presbyterian–St. Luke's Medical Center in Chicago. In fact, future generations will never get age spots if they slather on the sunscreen.

LIFETIME

Effective sunscreens weren't available until the early 1980s, Dr. O'Donoghue says. "So anybody born before 1980 is likely to get age spots. People born after 1980 have a good chance of never getting them." If you don't have a single age spot, count yourself lucky. To keep your skin spot-free, follow these do's and don'ts.

❐ Buy sunscreen and use it liberally. Look for products that have a sun protection factor (SPF) of 15 or higher and that protect the skin from two types of radiation: ultraviolet-A (UVA) and ultraviolet-B (UVB), says Dr. O'Donoghue. UVB rays are the main cause of sunburn and immediate skin damage. UVA rays have lower intensity, but they penetrate below the skin's surface and cause long-term damage.

❐ Lose the tanning mentality. Sorry, but wearing a sunscreen does not mean more time to bask in the sun. "Even with the best of sunscreens, you are still getting some sun damage, so lying in the sun and baking is a mistake," says Dr. Bondi.

❐ Stay out of direct sunlight from 10:00 A.M. to 3:00 P.M., when the sun's rays are strongest.

DAYTIME

❐ Cover up. Clothing provides some protection from the sun's harmful rays, so try to wear longer shorts, shirts with longer sleeves, and a wide-brimmed hat. If you have very fair skin, you may want to consider special lightweight clothing with an SPF of 30 that blocks out ultraviolet light, suggests Dr. Bondi. The best-known brand is Solumbra. A catalog of available Solumbra clothing can be ordered from Sun Precautions by writing to 2815 Wetmore Avenue, Everett, WA 98201.

❐ Wash your hands. Believe it or not, touching certain foods such as celery and lime can increase your sensitivity to the sun, says Dr. Vidimos. These foods contain psoralens, chemicals that, when exposed to ultraviolet light, cause a sunburnlike reaction that eventually blisters and heals with hyperpigmentation (darker skin). The hyperpigmentation persists for weeks to months, she says.

Psoralens are also found in carrot greens, fresh dill, figs, fresh parsley, and parsnips, among other things. So it is a good idea to wash your hands after handling these foods if you are going to be out in the sun.

❐ Skip the perfume. Some perfumes may contain a potent photosensitizer called oil of bergamot. This oil can cause a peculiar dark discoloration of the skin known as berloque dermatitis after exposure to sunlight. Oil of bergamot has been removed from most perfumes and lotions, so this condition is now rare.

❐ Be on the lookout for other photosensitizers. A number of drugs (like Retin-A, used for acne or wrinkles; antibiotics such as tetracycline; and blood pressure and diabetes medications) can render your skin more sensitive to sunlight. The most likely reaction is something resembling a sunburn. But photosensitizing drugs may make you more likely to develop age spots with repeated unprotected sun exposure, says Dr. Vidimos.

Prescriptions
TO FADE AGE SPOTS

Rx

If several birthdays and summers in the sun have left you with age spots, over-the-counter fade creams can help. But be patient—age spots don't develop overnight, and you are not going to lose them that quickly either. Here is what doctors recommend.

❐ Select a fade cream containing 2 percent hydroquinone. (The best-known brand is Porcelana.) While not 100 percent effective, these creams can help diminish age spots, especially darker ones, says Dr. Bondi. Apply the cream according to the package directions, and after one to two months, the spots should begin to fade. Age spots will return once exposed to sunlight, however, even if you are wearing sunscreen. So stay out of the sun.

❐ Try alpha hydroxy acids. Better known as AHAs, these naturally occurring mild fruit acids can help fade age spots by exfoliating dead skin cells and speeding up cell renewal. Incorporated in skin creams and lotions in concentrations of up to 8 percent, alpha hydroxy acids strip away dead skin cells and prompt growth of fresh, new cells. For best results, Dr. Vidimos advises looking for an AHA product containing glycolic acid, the most commonly used alpha hydroxy acid.

❐ For the sensitive areas around the eyes, use an AHA preparation containing no more than 5 percent acid, says Mary Lupo, M.D., associate clinical professor of dermatology at Tulane University School of Medicine in New Orleans. And don't use AHA products directly on the eyelid, which is particularly sensitive.

TIME IT RIGHT   ❐ Protect, fade, and exfoliate. Creams combining hydroquinone, glycolic acid, and sunscreen attack age spots on three fronts—but they are available by prescription only. Dr. Vidimos says that you can enjoy some of the same benefits, however, by applying sunscreen throughout the day, plus a 2 percent hydroquinone over-the-counter fade cream in the morning and an over-the-counter AHA lotion or cream at night.

Medical **Alert**

Unlike moles, age spots pose little health risk, says Dr. Bondi, and rarely develop into skin cancer. But be alert for changes in their appearance. "Technically, any pigment-forming cell, anywhere on the body, has the potential to turn into melanoma, which is the dangerous form of skin cancer," he says. So any pigmented spot that seems to be changing in size, color, or shape should be evaluated by your dermatologist.

Blemishes

Like bad-hair days, bad-skin days can make any woman feel self-conscious. One angry red pimple is all it takes to lower self-esteem and send a woman to the makeup counter for cover. Call them blemishes, pimples, or breakouts, skin eruptions of this sort are all variations of acne.

Acne develops when a tiny hair follicle pore becomes plugged with dead skin, even on seemingly hairless areas such as the face, says John Collins, N.D., a naturopathic physician who is board-certified in homeopathy, associate professor of homeopathy at the National College of Naturopathic Medicine, and co-owner of Rockwood Natural Medicine Clinic, both in Portland, Oregon. The plugged pore produces a closed pimple, or whitehead. If the plug breaks through the skin's surface, exposure to air will darken it, causing a blackhead.

As for those angry red pimples lurking just below the surface, they form when bacteria living in the follicle multiply and alert the immune system that there is going to be trouble. Infection-fighting white blood cells move in to counteract bacteria, a battle breaks out, and you, the victim, are left with redness, swelling, and soreness, typically on your face, chest, back, or shoulders.

For some women, acne flares up around midcycle—that is, with ovulation—and lingers until the menstrual period ends. For other women, doing a big presentation first thing in the morning—or coping with any other stressful situation—can provoke acne and send bumps rising to the surface. In both instances, the culprit is an increase in androgens, or male hormones, says D'Anne Kleinsmith, M.D., a dermatologist in private practice in West Bloomfield, Michigan. "Hormone production peaks at midcycle, when women ovulate, and when we are under stress," she says. "That in turn makes the skin more oily and increases acne at that time."

You might expect a prescription for acne to include advice to avoid greasy food, cleanse your skin vigorously, or get out in the sun to "dry out" your skin. But doctors say that those strategies are groundless.

"Fatty food is really not a factor in acne," says Dr. Kleinsmith. "Eating greasy food like french fries isn't good for your diet and cholesterol level, but it probably won't make a difference in whether or not you are going to get a zit tomorrow."

MONTHLY

Don't blame acne on poor hygiene either. Acne has nothing to do with dirt. In fact, washing too often can irritate the skin and aggravate acne.

The notion that the sun cures acne is also false, says Nelson Lee Novick, M.D., associate clinical professor of dermatology at Mount Sinai School of Medicine of the City University of New York in New York City and author of *You Can Look Younger at Any Age*. Although a tan will temporarily disguise your blemishes, the sun may actually make acne worse in the long run, he explains.

The sun's ultraviolet rays penetrate the skin's surface and damage hair follicle walls, which may ultimately lead to clogged pores and acne. "People don't blame the sun for their breakout since the breakout is about three weeks after sun exposure. So they continue to get more sun in hopes of getting better. It is a vicious cycle," says Dr. Novick.

Rx ——— *Prescriptions*
TO CARE FOR ACNE-PRONE SKIN

To be honest, nothing will make pimples disappear overnight. Benzoyl peroxide—available without a prescription in concentrations of up to 10 percent—can stop breakouts before they occur and prevent new blemishes from cropping up. Same goes for over-the-counter products containing salicylic acid (such as Fostex). Applied directly to pimples and acne-prone areas, these drying agents can make pimples disappear more quickly by acting as mild peeling agents, says Dr. Novick.

The problem is that benzoyl peroxide may be too harsh for some. And it can bleach colored clothing, so you need to drape an old towel or white pillowcase over your clothes before using it, advises Dr. Novick.

Here are some tips for taking care of your skin.

❏ Wash gently with a pH-balanced sensitive-skin cleanser and warm, not hot, water, advises Dr. Novick. Don't forget to wash from beneath the jaw to the hairline, as these places are often overlooked. Rinse thoroughly.

❏ Use your hands, not a washcloth. Scrubbing with a washcloth can make inflammation worse.

❏ Just say no to polyester scrub sponges, which aggravate acne, explains Dr. Novick. Ditto for abrasive skin gels.

❐ Wash your face no more than twice a day, once in the morning and once in the evening. Too-frequent washing can aggravate acne, says Dr. Novick.

❐ If oiliness tempts you to wash more often, wipe oily patches with a plain white tissue throughout the day, recommends Dr. Novick.

❐ If that doesn't help, dab a mild astringent (such as Sea Breeze) onto a two- by two-inch gauze pad. Then gently pat the astringent onto the oily spots only, suggests Dr. Novick.

❐ Use water-based or oil-free lotions and gels containing alpha hy- droxy acids (AHAs), advises Dr. Kleinsmith. These mild fruit acids help fight acne and clogged pores by preventing older skin cells from piling up on the skin and blocking pores. Use twice a day or alternate it with a benzoyl peroxide product—one at morning, the other at night.

❐ Check the concentration. The percentage of alpha hydroxy acids in nonprescription AHA products bought in stores or salons varies from a negligible amount to about 8 percent. If the product doesn't give a percentage, don't buy it, says Andrew Scheman, M.D., assistant professor of clinical dermatology at Northwestern University in Chicago and author of the *Cosmetics Buying Guide*. Some dermatologists will let you buy nonprescription AHA products with higher concentrations (12 to 15 percent) at their office without an appointment, he says.

❐ Apply a sunscreen or moisturizer with a sun protection factor (SPF) of at least 15 every day from April to October, when the sun's rays are most intense, advises Dr. Novick. Oil-free sunscreens are less likely to clog pores than oil-and-lotion formulations.

❐ If your hair tends to be oily, shampoo once a day, says Dr. Kleinsmith. And keep your bangs away from your face.

❐ Use a shampoo that you can see through and a conditioner labeled "oil-free." "If you are prone to breakouts, rich and creamy shampoos and conditioners are probably not the best thing to have next to your skin," says Dr. Kleinsmith.

❐ Use oil-free cosmetics and oil-free moisturizers. Look for products labeled noncomedogenic (won't promote blackheads and whiteheads) and nonacnegenic (won't provoke pimples).

❐ Avoid a diet high in iodine. In large quantities, iodine has been shown to worsen acne, explains Dr. Collins. Watch your intake of iodized salt and foods high in iodine such as lobster, shrimp, and cooked oysters.

❐ Keep your face away from the phone. Resting the receiver against your chin can cause a breakout because the receiver presses against hair follicles and prevents facial oils from escaping. (For the same reason, breakouts also happen from resting your chin in your hands.) Clean the

A Nutrition Prescription for Problem Skin

Take your vitamins, our mothers used to say. Now, we may have another reason to heed mom's advice. Certain vitamins can help clear up problem skin, according to John Collins, N.D., a naturopathic physician who is board-certified in homeopathy, associate professor at the National College of Naturopathic Medicine, and co-owner of Rockwood Natural Medicine Clinic, both in Portland, Oregon. Here is his nutrition prescription.

Vitamin A. This vitamin acts as an antioxidant, counteracting environmental damage and boosting the skin's natural ability to shed dead skin cells. Here is how to use this vitamin safely and effectively.

❐ Limit supplements of vitamin A to no more than 10,000 international units daily. Higher doses have been shown to cause side effects, including severe headaches, swelling in the brain, and skin rashes, says Dr. Collins. Pregnant women should be especially careful: More than 10,000 international units can cause birth defects.

❐ To play it safe, consume foods rich in beta-carotene, a plant substance converted into vitamin A in the body. Beta-carotene is plentiful in carrots, sweet potatoes, cantaloupe, tomatoes, and dark green leafy vegetables such as spinach.

receiver regularly with rubbing alcohol and hold the phone away from your face when talking, advises Dr. Kleinsmith.

❐ Replace cosmetic aids often. Dirty makeup implements such as sponges and brushes can cause acne, explains Dr. Kleinsmith. Replace or wash makeup sponges weekly, rinsing thoroughly. Likewise, wash your makeup brushes in soapy water once a week, and rinse well. Replace makeup brushes when the bristles get stiff or break off.

Vitamin B$_6$. This vitamin helps control acne, especially for women whose acne worsens with their menstrual cycles, says Dr. Collins. Limit your intake to no more than 50 milligrams daily. Taken in excess, vitamin B$_6$ can cause numbness and nerve damage.

Vitamins C and E and selenium. These antioxidant vitamins and selenium (a trace mineral) help the body fight inflammation and promote healing. For acne control, recommended daily doses from food are 1,000 milligrams of vitamin C, 400 international units of vitamin E, and 200 micrograms of selenium (no more than 100 micrograms in supplement form).

Zinc. "Many people with acne have lower levels of zinc," notes Dr. Collins. "When zinc levels increase, acne often improves." He recommends the following dosage.

❐ Take 50 milligrams of zinc a day for three months, then reduce the amount to 30 milligrams for the next 12 months.

Note: You should consult your doctor before taking zinc in amounts that exceed the Daily Value of 15 milligrams.

❐ Take 1 milligram of copper for every 15 milligrams of zinc. That is because zinc can interfere with copper absorption, says Dr. Collins.

❐ When a breakout occurs, don't pick, pop, or squeeze, says Dr. Kleinsmith. Squeezing your acne can press the accumulated debris more firmly into the clogged pore and increase the chance of inflammation. Picking at your acne can lead to permanent scarring.

Cellulite and Stretch Marks

Ah, summer. Time to trade in baggy pants and bulky sweaters for leg-baring shorts and scarcely there swimsuits. Time to expose parts of the body that haven't seen daylight for three months or more. Time to show the world square inches of skin that have been under wraps all winter long. *Eek!* Summer!

Many a woman would prefer to run for cover—or at least a cover-up—rather than reveal that she has cellulite or stretch marks. While these conditions may leave you feeling self-conscious or embarrassed, from a health perspective they are harmless.

Cellulite is nothing more than body fat, says Joseph P. Bark, M.D., a dermatologist in Lexington, Kentucky, and author of *Your Skin*. It looks different from other body fat because of the way your body stores it.

Think of cellulite as a bunch of fat cells packed into a storage room. When too many cells enter the room, the walls bulge and push against the skin, explains Melvin L. Elson, M.D., director of the Dermatology Center in Nashville. This creates the characteristic dimpling or cottage-cheese look of cellulite.

Cellulite usually shows up on your thighs, hips, or backside. If you have it, you may want to blame your genes. Research suggests that cellulite is inherited, according to Dr. Elson. This helps explain why some women—even those who are considered thin—develop cellulite, while others don't.

While cellulite takes shape beneath the skin, stretch marks occur right on the surface. They initially appear as pinkish or purplish lines on the breasts, abdomen, buttocks, thighs, and sometimes even the arms. Eventually, they turn white or lighter-colored but will still have the appearance of shiny, stretched skin.

Most women associate stretch marks with pregnancy. But the scar-like lesions can result from weight gain or exercises that bulk up the muscles—or anything that makes the skin's elastic tissue stretch and tear. They have also been linked to prolonged use of high-potency cortisone creams and other corticosteroid medications, which cause the skin to become thin. Once you have cellulite or stretch marks, they stick around for a lifetime. That's the bad news. The good news is that you can take steps to make cellulite or stretch marks less noticeable so that you feel more comfortable and confident about your appearance. Even better news: With good nutrition, regular exercise, and a handful of other self-care strategies, you may never develop cellulite or stretch marks in the first place.

LIFETIME

Prescriptions
FOR DEALING WITH DIMPLING

Rx

Fighting cellulite has become a cottage industry, producing all sorts of miracle creams and clever devices that promise to break up or squeeze out fat. But the fact is that nothing can cure cellulite. You can minimize or prevent its appearance by maintaining a healthy, fat-fighting lifestyle that includes the following measures.

❏ Limit your intake of dietary fat to no more than 25 percent of your daily calories. You can start by replacing fried foods, fatty meats, and oily dressings with pasta, fruits, vegetables, and other nonfat and low-fat options. The less fat you consume, the less fat your body has available for storage, explains Dr. Elson. And without those fat cells, cellulite can't form.

❏ Exercise aerobically for 30 minutes at least three times a week, ideally on alternating days. Aerobic exercises are activities that require your body to use oxygen at a rate higher than daily living, explains Amy Nelson, president of Heart Aerobics, a Los Angeles–based fitness company, and a certified health and fitness instructor. She recommends jogging, swimming, cycling, or even brisk walking at a level that should be exerting but still allow you to carry on a conversation without shortness of breath. This type of activity revs up your metabolism, your body's calorie-burning mechanism. And the more calories your body burns, the fewer it stores as fat.

TIME IT RIGHT

❐ On days off from your aerobic workouts, do strength training instead. Strength training—exercising with weights or using your body as the resistance weight—replaces body fat with muscle. "As you increase your muscle mass and decrease your fat mass, your cellulite becomes less apparent," says Dr. Elson. And don't worry about developing an Arnold Schwarzenegger–type physique—the idea is to tone and not to bulk up. For toning exercises, a woman should strive to increase her number of repetitions at a minimal weight, rather than trying to increase her maximum weight, as in weightlifting. Exercises from the waist down are best for cellulite-fighting, such as leg curls, leg presses, knee bends, and even situps and crunches.

Rx ——— *Prescriptions*
FOR SIDESTEPPING STRETCH MARKS

For stretch marks, prevention is the best medicine. Because once you have them, all the cocoa butter, olive oil, and vitamin E gel in the world won't make them disappear. Some women have tried the prescription acne medication tretinoin (Retin-A) and over-the-counter products containing alpha hydroxy acids (AHAs) with modest success, according to Wilma F. Bergfeld, M.D., a dermapathologist for the Cleveland Clinic Foundation, head of clinical research in the department of dermatology at the Cleveland Clinic in Cleveland, and author of *A Woman Doctor's Guide to Skin Care*. (AHAs are the active ingredient in Vaseline's Intensive Care Lotion for Dry Skin and St. Ives Alpha Hydroxy Renewal Lotion.)

To keep stretch marks from scarring your skin, heed this advice from the experts.

MEALTIME

❐ Keep a lid on your weight by eating a sensible diet that gets no more than 25 percent of its calories from fat and exercising for 30 minutes at least three times a week. Packing extra pounds can lead to the formation of stretch marks, says Diane Madlon-Kay, M.D., a family physician for the St. Paul–Ramsey Medical Center in St. Paul, Minnesota.

While there are a number of complex formulas for figuring out your ideal weight, one simple formula used by some experts can tell you if you are close: If you are five feet tall, you should weigh 100 pounds. If you are taller, add 5 pounds for each additional foot of height. To that number, add

10 percent if you have a large frame, or subtract 10 percent if you have a small frame.

☐ If you are pregnant, follow your doctor's guidelines for weight gain. A typical maternity weight gain is about three to four pounds during the first trimester, and about a pound a week during the second and third trimesters. In her own research, Dr. Madlon-Kay has found that women who put on only as many pounds as their doctors advise tend to get stretch marks less often. "But that's not absolute," she adds. "Some women who gain an appropriate amount of weight during pregnancy may still get stretch marks."

LIFETIME

☐ During pregnancy, apply moisturizer to your abdomen twice a day, advises Dr. Bergfeld. Your skin's elastic tissue stretches more and tears less when it is moisturized, she explains.

LIFETIME

Note: Mothers-to-be should reduce their exposure to strong drugs and chemicals—including some topical drugs, such as tretinoin—while they are pregnant or nursing, cautions Dr. Bergfeld. Be selective about lotions and creams—the most natural is usually the safest.

☐ Apply a sunscreen with a sun protection factor (SPF) of 15 or higher at least 30 minutes before heading outdoors, to allow for absorption. Remember to reapply every few hours, and immediately if washed, rinsed, or sweated off. "Anything that damages the skin—including the sun—makes the skin more fragile and prone to stretch marks," says Dr. Bergfeld.

TIME IT RIGHT

☐ If you can, stay out of the sun entirely between the hours of 10:00 A.M. and 3:00 P.M. That's when the sun's ultraviolet rays are at their strongest and can do the most damage to your skin.

DAYTIME

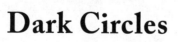

Dark Circles

Go ahead and blame Mom, Dad, or some other leaf on the family tree for those dark circles under your eyes. Contrary to popular belief, heredity, not lack of sleep, typically paints that bluish black or brownish tinge on the skin.

"Fatigue will accentuate, not precipitate, dark circles," says Alan Boyd, M.D., assistant professor of dermatology and pathology at Vanderbilt University in Nashville. "Dark circles are almost always an inherited family trait."

Sometimes, dark circles are caused by hyperpigmentation—the skin produces too much melanin, or brown pigmentation. Dark circles tend to appear in people of Mediterranean and Indian descent.

But in others, dark circles are caused by dilated blood vessels beneath the skin, explains Allison T. Vidimos, M.D., a staff dermatologist at the Cleveland Clinic Foundation in Cleveland. The skin under the eyes is thin and transparent, she says, and "a network of blood vessels underneath the eyes can give a blue-black appearance to the skin."

And in some people, dark circles are due to both pigmentation and dilated blood vessels.

NIGHT-TO-DAY Rx

Prescriptions
FOR DARK CIRCLES

Aside from fatigue, such things as allergies, illness, menstruation, and even pregnancy can aggravate the under-eye area and accentuate dark circles. Also, dark circles become more pronounced with age, as skin loses tautness, says Mary Lupo, M.D., associate clinical professor of dermatology at Tulane University School of Medicine in New Orleans. Overexposure to the sun only aggravates the problem, since sunlight breaks down collagen (the supportive structure of the skin) and elastin, which helps skin spring back after it is stretched.

Try the following prescription recommended by Dr. Lupo to minimize and, in some cases, prevent dark circles.

NIGHTTIME

❐ Get to bed. Staying up late and watching Jay Leno may put a smile on your late-night face, but it can also aggravate those dark circles under your eyes. Sleep needs vary for individuals, but try to get at least six hours.

MORNING

❐ While you are waiting for your morning cup of coffee to brew, lie back down on your bed and apply a cold compress underneath your eyes for 10 to 20 minutes. The cold helps reduce swelling and soothes the skin. Homemade compresses include an ice cube wrapped in a damp facecloth, cotton balls soaked in witch hazel, chilled iced-tea spoons, and moistened and chilled chamomile tea bags (after 5 minutes, tea bags lose their coolness). Chamomile helps minimize dark circles by constricting the blood vessels underneath the eyes. (Some pollen-sensitive people have an allergic reaction to chamomile's pollen-rich flower heads and, sometimes, to chamomile tea as well. Discontinue use if you develop any negative reaction.)

❐ Slather on the sunscreen. Look for a sun protection factor (SPF) of 15 or greater. In addition, wear wraparound sunglasses to protect the entire eye area.

DAYTIME

Prescriptions
FOR LIGHTENING THE DARKNESS

If hyperpigmentation—not dilated blood vessels—is to blame for your dark circles, you might be able to lighten them with bleaching creams. Skin creams containing natural fruit derivatives known as alpha hydroxy acids (AHAs), ascorbic acid (vitamin C), or Retin A may also help. But don't expect a miracle, says Dr. Vidimos. "You can lighten the dark circles somewhat, but I've never seen them disappear 100 percent."

Also, lightening takes time. Expect to wait three to six months before you notice improvement in the color and texture of your skin.

MONTHLY

❐ Reach for an over-the-counter bleaching cream containing 2 percent hydroquinone (such as Porcelana), suggests Dr. Vidimos.

❐ Give AHAs a try. Derived from sugarcane (glycolic acid), fruits (citric, malic, and tartaric acids), and sour milk (lactic acid), these mild natural acids can improve the appearance of dark circles by sloughing off dead cells on the skin's surface and speeding up cell renewal. Because the skin around the eyes is so sensitive, choose an AHA product made especially for use on this area, advises Dr. Vidimos.

❐ If a skin bleaching cream or an AHA product alone doesn't get results, try a combination, says Dr. Vidimos. Apply an AHA lotion or cream suitable for use around the eyes. Next apply a 2 percent hydroquinone product (be careful not to get any in your eyes) and let it dry. Using the two products together actually works faster than using either

NIGHTTIME

one alone. But if the combination irritates your skin, alternate products by applying hydroquinone in the morning and AHAs at night.

❏ Try a topical cream containing the vitamin C derivative magnesium ascorbyl phosphate. Make sure the product you choose has been labeled for use around the eyes, says Dr. Lupo. (One brand is Vivifying Serum C. You can receive ordering information for this product by writing to Skin Care System, P.O. Box 24220, New Orleans, LA 70184.)

DAYTIME

❏ Whatever method you try, be sure to apply sunscreen whenever you go outdoors. Otherwise, dark circles will reappear.

PROFESSIONAL
Rx

Prescription
FOR UNDER-EYE SHADOWS

If you have dark circles, chances are that you have tried wearing a concealer cream. The right cream, when used correctly, can help, according to Cynde Watson, the national makeup artist for Bobbi Brown Essentials in New York City. Still, many women choose the wrong color for their skin tone or use a concealer that is too chalky or too dry.

To conceal dark circles like the pros, Watson recommends the following steps.

❏ Before applying concealer, use a moisturizer or eye cream to hydrate the area under the eye.

❏ Choose a yellow-based concealer. The yellow base neutralizes red, pink, and purple colors in the skin and conceals almost anything, including dark circles. "I'm sold on yellow-based concealer," says Watson. "I use it on all skin tones."

❏ Stay close to your natural skin color, especially if you don't wear foundation. Otherwise, use a concealer that is one shade lighter than your skin tone, but no lighter. "Most women choose a concealer that is too light. Or its undertones are too pink or too white for their skin tone," Watson explains.

❏ Use a *stick* concealer. "Concealers come in sticks, tubes, and pots, but the best concealer is the stick concealer because it is creamier and easier to apply," says Watson. Concealers in tubes are water-based and tend to be drier than stick concealers, she adds. And concealers in pots are "usually very, very dry and don't move as well."

THE CONCEALER TRICK

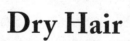

Using a thin, firm brush, apply concealer within the dark circle. Apply more near your nose, where the circle is darker, and less toward the outer corner of your eye, as shown. Using a brush enables you to get underneath the eyelashes and into the crease of the eye near the nose. Gently pat the concealer into your skin with one or two fingertips. Don't rub—rubbing removes the concealer.

❐ Use a brush to apply the stick concealer underneath the eyelashes and toward the nose, an area most women forget to cover, says Watson.

❐ Apply foundation. Use a sponge to apply a yellow-based foundation—one shade darker than your concealer—to your face. Pat the foundation over the concealer, taking care not to rub the under-eye area.

❐ After applying the foundation, dust lightly with a yellow-based powder.

❐ Play up your other features. To draw attention away from your dark circles, apply eyeliner and mascara to the upper lids only. Groom your eyebrows. And shun blue and purple eye shadows and mascaras in favor of earthier tones.

Dry Hair

When salon owner Salvador Calvano moved from Chicago to Phoenix, he was amazed by the dryness of people's hair and skin. Much to his dismay, he found his own normally well-oiled hair behaving badly for the first time in his life, courtesy of the arid climate.

Now, thanks to a hair-care regimen that includes daily cleansing with a moisturizing shampoo and frequent deep conditioning, Calvano's hair has regained its healthy shine and feel. His clients at Cutter's Hair Salon and Day Spa in Phoenix have adopted his regimen, too—with fantastic results.

An arid climate is just one of many causes of dry hair, which lacks shine and feels brittle or coarse to the touch, says Diana Bihova, M.D., a dermatologist in New York City and author of *Beauty from the Inside Out*. Other culprits include exposure to the sun or chlorine, overprocessing with chemicals, overuse or misuse of styling implements such as blow-dryers and curling irons, and poorly made brushes and combs.

These things dry out your hair by damaging the outer layer of each hair shaft, called the cuticle. The cuticle is made up of cells that overlap, kind of like shingles on a roof. Normally, these cells lie flat, which holds in moisture and reflects light. Your hair feels and looks healthy and shiny. When the cuticle cells get roughed up, the hair shaft loses moisture and doesn't reflect light as well. The result is hair that looks dull and feels coarse to the touch.

Rx —— *Prescriptions*
TO CARE FOR DESERT-DRY HAIR

These days, you can choose from among dozens of commercial shampoos and conditioners. Each one claims to fix a specific hair problem, such as dryness. How do you know which one will work best for you?

One way to find out is through trial and error: Purchase sample-size bottles of various products and try them until you find a shampoo and conditioner that you like. To narrow your search—and to get the most benefit from the products you choose—heed this advice from the experts.

❒ Select a shampoo that lists aloe among the first five items in its ingredient list. Calvano swears by aloe's moisturizing properties.

❒ Look for shampoos that contain natural oils, glycerin, honey, or amino acids. Like aloe, these ingredients are moisturizers. Shampoos that contain them will gently cleanse your hair without drying it out, explains Dr. Bihova.

❒ Each time you shampoo, follow with an instant conditioner specially formulated for dry hair. A conditioner coats your hair and minimizes damage from brushing, combing, and drying, says David Cannell, Ph.D., senior vice president of research and development for Redken Laboratories in New York City. It may add shine to your hair, too.

❏ Deep-condition your hair for 20 minutes every 7 to 10 shampoos, suggests Dr. Cannell. How often you do it depends on how dry your hair is. Deep-conditioning products restore shine to your hair and help fill in nicks and chips in each strand's damaged outer layer. Look for a product that contains lanolin, vitamin E, balsam, or protein.

❏ If you choose a hot-oil treatment as your deep conditioner, apply moist heat to your hair for 20 minutes to improve the oil's penetration. The heat provides energy, which increases the speed at which the oil seeps into the hair shaft.

If you have access to a steam room, spread the oil onto your hair and then sit in the steam with your head uncovered. Otherwise, apply the oil, then wrap a comfortably hot, wet towel around your head and leave it on during your bath. "Especially if you have really dry hair, you need to allow at least 20 minutes for the oil to penetrate," says Dr. Cannell.

Prescriptions
for a Dry-Defying Do

Rx

Of course, washing and conditioning is merely a prelude to the "mane" event: styling. But blow-dryers, curling irons, and harsh chemicals can conspire to sap the moisture from your hair, leaving it brittle and unmanageable. With the right styling implements and products, used in the right way, you can have healthy, head-turning tresses. These tips will help.

❏ Choose a boar-bristle brush. This type of brush works best for styling because the smooth, natural bristles are kinder to and gentler on dry hair, according to Dr. Cannell. Be aware, though, that a boar-bristle brush is a lot pricier than a plastic-bristle brush.

❏ If you opt for a brush with plastic bristles, make sure that the bristles have beads on the ends. Steer clear of brushes whose bristles have rough edges, advises Dr. Cannell.

❏ As for a comb, look for one that is carved from a solid piece of hard rubber. This design—called saw cut—prevents the hair from

Prescriptions to Moisturize Your Mane

Can't find a commercial conditioner you like? Make your own instead. The following two recipes can help rehydrate dry tresses, according to Kathi Keville, director of the American Herb Association in Nevada City, California, and author of *Herbs for Health and Healing.* You will find most of these ingredients in health food stores (the exception is burdock root, which you may have to special-order).

TIME IT RIGHT

❐ Add six drops each of lavender, bay, and sandalwood essential oils to six ounces of warm sesame or soy oil, suggests Greenwich, Connecticut, aromatherapist Judith Jackson, author of *Scentual Touch: A Personal Guide to Aromatherapy* and *The Magic of Well-Being.* Part your hair into one-inch sections and apply the oil blend to your scalp with a wad of cotton. Wrap your head in a towel and leave it on for about 15 minutes. Then uncover your hair and shampoo it twice.

❐ Combine one teaspoon of each of the following herbs: burdock root, calendula flowers, chamomile flowers, lavender flowers, and rosemary leaves. Pour one pint of freshly boiled water over the herbs and allow them to steep for about 30 minutes. Strain the mixture and add one tablespoon vinegar to it. Shampoo your hair, then pour the herbal conditioner over it, suggests Keville. Don't rinse your hair, she adds—simply dry and style it as usual.

catching, sticking, and breaking, says Dr. Cannell. Most hairstylists use saw-cut combs, so if you can't find one or don't know what to look for, ask your stylist for assistance.

❐ Use a comb to untangle wet hair, starting at the ends and slowly working toward the roots. Wet hair stretches by as much as 40 to 50 percent. So if you comb your hair too vigorously, you can snap it like a rubber band, says Philip Kingsley, owner of Philip Kingsley Trichological Centres in London and New York City and author of *Hair: An Owner's Handbook*.

❏ If you blow-dry your hair, spray it first with a thermal styling conditioner such as HeatSafe or Redken's Airset or One 2 One Smooth. The moisturizers in these products protect your hair from the dryer's hot air.

❏ To blow-dry your hair, start by gently squeezing your hair with a towel to remove as much water as possible. Turn your blow-dryer on high to remove the water from the surface of your hair and from in between the strands. As your hair begins to feel dry, switch to a low setting to style your hair. Keep the blow-dryer six to eight inches from your head at all times. This technique protects your hair from heat damage, and the cool air helps fix the style, says Dr. Cannell.

❏ Put two drops of sandalwood or rosemary essential oil on your fingertips and massage it into the ends of your hair. These oils help tame dry, wispy hair without leaving your hair greasy, says Kathi Keville, director of the American Herb Association in Nevada City, California, and author of *Herbs for Health and Healing*.

❏ If you have your hair permed, straightened, or colored, consider switching to a new, chemical-free hairstyle. Treating your hair with chemicals can leave it dry, drab, and lifeless, says Calvano.

❏ Trim your hair once a month. This removes dry, dull ends and keeps hair looking healthier, says Calvano.

MONTHLY

Prescriptions
FOR REVIVING DEHYDRATED LOCKS

Rx

Besides adjusting your daily hair-care routine, you can take other steps to keep your tresses in tip-top shape. They include the following strategies.

❏ Eat fish rich in omega-3 fatty acids at least twice a week, suggests Earl Mindell, R.Ph., Ph.D., professor of nutrition at Pacific Western University in Los Angeles and author of *Earl Mindell's Secret Remedies*.

Salmon, trout, whitefish, and fresh tuna all have abundant supplies of omega-3's, which help replenish moisture in dry hair.

❐ Massage your scalp with your fingertips for at least three minutes every day. Massage increases circulation to your scalp and may help redistribute the existing oils on your scalp, says Dr. Cannell.

❐ When you spend time in the sun, wear a lightweight, tightly woven hat with a wide brim that wraps around your entire head. A hat protects your hair from the sun's ultraviolet rays, which make your hair dry and brittle and reduce its shine.

❐ For additional protection from the sun, use a hair spray or another styling product that contains sunscreen or a sun filter, such as octyl-dimethyl PABA. Check the product labels for specific sun protection factors (SPFs).

❐ If you swim in a chlorinated pool, apply conditioner to your hair before you get in the water, then tuck your hair into a swim cap. When you get out of the pool, thoroughly rinse your hair and shampoo as usual. This not only safeguards your hair against the drying effects of the chlorine but also gives your hair a good conditioning, says Ted Gibson, global hair-care educator for Aveda Lifestyle Products, based in New York City.

Expression Lines

The more we experience life's ups and downs, it seems the more the results show up on our faces in the form of laugh and frown lines, brow furrows, lip lines, and crow's-feet. In fact, expressive people tend to get deeper lines than others, says William P. Coleman III, M.D., clinical professor of dermatology at Tulane University in New Orleans. Conversely, people who go through life with straight faces keep their skin looking smoother longer.

"If you look at people who are never animated, who rarely express their emotions, they tend to have beautiful skin," Dr. Coleman says.

Expression lines begin to appear on a woman's face when she is in her late twenties. Typically, they are visible only when she is smiling, squinting, or otherwise moving her face, according to Nelson Lee Novick, M.D., associate clinical professor of dermatology at Mount Sinai School of Medicine of the City University of New York in New York City and author of *You Can Look Younger at Any Age*. By the midthirties, wrinkles begin to show up around her mouth, eyelids, and across her forehead; by the end of the decade, smile lines may emerge.

In the forties, crow's-feet appear, and forehead worry lines and brow furrows become more prominent. This is the decade when the results of past sun damage appear. By her fifties and sixties, a woman's skin is drier and less elastic, and facial lines and furrows deepen and curve downward.

While expression lines are unavoidable, how deep and obvious they become depends on heredity (which we can't control) and other factors (which we can control).

Prescriptions Rx
FOR CROW'S-FEET AND LAUGH LINES

If you never cracked a smile, you wouldn't have any laugh lines. You also wouldn't have any fun. And that's no way to go through life. Thankfully, there are some things that you can do to keep expression lines from deepening.

❏ Slather on sunscreen daily. "Over time, the sun damages collagen and elastin (skin proteins that make the skin firm and stretchy), causing skin to become thinner and more lax," explains Lorrie J. Klein, M.D., a dermatologist in private practice in Laguna Niguel, California. So with repeated facial expressions, tanned skin wrinkles more easily. Daily use of a sunscreen with a sun protection factor (SPF) of at least 15 not only prevents further damage to your skin but it also allows the skin to continue its normal active renewal process, she says.

DAYTIME

❏ For extended protection while you are outside, apply a sunscreen with an SPF of 30 or higher *before* you head out the door, advises Jonathan Weiss, M.D., assistant clinical professor of dermatology at Emory University in Atlanta and a dermatologist in Snellville, Georgia. Smooth it over all exposed areas. The higher SPF means that you may not have to reapply the sunscreen as frequently.

TIME IT RIGHT

❏ If you stay cool and dry, you can wait about three hours before reapplying sunscreen.

TIME IT RIGHT

❏ If you sweat, swim, or towel off, reapply the sunscreen after 80 minutes.

MORNING

❏ To save a step in your beauty routine, choose a moisturizer with a built-in SPF of 15 and smooth it on in the morning under your makeup. Even if you know that you are going to spend most of your day indoors, you still need sun protection for those infrequent trips outside, says Dr. Weiss.

❏ Keep your hands away from your eyes. The delicate skin around the eyes tends to stretch and wrinkle in response to rubbing. "The eyes are the first area where people begin to show aging," says Margaret Weiss, M.D., a dermatologist and assistant professor of dermatology at the Johns Hopkins Medical Institutions in Baltimore.

DAYTIME

❏ Always wear wraparound sunglasses in bright or hazy outdoor light. Sunglasses may help prevent crow's-feet because they stop you from squinting, says Dr. Klein. They also cover and protect the delicate skin around the eyes.

❏ Wear a broad-rimmed hat to shade out the sun. This, too, will help you avoid squinting, but it will also protect your face from overall sun damage.

❏ Toss the cigarettes. Pursing your lips repeatedly as you smoke forms permanent pucker lines above the lips. "Smokers ages 40 and over often have severe pucker lines," says Dr. Coleman. Smoking also worsens crow's-feet because smokers squint to keep irritating smoke out of their eyes.

Rx —— *Prescriptions*
FOR SMOOTHING OUT FACIAL LINES

While you can't wipe expression lines completely off your face, using the right skin-care products can lessen their appearance.

❒ Use a moisturizer with alpha hydroxy acids (AHAs). "Alpha hydroxy acids provide an important means of reversing some of the changes that we see in aging and sun-damaged skin," says Dr. Margaret Weiss. AHAs are a group of naturally occurring acids that are derived from plants, fruits, and other food products, such as sugarcane (glycolic acid), apples (malic acid), and sour milk (lactic acid). Available over the counter in lotions, creams, and gels, alpha hydroxy acids smooth the skin by sloughing off dead skin cells and exposing the younger ones underneath. They also plump the skin and restore its ability to retain moisture.

MORNING

To smooth out skin texture, use an 8 percent AHA preparation twice a day, suggests Dr. Klein. Apply the cream to your face in the morning after you bathe, while your skin is still wet, to trap moisture. Then reapply it at night.

❒ For the areas around your eyes, use a 5 percent AHA eye cream. (Don't apply it directly to your eyelids.) And if the skin around your eyes is especially sensitive, choose a fragrance-free AHA cream, says Dr. Klein.

❒ Try beta hydroxy acids. In some women, alpha hydroxy acids can sting or irritate sensitive skin. A milder alternative is a salicylic acid called beta hydroxy acid, found in products such as Clinique's Turnaround Cream. Like AHA, beta hydroxy acid reduces the signs of fine lines and wrinkles by exfoliating the skin, but with less irritation, says Debra Price, M.D., clinical assistant professor of dermatology at the University of Miami School of Medicine and a dermatologist in South Miami.

Fine Hair

Soon after *Charlie's Angels* made its television debut in 1976, women were begging their stylists for hair that looked just like Farrah Fawcett's: thick and voluminous, with long, cascading curls. For some, the style worked. But for those with fine hair, all the primping in the world couldn't make their locks even remotely resemble those of the prime-time goddess.

Hair has endured many fads and trends since then. And through it all, fine hair has insisted on doing its own thing. What makes this hair type so difficult to control is the thinner-than-normal hair shaft. Yes, it gives fine hair a baby-soft, silky feel. But it also makes fine hair very difficult to style.

These days, you can arm yourself with an entire arsenal of hair sprays, mousses, and volumizers that promise to fluff up fine hair. But these products will do you little good if you don't pay attention to the basics of fine-hair care, says Carmine Minardi, owner of Minardi Salon in New York City.

What are these basics? Minardi cites three: appropriate products, proper styling techniques, and a flattering cut.

Rx —— *Prescriptions*
FOR HAIR HYGIENE

Fine-hair care begins the moment you lather up. The right shampoos and conditioners give your hair body and volume. The wrong ones weigh down hair and make it more difficult to manage, says Minardi. To choose your products wisely and use them properly, follow this advice from the hair-care professionals.

❑ Wash your hair every day. This prevents oil from building up on your scalp, so your hair looks healthy rather than flat and limp, explains Minardi.

❑ Use a shampoo that is protein-based. Protein coats the hair shaft and makes hair appear fuller and thicker. You can identify protein-based shampoos by words such as *body-building*, *thickening*, and *volumizing* on their labels.

❑ If you wash your hair more than once a day, switch to a mild baby shampoo after the first time. Baby shampoo cleans your hair without stripping away its natural oil. Your hair won't become overly dry and prone to breakage. This is especially good for people who work out a lot and who wash their hair a couple of times a day, says Diana Bihova, M.D., a dermatologist in New York City and author of *Beauty from the Inside Out*.

❐ Avoid shampoos that also condition. They tend to coat and flatten fine hair with a slick film.

❐ Use a light instant conditioner each time you shampoo. Look for a product labeled as "detangling" or "lightweight." Heavier products can make fine hair look limp and feel greasy, says Minardi.

Prescriptions
for Fail-Safe Styling

Rx

While clean, conditioned hair cooperates better, getting it to do what you want it to still presents a challenge. Fine hair can pouf out perfectly, only to fall flat an hour later. For a more enduring coif, try these styling secrets.

❐ After washing your hair, vigorously dry it with a towel to remove excess water. Vigorous rubbing will rough up the hair cuticle to add body, says Minardi.

❐ Use a wide-tooth comb to remove tangles from wet hair. A brush stretches wet hair, causing it to break more easily, explains Dr. Bihova.

❐ Scrunch your hair with your fingers, then let it air-dry. This technique gives your hair extra lift, so it appears fuller, says Ted Gibson, global hair-care educator for Aveda Lifestyle Products, based in New York City.

❐ For even more volume, air-dry or blow-dry your hair until it is just the slightest bit damp. Then set your hair with rollers, spritz it with hair spray or a thermal styling conditioner such as Neutrogena HeatSafe or Redken Hot Sets, and give it a quick blast of heat with your blow-dryer. Remove the rollers and style your hair as usual. Refrain from smoothing out a blow-dried style with a curling iron. This just robs hair of the volume that blow-drying creates, says Minardi.

❐ Apply a cream remoisturizer to add shine to fine hair without adding weight. Steer clear of silicone products, which weigh down fine hair, according to Minardi.

All the Right Fluff

Blow-drying can give lift and volume to fine hair—if you do it properly. The following styling sequence can work wonders for fine hair, according to Carmine Minardi, owner of Minardi Salon in New York City. All you need (besides a blow-dryer, of course) are mousse or styling gel, maybe a thermal blow-dry setting lotion, and a medium or large, round boar-bristle brush. The size brush you choose depends on the length of your hair and the amount of body desired. A medium brush produces more body, while a large brush produces less. With patience and practice, you will be wielding your blow-dryer like a pro in no time.

▶ Vigorously towel-dry just-washed hair to remove excess water.

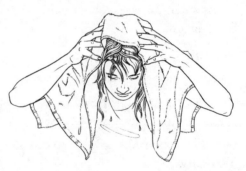

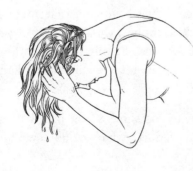

◀ Bend forward so that your hair hangs down, then apply mousse or styling gel at the roots. Massage the mousse or gel into your entire scalp, covering the back and top of your head. Pay special attention to the crown and temples. Return to an upright position.

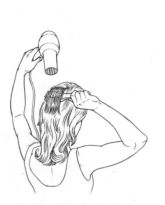

▶ Starting at the back of your neck, place your brush underneath a section of hair. Set your blow-dryer on medium and direct the air away from your scalp, from the roots toward the ends. Continue until your hair feels dry to the touch. (Overdrying leads to static electricity and diminished volume.) Then roll your brush under one time at the ends and dry your hair for five seconds. Remove the brush and repeat these two steps with the next section of hair. Once you finish all of the hair at the back of your neck, move on to your head's midsection, working out toward your ears. Then proceed to the crown area and the temples. Continue working the sections until your hair is dry.

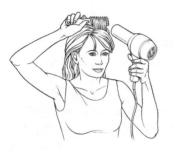

◀ You're now ready to move to the top of your head in front of the crown. Pull your hair straight up with your brush and dry it. Make sure that the dryer nozzle is always directing the air from the roots to the ends. When you reach the ends, turn the brush backward one time and dry for five seconds. Your goal is to lift your hair at its roots and make it "bend" at the ends. When you're finished, allow your hair to cool.

▶ For extra height or lift at the front hairline, lightly spritz your hair with thermal blow-dry setting lotion or spray mousse. Then using your fingers or your brush, lift your hair at the roots in the direction you want it to go. Set the style with a quick blast of air from your blow-dryer at its lowest heat. After your hair is dry, you can add even more body with the help of hot rollers. Set your hair with the rollers and then lightly mist it with a mild hair spray.

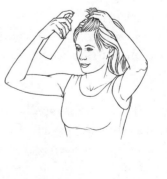

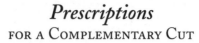

Rx

Prescriptions
FOR A COMPLEMENTARY CUT

If you still find your hair hard to manage, you may want to consider a new style. The right cut naturally gives your hair lift and volume, so you don't have to fuss with it so much, says Minardi. The next time you visit your stylist, mention the following options to help her create the ideal do for you.

❏ If you have a narrow or thin face, try wearing your hair in a blunt bob. This cut adds width to your face, notes Minardi.

❏ If you have a round face or broad cheekbones, wear your hair in short, two- to four-inch layers. Your hair appears higher on top, longer at the back of your neck, and less poufy on the sides. As a result, your face looks longer and less round, says Minardi.

❏ Avoid hairstyles that are shoulder-length or longer. The weight of your hair drags down the style, explains Minardi. That means your hair appears even flatter and finer.

❏ To tie back fine hair, use cloth bands with plenty of give, like scrunchies. Rubber bands damage all hair types, but fine hair is especially vulnerable, says Gibson.

❏ For longer-lasting body and bounce, consider getting a loose perm. A tight perm could cause problems. "When you curl fine hair too tightly, you get volume, but you also rough up each hair's cuticle (its protective outer layer) too much," says Minardi. "That makes your hair appear frizzy."

❏ To give hair extra volume, color it. The color penetrates the cuticle, causing it to swell. Your hair looks and feels thicker. "In my experience, coloring gives hair 30 to 50 percent more body than what it normally would have," notes Minardi. Use a product that is ammonia- or peroxide-based.

Medical **Alert**

If your hair is rapidly thinning or falling out, see your dermatologist as soon as possible. Either condition may signal an underlying health problem, such as iron-deficiency anemia or a thyroid disorder. Thinning hair and hair loss have also been linked to crash dieting, stress, and certain medications, according to Dr. Bihova.

Frizzy Hair

When it comes to hair, genes don't always play fair. Women with stick-straight strands may spend a small fortune on perms in pursuit of natural-looking curls. Women with natural curls may spend a small fortune on contraptions and concoctions in pursuit of stick-straight strands. Either way, the end result is usually the same: a bad case of the frizzies.

Women have frizzy hair for one of two reasons, according to David Cannell, Ph.D., senior vice president of research and development for Redken Laboratories in New York City. First, your hair can have a natural-wave pattern that lends itself to frizziness. When you are in damp or humid conditions, your hair absorbs too much moisture. The curls push away from each other, giving them a frizzy appearance.

Second, your hair can become frizzy from overprocessing, says Dr. Cannell. "If you have had three or four perms, for example, your hair develops a tighter wave pattern at the ends. As a result, your hair takes on a flyaway look."

Just because your mane has a mind of its own doesn't mean that you should let it have its way. "People think their hair is wild, unruly, and unmanageable because they don't really know how to work with it," says Ouidad, owner of Ouidad Salon in New York City and Ouidad Hair Care Division, a mail-order service specializing in products formulated for frizzy hair. "Once you have your hair in top condition, it's so easy to maintain. It's carefree."

You can liken controlling the frizzies to caring for a houseplant, according to Ouidad. "You have to wipe the leaves of a plant (shampoo your hair and scalp) to keep them clean, feed the plant (condition your hair) to give it the nourishment it needs, and remove dead leaves (trim your hair) to weed out unhealthy growth."

Prescriptions
FOR CLEANSING YOUR CURLS

Calming your hair's wild side begins with proper shampooing and conditioning techniques, says Ouidad. Try incorporating the following strategies into your personal hair-care routine.

❒ Wash your hair in the morning. "If you wash it at night, you are going to get that matted look known as bed head," says Ouidad. "You'll have to rewet your hair in the morning before you can do anything with it. That defeats the whole purpose of shampooing it at night."

❒ Place a quarter-size dollop of shampoo in the palm of one hand, then massage it onto your scalp and through your hair with your fingertips. If your hair is either very long or very short, you can adjust the amount of shampoo accordingly. Just remember that your goal is to remove sebum (a mixture of fatty acids that prevents your scalp from drying out), not to scrub every strand of hair, root to tip. Use what Ouidad calls a piano technique—that is, move your fingers downward through your hair as though you were playing a piano. Avoid scratching your scalp with your fingernails. Any shampoo specifically formulated for dry or damaged hair will work. These products often contain ingredients such as vitamin E, mineral oil, glycerin, and aloe vera.

❒ Allow your hair to hang down as you wash it. Bunching your hair on top of your head, as many women do, causes breakage, according to Ouidad. Remember that frizzy hair is often baby-fine and extremely delicate.

❒ Apply a daily detangler after each washing. Place a quarter-size amount of the detangler in the palm of one hand, rub your hands together, and work it into your hair. Then run a wide-toothed comb through your hair to gently detangle your hair while it is still wet. Work in small sections, beginning at the ends and moving toward your scalp. Allow your hair to hang behind you so that the water helps shape the curls. Stop when you are about one inch from your scalp. This gives your scalp a chance to breathe, explains Ouidad. Leave the detangler on for two to three minutes so that it has time to plump each strand with protein moisture. Then rinse your hair, leaving a little of the detangler in.

When you are shopping for a detangler, be sure to steer clear of those that are heavy, waxy, or silicone-based.

❒ Use a protein-based deep conditioner twice a month until you notice improvement in your hair. Then cut back to once a month. "A daily conditioner is designed to detangle hair," notes Ouidad. "A deep conditioner may help repair damage." A good protein-based deep conditioner penetrates the hair shaft and fills the hair from the inside with protein. This enhances the hair's ability to repel moisture. She recommends using a product that has wheat germ or soybean protein as its main ingredient rather than wax, paraffin, or animal fat, which merely coats the exterior of the hair shaft.

You will find an array of deep conditioners on the market. Experiment until you find one that is right for you.

Note: If you apply color to your hair, refrain from using "heated" deep conditioners (such as hot-oil treatments) for at least 10 days afterward, cautions Ouidad. Heat relaxes the outer layer of the hair shaft, called the cuticle, causing the color to seep out of the hair follicle. As a result, the color fades or turns brassy.

Prescriptions
FOR FRIZZ-FREE STYLING

Rx

Call it the law of the unmanageable mane: The more you handle and manipulate your hair, the more uncooperative it becomes. But as Ouidad points out, the opposite also holds true: The less you fuss with your hair, the less it will frizz. The following tips will help you achieve the hairstyle you want with minimum effort.

❒ After washing and conditioning, drape a towel over your head and gently squeeze your hair to remove excess water. Refrain from creating a "towel turban": It can weaken your hair and lead to breakage, says Ouidad.

❒ Apply molding gel to your hair. Molding gel acts like a raincoat for your hair, protecting it from environmental elements and keeping out excessive moisture, says Carmine Minardi, owner of Minardi Salon in New York City.

❒ For extra shine and control, add six to eight drops of a silicone product, such as Frizz-Ease, to a quarter-size dollop of molding gel. Combine the two in the palm of your hand, then work them through your hair while it's still damp. This seals in the good, protein moisture of your hair while sealing out bad, frizz-causing moisture from environmental elements such as humidity, rain, and wind. Your curls look curly rather than frizzy, explains Minardi.

If you have fine hair, don't use silicone products. They are too heavy and make fine hair look limp and dull.

❏ Work gel into wet hair in sections. Start at the nape of your neck, working toward the center of your head. Then spread out from ear to ear, paying careful attention to the crown area at the center of your head. Finally, work your way to your forehead and hairline area, distributing the gel evenly throughout the hair. "I find that a lot of people tend to apply gels wrong," says Ouidad. "They rub from front to back, then flip their hair forward and rub from back to front. They do the sides of their heads, and that's it. The center never gets touched, yet that's the curliest spot. Then during the day, their hair expands and frizzes, and they think the gel isn't working."

❏ While your hair is wet, use long clips to position curls. Lift your hair at the roots and insert the clips wherever you want to create height. "When hair is wet, it has a memory," notes Ouidad. "You can manipulate it to create a shape that frames your face."

❏ Allow your hair to air-dry. Blow-drying dehydrates hair, which causes it to frizz. And don't worry about arriving at the office with wet hair: Curly hair, when conditioned properly, dries rapidly, according to Ouidad.

❏ Steer clear of diffusers, too. A diffuser creates volume by opening the hair cuticle, according to Minardi. And that, in turn, creates frizz.

❏ Use a boar-bristle brush to style your hair. Boar bristles are very soft and, in combination with a light gel, help keep the hair cuticle lying flat. "The flatter the cuticle, the less frizz you'll have," explains Minardi.

❏ To reduce the bushiness of your hair, use a straightening or flattening iron. This newfangled contraption, available in drugstores and beauty supply stores, looks like a pair of tongs with two plates attached. Place your hair between the plates, then gently glide the iron over the surface of your hair to straighten curly strands, says Minardi. But be careful. Although these irons have heat governors on them, if your hair has been overprocessed or severely damaged, it may become more dehydrated and frizzy. Your hair may also snap and break because of the loss of elasticity. Minardi cautions people with shorter hair to keep the iron away from the scalp and hairline area to prevent a burn.

❏ If you have naturally frizzy hair, consider a mild chemical relaxer. A chemical relaxer may actually tame naturally frizzy hair because it relaxes the hair shaft and weakens the curl pattern, explains Minardi. The hair cuticle becomes softer, which means less frizz.

Ask your hairstylist to apply a solution made from sodium hydroxide and a good protein-based deep conditioner. The solution softens the effect of the curls and helps to tame frizz, says Ouidad.

❏ Choose a hairstyle that complements the texture of your hair. Avoid layered cuts, blunt cuts, and cuts that are short on top. These make curls shrink up and stick out, so your hair has a poufed appearance, says Ouidad. Frizzy hair behaves better when it is worn longer because the weight of the hair helps to tame the frizz. A close crop is both easy to manage and stylish, if you have the courage to go short.

It is a good idea to see a stylist who has experience working with frizzy, curly hair. She may be able to cut your hair in such a way that it meshes together and appears less bulky. The result is a soft, light style that allows your curls to flow like a waterfall.

Melasma (Mask of Pregnancy)

Pregnant women are sometimes surprised to find that they develop pigmented blotches on their cheeks, foreheads, upper lips, and necks. Called melasma, or mask of pregnancy, this condition may also affect women who take the Pill or hormone-replacement therapy (HRT).

Rarely seen in men, melasma can result from excess levels of the female hormone estrogen (whether prompted by pregnancy, oral contraceptives, or HRT) and sun exposure, says Edward Bondi, M.D., professor of dermatology at the University of Pennsylvania Medical Center in Philadelphia. "But one out of three women with melasma has no evidence of estrogen excess. For her, any estrogen plus sunlight will do it."

For some women, the patchy pigmentation fades away following pregnancy or once oral contraceptive use or hormone therapy ends. But for others, melasma may be permanent or may come and go. It may disappear after one pregnancy, for example, then return with the next. Also, women who have had melasma during pregnancy are more likely to get it again while taking oral contraceptives or HRT than are women who have never had melasma.

If you are on birth control pills or HRT and have melasma, talk to your doctor. A change in your prescription may help. You may be reacting to the dose of estrogen or the type of progesterone in your prescription, says Wilma F. Bergfeld, M.D., a dermapathologist for the Cleveland Clinic Foundation, head of clinical research in the department of dermatology at the Cleveland Clinic in Cleveland, and author of *A Woman Doctor's Guide to Skin Care*.

Rx — *Prescriptions*
FOR EVADING SOLAR-INDUCED SPOTS

Doctors don't have a really good medical treatment for melasma, says Dr. Bondi. So the best prescription for melasma is prevention, he says. That is, stay away from the sun's harmful rays, especially when you are pregnant, on the Pill, or taking HRT. Here's how.

❏ Stay indoors or under shade—especially if you are pregnant. Many women soak up the sun for comfort and cosmetic reasons, says Dr. Bondi. "I think that's a mistake. Getting a lot of sun while you are pregnant is inviting melasma."

❏ Use a sunscreen with a sun protection factor (SPF) of 15 or higher, especially on your face. Look for sunscreens that protect the skin from ultraviolet-A (UVA) and ultraviolet-B (UVB) forms of sunlight, advises Dr. Bondi.

❏ Even with sunscreen, exposure to sunlight can darken melasma. So for added protection, apply an opaque foundation over your sunscreen, says Dr. Bondi. Then top it off with a powder.

❑ Watch the clock, and avoid direct sunlight from 10:00 A.M. to 3:00 P.M., when the sun's rays are most intense.

DAYTIME

❑ Whenever you go outdoors, wear a broad-brimmed hat to further minimize exposure.

DAYTIME

Prescriptions
FOR UNMASKING MELASMA

Rx

"If you already have melasma, the mainstay of treatment is use of products with hydroquinone (a bleaching agent) plus sunscreens that block against UVA and UVB rays," says Dr. Bondi. "Hydroquinone helps fade the pigmented blotches, while sunscreen helps prevent further darkening." To make stubborn patches disappear, he suggests these steps.

❑ Apply a 2 percent hydroquinone cream (such as Porcelana) twice a day. Be sure to cover the cream with a sunscreen with an SPF of 15 or higher, says Dr. Bondi. It may take three to six months of treatment to see improvement. If dark patches persist, the treatment can be continued indefinitely.

❑ Add a moisturizing cream containing alpha hydroxy acids (AHAs) to your daily beauty routine. Derived from sugarcane, fruit, or milk, AHAs are mild natural acids that exfoliate dead cells on the skin's surface and speed up the skin's ability to replace them with newer, fresher ones underneath. You can buy AHA creams without a prescription in strengths of up to 8 percent. But they are weaker than the 10-percent-or-higher versions that your doctor may prescribe, and they show only modest success at fading melasma patches, says Dr. Bondi.

MORNING

To help optimize the effectiveness of an over-the-counter AHA cream, Dr. Bondi suggests alternating it with a hydroquinone fade cream. Apply one in the morning (always cover it with sunscreen) and the other at night.

❑ For the sensitive area around the eyes, use an over-the-counter AHA preparation containing no more than 5 percent acid, says Mary Lupo, M.D., associate clinical professor of dermatology at Tulane University School of Medicine in New Orleans. Discontinue use if irritation occurs anywhere on the face.

❐ Stay out of the sun until melasma disappears. Even if you wear sunscreen, the discolored patches of skin will darken with exposure to sunlight, according to Dr. Bondi.

Oily Hair

If John Corbett, Ph.D., had his way, the phrase "oily hair" would be banned from our vocabulary. The reason? Contrary to popular belief, "it's not your hair that gets oily, it's your scalp," explains Dr. Corbett, vice president of scientific and technical affairs for Clairol in Stamford, Connecticut.

Like the oil on your skin, the oil on your scalp comes from sebaceous glands, oil-secreting sacs attached to the hair follicles. These glands excrete sebum, a mixture of fatty acids that prevents the scalp from drying out. Too much sebum weighs hair down and prevents strands from lifting at the roots. As a result, hair looks flat, dull, and lifeless.

LIFETIME

Your hormones control how much sebum your sebaceous glands produce. That explains why hair tends to become oilier during puberty, pregnancy, and menopause, when hormonal changes shift sebum production into overdrive, says Diana Bihova, M.D., a dermatologist in New York City and author of *Beauty from the Inside Out*. In fact, women who have oily hair often find that the problem literally dries up once they pass through menopause. Birth control pills that contain mostly androgen, a male sex hormone, tend to stimulate oil production in women and can also cause hair to feel and look greasy, according to Dr. Bihova.

Rx

Prescriptions
TO DEPLETE YOUR HAIR'S OIL SUPPLY

Of course, waiting to go through menopause isn't the most timely means of decreasing the oiliness of your hair. Thankfully, other, more practical remedies exist. "And nowadays, people wash their hair so often that it seldom has a chance to get oily in the first place," says Philip Kingsley, owner of Philip Kingsley Trichological Centres in London and New York City and author of *Hair: An Owner's Handbook*.

To keep your locks looking clean and oil-free, follow this hair-care advice from the pros.

❏ Wash your hair every day, preferably in the morning. You can work up a sweat while you sleep. And sweat leaves your hair looking oily—not to mention matted and unkempt, says Ted Gibson, global hair-care educator for Aveda Lifestyle Products, based in New York City.

MORNING

❏ Find a shampoo that you like. "You want a product that is gentle on your hair, but strong enough to thoroughly cleanse your scalp," says David Cannell, Ph.D., senior vice president of research and development for Redken Laboratories in New York City.

❏ If you can't find a brand that works well on your hair, make your own gentle, herbal shampoo. Just add four drops each of rosemary and lavender essential oils (available in health food stores) to two ounces of any unscented shampoo. Shake the mixture well, then wash your hair as usual. Start off with a quarter-size dollop, adjusting the amount to the length of your hair. Both rosemary and lavender essential oils tone your scalp and add shine to your hair, says Kathi Keville, director of the American Herb Association in Nevada City, California, and author of *Herbs for Health and Healing*.

❏ If your hair is prone to buildup of conditioners and styling products, use a clarifying shampoo every other day, switching between it and your regular shampoo. Clarifying shampoos (also called buildup removers) are rich in cleansers but low in conditioners. They strip oil from your scalp as well as your hair shaft. Look for a product that is high in cleaning agents, such as sodium lauryl sulfate, and low in any kind of conditioner, such as lanolin, suggests Dr. Cannell. Two to try are Neutrogena's Anti-Residue Shampoo and Pantene's Pro-Vitamin Clarifying Shampoo.

❏ If you wash your hair more than once a day, choose a mild baby shampoo for those subsequent soapings. Overusing a clarifying shampoo can actually strip your scalp and hair of too much oil, leaving it dry and damaged.

❏ Avoid protein and balsam shampoos. These products tend to increase oiliness, make hair heavy, and attract dirt, says Keville.

A Prescription for Diminishing Dandruff

Most people think of dandruff as a dry-hair problem. But it occurs with oily hair as well, says Diana Bihova, M.D., a dermatologist in New York City and author of *Beauty from the Inside Out.* "Dandruff results from the abnormally accelerated maturation of skin cells on your scalp," she explains. Essentially, the cells grow up too fast and reach the surface of your scalp too soon. There they build up until they are finally shed in clumps. That's what you see as tiny white flakes.

To banish dandruff and dry out oily hair, choose a dandruff shampoo that contains coal-tar derivatives, such as Neutrogena T/Gel or Sebutone. Both are available over the counter in your local drugstore. The naturally derived coal tar not only reduces oiliness but also adds softness and shine to your hair—without the oils found in conditioners, says Dr. Bihova.

Coal-tar dandruff shampoo may be too harsh for daily use, so be sure to alternate it with your regular shampoo, advises Dr. Bihova.

❒ After shampooing, rinse your hair with vinegar. Vinegar may wash excess oil from your hair and discourage dandruff. It also reduces soap and hard-water residues, leaving your hair shiny, smooth, and soft, says Keville. Simply mix one cup vinegar with one cup water, then pour the solution over your hair as your final rinse. And don't worry about smelling like a salad; vinegar's aroma subsides quickly, she says.

❒ As an alternative to vinegar, rinse your hair with sage tea. Like vinegar, sage may help remove excess oil from your scalp and may reduce dandruff, says Keville. Simply add one teaspoon sage leaves to one cup freshly boiled water and steep for 15 minutes. After the tea has cooled, strain and pour it over your hair. You can buy sage leaves in health food stores and gourmet markets.

❑ If you have fine hair and an oily scalp, try conditioning only the ends of your hair after each washing. Any conditioner will do the trick. "You don't want to put more oil on the surface of your scalp," notes Dr. Cannell. "It only adds to the perception of oiliness."

Prescriptions
FOR GREASELESS GROOMING

While everyday washing keeps oiliness to a minimum, proper grooming counts, too. Try these strategies to keep your hair healthy-looking from breakfast to bedtime.

❑ Brush your hair less often. Depending on your hair type, once or twice a day is plenty. "The more you brush, the more you spread the oil from your scalp to your hair," says Dr. Corbett.

❑ Clean your brushes and combs at least twice a week. You can make your own cleaning solution by adding a capful of shampoo and a few drops of ammonia to a sinkful of water. Soak your brushes and combs in the water, then rinse them thoroughly. This regimen prevents you from re-cycling the dirt and oil on your scalp, says Kingsley.

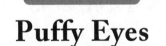

Puffy Eyes

Perhaps it was a sad movie that led to a good, long cry. Or maybe it was a fight over chores with the hubby. Whatever the reason, yesterday's tears have caused today's puffy eyes. And the sight ain't pretty.

Aside from crying, such things as fatigue, allergies, eating salty foods, and even menstruation can prompt your body to collect and retain fluid under the eyes, says Mary Lupo, M.D., associate clinical professor of dermatology at Tulane University School of Medicine in New Orleans. So sometimes—thankfully—puffiness is temporary.

Herbal Prescription for Puffy Eyes

Next time your eyes decide to swell up like a prizefighter's, try applying wet, chilled chamomile tea bags for 10 to 20 minutes. (Squeeze out the excess water first, though.) Chamomile has a constricting effect on the blood vessels, which may help minimize puffiness, says Mary Lupo, M.D., associate clinical professor of dermatology at Tulane University School of Medicine in New Orleans. One caution: If you are allergic to pollen, you may react to the pollen-rich flower heads found in chamomile and, sometimes, chamomile tea. If that's the case, or if this remedy makes your eyes worse instead of better, skip it or discontinue its use.

LIFETIME

But puffy eyes also can develop with age, notes Alan Boyd, M.D., assistant professor of dermatology and pathology at Vanderbilt University in Nashville. As we grow older, the muscles under our eyes weaken and the skin becomes less elastic. Fat tissues push through and around the weakened muscles, creating a puffy appearance that can be aggravated at intervals by fatigue, allergies, and other temporary influences.

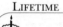

Prescriptions
FOR UNPACKING THOSE BAGS

You can minimize under-eye puffiness—and in some cases, prevent puffiness—with the following strategies recommended by Dr. Lupo.

❐ Steer clear of the saltshaker and salty soups and snacks. As mentioned, too much salt can cause you to retain water under the eyes.

NIGHTTIME

❐ Get plenty of sleep, somewhere between six and eight hours.

❐ Sleep with two standard-size pillows to keep your head slightly elevated. "Lifting your head helps drain any fluids from that pocket underneath your eye," explains Dr. Lupo.

❐ Sleep on your back. Sleeping on your face accentuates puffiness, says Dr. Lupo.

❐ Apply something cold underneath your eyes for 10 to 20 minutes first thing in the morning. "Cold reduces swelling and inflammation, so any type of compress should work," says Dr. Lupo. She suggests an ice cube wrapped in a damp facecloth or chilled iced-tea spoons (keep them in the refrigerator).

MORNING

❐ Act fast. The trauma of crying causes under-eye swelling that can take up to 24 hours to go down, says Dr. Lupo. "If you have cried, start icing the area as soon as you can for about 10 to 20 minutes. The faster you do it, the faster the swelling will go down." If you happen to cry just before sleep, prop yourself up with three or four pillows, and apply a cold compress over your eyes.

TIME IT RIGHT

❐ Use an eye gel. These products contain cucumber or chamomile extracts that penetrate quickly to cool and tone the skin and temporarily relieve puffiness. Using the tip of your finger, apply a thin layer of gel under your eyes twice a day.

Prescriptions
FOR CONCEALING PUFFINESS

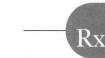

When it comes to hiding puffy eyes, nothing beats a dark pair of wraparound sunglasses for total concealment. And that's not a bad strategy: The last thing you need is an assault of sunlight to further strain delicate skin around the eyes. But what about concealer creams to help camouflage puffiness in indoor light?

"The natural tendency is for women to use a light-shaded cover-up cream on under-eye puffiness," says Carole Walderman, president of Von Lee International School of Aesthetics and Makeup in Baltimore. "But actually, you don't want to put light shades of cover makeup on anything that you are trying to hide—it draws attention to the problem."

The solution? Try the following strategies.

❐ Lighten the nonpuffy area only. With a small, firm brush and a concealer that is a shade lighter than your natural skin color, draw a thin line along the crease, Walderman advises. Gently pat the concealer into the crease with the tip of your ring finger.

❐ After applying the concealer, apply foundation directly to the puffy area. Select a foundation that's close to your skin color, about one shade darker than the concealer. Use your ring finger to dab it onto the puffy area and blend.

❐ If your foundation is oil-based, add a translucent powder to cut the sheen.

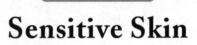

Sensitive Skin

One woman breaks out in an angry, red rash when she dabs on her new cologne, a Valentine's Day gift from her husband. Another gets dry, itchy hands when she switches to a new brand of soap. Yet a third discovers that the makeup she has used without incident for years leaves her face itchy and blotchy.

So it goes with sensitive skin, which can itch, burn, sting, or break out into a red, swollen rash or tiny blisters at the least provocation. Sensitive skin commonly occurs when certain ingredients in cosmetics, skin-care products, and household cleaners irritate the skin. Products that don't bother others—soaps, detergents, shampoos, deodorants, antiperspirants, cosmetics, and bubble baths—can rile women with sensitive skin.

Some women find that their skin is more sensitive at certain times rather than others. Cold, dry weather and allergens in the environment can aggravate sensitive skin and leave it vulnerable to breakouts, says Michael Ramsey, M.D., associate in dermatology at the Geisinger Medical Center in Danville, Pennsylvania.

"When women say that they have sensitive skin, they are usually talking about skin that dries out easily, gets itchy in the winter, or is more prone to react to allergens in the environment," Dr. Ramsey explains. Some women find that the skin on their faces, especially around the eyes, is more sensitive than the skin on the rest of their bodies.

"We don't fully understand why someone gets sensitized to an ingredient that she didn't find irritating before," says Andrew Scheman, M.D., assistant professor of clinical dermatology at Northwestern University in Chicago and author of the *Cosmetics Buying Guide*. Perhaps a lower-grade problem has gradually worsened over time, or an irritating substance gets into the skin through a cut, burn, or infection. A bad sunburn can increase sensitivity by reducing the skin's protective properties. And the hormonal changes of menopause cause the skin to be drier, and thus more susceptible to the environment. "Usually, if a problem starts where there never was one before, it is due to allergy rather than irritation," he adds.

Sensitive skin reacts in one of two ways. Your skin may be irritated by a new brand of shampoo or harsh household detergents. Or you may be allergic to a fragrance, the formaldehyde resin in nail polish, or any one of a number of possible allergens. Without patch testing by your dermatologist, you may never know whether an irritation or an allergen is behind that red, itchy, dry patch on your skin. You just know that you want it to clear up.

If an allergy is the culprit, you will know to avoid the offending ingredient. If it is irritation, however, the only "cure" is to move on to a milder product and minimize your discomfort.

Prescriptions
FOR IRRITATION-FREE SKIN

Women with sensitive skin approach new products warily, worried lest the newest moisturizer or antiaging cream will cause more problems than it solves. Consider being tested by a dermatologist before wasting time and money in trial and error at the cosmetics counter. To help you along those lines, keep in mind the following precautions.

❒ Use as few skin-care and cosmetic products as possible. Keeping your skin-care regimen simple limits the number of potential irritants that you encounter.

❒ Avoid products with fragrances if you have not been tested by a dermatologist. Fragrance is a number one sensitizer. Read labels and steer clear of products that use words such as *perfume, fragrance,* or *aromatherapy* or that contain any of the botanicals, including chamomile, rosewood, lavender, lemon, and rosemary. An unscented or fragrance-free product may actually contain fragrances to mask the odor of other ingredients, according to Dr. Scheman.

❒ Avoid other top sensitizers. "While virtually anything can cause irritation or an allergic reaction in someone, there are a few agents that I commonly advise sensitive-skin patients to avoid," says Dr. Ramsey. His hit list includes lanolin (derived from sheep wool); benzocaine (a commonly used topical anesthetic found in some sunburn remedies and anti-itch medications); neomycin (a topical antibiotic found in Neosporin and triple-antibiotic ointments); and formaldehyde (found in shampoos, makeup, and many skin-care products). You probably won't see formaldehyde, the second most common sensitizer, listed as an ingredient. Look instead for quaternium #15, DMDM hydantoin, imidazolidinyl urea, diazolidinyl urea, or Bronopol—chemical additives that release formaldehyde over time.

❒ Try hypoallergenic products, which contain fewer skin-irritating fragrances and preservatives. But don't be fooled by the language: Hypoallergenic does not mean nonallergenic. "It simply means that the manufacturer has made a concerted effort to eliminate those ingredients in the product that are well-known allergens or irritants," says Nelson Lee Novick, M.D., associate clinical professor of dermatology at Mount Sinai School of Medicine of the City University of New York in New York City and author of *You Can Look Younger at Any Age.*

❒ Stay away from products with labels that list "and other ingredients." An irritating ingredient could be lurking within.

❒ Steer clear of medicated soaps. These soaps, which may contain alpha hydroxy acids, benzoyl peroxide, antibacterial agents, or other ingredients, tend to be more irritating and drying than conventional cleansers, Dr. Novick says.

❒ Wear cotton glove liners inside rubber gloves or cotton-lined rubber gloves when washing the dishes or using any household chemicals. The rubber gloves provide a protective barrier between you and irritating detergents. The cotton liner helps absorb perspiration, which can further irritate the skin.

❐ Use fragrance-free detergents when washing clothes. If irritation persists, run clothes through an extra rinse cycle to remove any lingering detergents, says Dr. Ramsey.

❐ Check out beta (not alpha) hydroxy acid. Alpha hydroxy acids (AHAs), such as glycolic acid and lactic acid, have been shown to improve sun-damaged skin by sloughing off dead skin cells and promoting new cell growth. But many women with sensitive skin can't tolerate AHAs, which can cause stinging, burning, and irritation. A gentler alternative is a salicylic acid called beta hydroxy acid, now available in moisturizers and cleansers such as Oil of Olay's Age-Defying Series. Like AHA, beta hydroxy acid exfoliates the skin and reduces the signs of lines and wrinkles, but with less irritation, says Debra Price, M.D., clinical assistant professor of dermatology at the University of Miami School of Medicine and a dermatologist in South Miami.

Prescriptions
FOR TOUCHY SKIN

BATHTIME
Rx

Ironically, hot baths or long showers can dry out your skin. As water, cleansers, and washcloths scrub away dirt, they also remove any invisible, protective film of oil that holds in moisture. To make your bath sensitive-skin friendly, follow these pointers from Dr. Ramsey.

❐ Choose a mild, fragrance- and preservative-free cleanser such as Cetaphil or Basis.

❐ Take short baths and showers in cool or lukewarm (not hot) water.

❐ Add a fragrance-free bath oil to your bathwater. Or try an oatmeal bath powder, which also soothes irritated skin. Be careful: Bath oils and powders make tubs slippery. To avoid slips and falls, put a bath mat or grippers in the bottom of the tub.

❐ Rinse well and pat your skin dry. Apply a fragrance-free, oil-based moisturizer while your skin is still damp, to help your skin trap and retain moisture.

TIME IT RIGHT

❐ If your skin becomes unbearably itchy, apply a 1 percent hydrocortisone topical cream (such as Cortaid) sparingly on dry patches twice a day. Don't use this product for more than two weeks, since hydrocortisone can thin out the skin with prolonged use. An alternative is to use a topical product such as Aveeno Anti-Itch cream or a lotion containing pramoxine, an anti-itch ingredient.

Rx ——————

Prescriptions
FOR WINTER ITCH

Men and women alike notice that their skin feels itchy and sensitive to irritation during the winter. Here's what you can do.

AUTUMN

❑ Moisturize early and often. If you know that your skin tends to break out in a flaky or scaly rash with the first hint of cold weather, start moisturizing before the irritation begins.

❑ Invest in a home humidifier to moisten the air. Central heat dries out the air indoors and takes moisture from the skin.

Split Nails

Brittle nails split easily. They are unattractive, but they are also hazardous. Catch a split nail on your new sweater, and it's likely to catch a thread and pull. Worse yet, you could scratch yourself and break the skin.

Some women seem to suffer split nails more than others. That's no accident. "Some people are simply born with brittle nails," says Paul Kechijian, M.D., chief of the nail section and associate clinical professor of dermatology at New York University in New York City and a dermatologist in Great Neck, New York.

LIFETIME

For years, women have been taking calcium supplements or drinking gelatin in hopes of growing longer, stronger nails that resist chips and tears. These remedies don't work. "One of the only things that can change the way your nail grows is the weather. Nails grow stronger and faster in warmer weather, and they grow more slowly and become more brittle in cold weather," says Dr. Kechijian. Pregnancy makes your nails grow faster, too.

Some women are dismayed to find that their nails break more easily as they get older. That's not their imagination. "In almost everybody, there is a tendency for nails to get more brittle with age," Dr. Kechijian says.

Nevertheless, even tough nails can become brittle and split if they are not properly maintained or if they are frequently immersed in water or harsh household detergents.

In fact, prolonged repeated contact with water is one of the leading contributors to split or brittle nails, according to Dr. Kechijian. That is because nails expand when they absorb water, then contract as the water evaporates. As water moves in and out of the nail, weak areas of the nail become weaker and tend to crack.

Prescriptions —— Rx
FOR TOUGH-AS-NAILS FINGERNAILS

Even if you were born with weak nails, you can minimize splits and tears. To keep your nails looking great, try these strategies.

❏ Wash dishes once a day. To spend less time with your hands in dishwater, Dr. Kechijian suggests keeping a plastic basin in the sink and letting rinsed dirty dishes accumulate until the end of the day.

❏ Wear protective latex gloves with separate, thin cotton gloves underneath when you wash dishes and use household cleansers. The cotton gloves help absorb perspiration. That's important, says Dr. Kechijian, because sweat makes hands soggy, further weakening the nails.

❏ After washing, pat your hands dry, then apply moisturizer to your hands and nails while they are still damp, advises Dr. Kechijian. This helps keep the water in your nails.

❏ To hydrate nails further, soak your fingertips in olive oil before you go to bed at night. Use a half-cup olive oil and soak for 15 to 30 minutes.

NIGHTTIME

❏ Cut your nails only after you bathe, when the nails are still moist and soft. Dry nails are more likely to crack when you cut them.

❏ File your nails only when they are damp. Otherwise, they could split, suggests Dr. Kechijian.

❏ File in only one direction, from side to center. Filing in a back-and-forth, seesaw motion weakens the nail, says Diane Hengstler, a nail instructor at Gordon Phillips in Philadelphia. Opt for a square shape. Nails are less prone to splitting when the corners are square.

❒ Go for the quick fix. If you split your nail, cut it or file it immediately so that you don't catch it on something and split it even more. If you are determined to save the nail, apply nail glue sparingly to the tear, then reinforce the tear with a small piece of tissue from a tea bag, suggests Hengstler. Lay the tissue over the top of the tear, let the glue dry completely, then buff the surface of the nail with a fine buffer. (Be sure to leave the tissue in place.) Finally, apply a top coat over the tissue.

❒ Keep 'em short. If your nails break easily, they are less likely to be injured if you wear them short.

❒ Don't pick at your polish. "Any time you pick at polish, you injure the nail by peeling off part of the nail's surface," says Dr. Kechijian. To curb the urge to pick at your polish, carry the bottle of polish with you and repair chips as soon as you notice them.

❒ Use polish remover sparingly, and no more than once a week, says Richard K. Scher, M.D., nail specialist and professor of dermatology at Columbia University Presbyterian Medical Center in New York City. Overuse of nail polish remover dries out the nail. To minimize drying, opt for an acetone-free remover. Apply a small amount to a cotton ball, press it against the nail for about two seconds to loosen the polish, then gently rub it off.

❒ Skip the nail hardeners. "They will make the nail harder in the short term, but over the long term, they may damage the nail by lifting the nail plate," says Dr. Scher.

❒ Shun artificial nails. They only mask the problem, and removing them tears off the nail surface, says Dr. Kechijian.

❒ Don't use your fingernails as tools. Using fingernails to peel off labels, remove staples, open canned soft drinks, and perform other mundane tasks can weaken or even break nails.

Trouble Zones

What makes a trouble zone so . . . well, troublesome is the unflattering, hard-to-lose flab. It can settle in anywhere on your body, although your abdomen, buttocks, hips, and thighs are the most likely sites.

Poor diet, lack of exercise, and pregnancy account for most of the weight gain associated with trouble zones, but aging also plays a role. Once women reach menopause, they tend to gain weight at the rate of 10 pounds per decade, says Brian Walsh, M.D., director of the Menopause Center at Brigham and Women's Hospital in Boston. Blame it on a slowing metabolism: Once you reach age 30, your body burns 2 to 4 percent fewer calories every 10 years. "So if you continue to take in the same number of calories but don't exercise to burn off the excess, at least some of those calories will get converted to fat," he says.

Fat accumulates on the body in two distinct patterns. In an apple-type distribution, fat cells set up shop in the abdomen and lower chest. A pear-type distribution, on the other hand, is characterized by fat on the hips, buttocks, and thighs.

How do you become an apple or a pear? Cells in certain parts of your body are specifically programmed for storing fat, explains Jack H. Wilmore, Ph.D., professor and department head for the department of health and kinesiology at Texas A & M University in College Station. The cells are assisted by lipoprotein lipase, an enzyme that sends fat their way. Lipoprotein lipase acts sort of like a traffic cop, he explains. It sees fat and says, "Stop, come in here."

In women, it seems, fat is generally directed toward the hips, buttocks, and thighs. There, it is safely stored for your body to use in the event of pregnancy. Unfortunately, a pear shape is hard to pare down because lower-body fat isn't as metabolically active as abdominal fat, says G. Michael Steelman, M.D., a physician in Oklahoma City and chairman of the board of the American Society of Bariatric Physicians.

Being a pear does have its advantages, however. Most notably, it doesn't present the serious health problems that being an apple does. In fact, apple-type fat distribution—which is more common among men than women—is considered a risk factor for heart disease, stroke, and diabetes.

Experts have yet to come up with an explanation for why abdominal fat is more of a health hazard than lower-body fat. Some theorize that abdominal fat sits dangerously close to vital organs and to the hepatic portal circulatory system, the network of blood vessels that directly links the intestines to the liver. "It could be that changes in or pressure on the circulatory pattern affects the flow of blood to the organs, impeding their function," says Dr. Steelman. "It could also be that because this fat has a different metabolic activity, it is more likely to generate metabolic toxins that create a problem."

So where does all this leave women who want to reduce the fat that has accumulated in their most troublesome areas? Unfortunately, you can't spot-reduce a trouble zone—that is, you can't make it go away by doing exercises that work that area only. "Spot-reducing absolutely does not work," says Kathleen Little, Ph.D., assistant professor in the department of human performance and exercise science at Youngstown State University in Ohio. "You can do 1,000 situps a day, and you won't take off any additional fat in your abdominal area. You will tone the muscle, and that area will look aesthetically more pleasing than it did before. But unless you do something to reduce overall body fat, the trouble-zone fat will still be there."

To effectively target a trouble zone, experts recommend a three-part plan that includes a sensible diet that keeps a lid on caloric and fat intake, aerobic exercise (to burn calories and fat), and resistance training (to tone and tighten muscles).

DIETARY
Rx ——— *Prescriptions*
FOR A SHAPELIER PHYSIQUE

Crash dieting is not part of the trouble-zone prescription. "Too often people look at losing weight as a temporary endeavor," says Neva Cochran, R.D., a nutrition consultant in Dallas. "If you want to keep it off, you are going to have to make some permanent lifestyle changes." Follow this checklist.

❏ Eat when you are hungry, and stop before you feel full. "Your body can be your best guide," says Debra Waterhouse, R.D., a nutritionist in Oakland, California, and author of *Outsmarting the Female Fat Cell*. "We need to start trusting our food messages and learn to eat in response to our body's needs."

MEALTIME

❏ Measure and weigh your food to get a clear picture of how much you are eating. "Watch your portions," says Cochran. "What you think is a half-cup might be one cup, so you are unknowingly getting twice as many calories."

❏ Switch to low-fat or nonfat dairy products for eating and cooking.

❏ Remove visible fat from beef before you cook it. Otherwise, the fat will absorb into the leaner part of the meat during cooking. Also, some experts suggest blotting the cooked ground meat with a paper towel, then rinsing it with hot water. The initial blotting removes the surface fat, so rinsing can penetrate to the inside of the beef.

❏ When possible, use pureed fruit instead of part or all of the oil in recipes for baked goods. Replace one cup oil with one cup puree, or whatever the equivalent measurement may be. Prune puree works well in dark-colored desserts, such as brownies. Try applesauce, apple butter, or mashed bananas in lighter-colored treats such as muffins and cakes.

❏ Add butter-flavored sprinkles to vegetables and popcorn instead of butter. Lightly coat the food with a butter-flavored spray like Pam to make the sprinkles stick.

❏ Don't overindulge in fat-free treats. Fat-free doesn't mean calorie-free, explains Waterhouse. "If you overeat, that food is going to be converted to fat anyway and stored as fat."

❏ Allow yourself an occasional treat—and don't feel guilty. If you crave brownies, eat one, but not two or three.

Prescriptions
FOR BURNING FAT AEROBICALLY

Rx

Mention the word *aerobic*, and most people envision a room full of super-fit women in skimpy leotards, steppin' and sweatin' to the music. In reality, aerobic exercise is any activity that increases your heart rate, works your heart and lungs, and, of course, burns fat. So walking and bicycling qualify, as do dancing and gardening.

When it comes to aerobic exercise, most experts prescribe at least 30 minutes a day, three times a week. To get started, try the following strategies.

TIME IT RIGHT

❏ Take long walks. Walking works miracles for your lower body, especially your lower abdominals, says Tedd Mitchell, M.D., medical director of the Cooper Wellness Program in Dallas. To maximize your walk, keep your back straight and pull your abdominal muscles tight. With each step, come down on your heel and push all the way off with your toes.

Swing your arms only slightly, maintaining control of your upper body. Work yourself up to a pace of 3½ to 4 miles per hour. (That's between 15 and 17 minutes per mile.)

❏ Walk in place. If your idea of fun is talking on the telephone, listening to books on tape, or watching TV, consider buying a treadmill.

❏ Try something new. Snowshoeing and cross-country skiing can really put your rear in gear. And skating—inline, roller, and ice—are great for thighs and hips. "The neat thing is that anybody can do these activities," Dr. Mitchell says.

❏ Pair up with someone who is equally committed to exercise. "Almost everybody does better with buddies," says Mary Leonard, co-owner of U.S. Athletic Training Center in New York City, and co-author of *Get a Gold Medal Butt*.

❏ To keep down the expense, rent, don't buy. Look into equipment rentals by calling specialty shops listed in the Yellow Pages under the specific sport that you are interested in.

❏ Borrow exercise videos from the library or friends. Or find an exercise program on TV, tape it while you are at work, and exercise at your convenience.

❏ Turn up the music and dance around your living room. Only the cats will know.

TIME IT RIGHT

❏ Exercise at the same time every day. And pick the time of day that works best for you. If you are the kind of person who leaps out of bed, start early. If you are a zombie until noon, consider an evening workout.

TIME IT RIGHT

❏ When you are done, s-t-r-e-t-c-h. "It's always best to stretch at the end of exercise, when your muscles are nice and warm," says Amy Nelson, a certified health and fitness instructor and president of Heart Aerobics, a Los Angeles–based fitness education company. "Hold a stretch from 30 seconds to two minutes, feeling the muscles relax and elongate with time. Never force to the point of pain."

❏ Give it time. "It took a while to get out of shape and become overweight, and it's going to take a while to get back in shape," says Judith S. Stern, R.D., Sc.D., professor of nutrition and internal medicine at the

University of California, Davis, and past president of the American Society for Clinical Nutrition.

Prescriptions
FOR TONING YOUR TROUBLE SPOTS

Rx

Okay, so you have been burning fat on your treadmill and cutting back on fat and calories—two major ingredients in the prescription for conquering trouble zones. The final, essential part of the prescription is resistance training.

Resistance training tones and strengthens muscle mass—the infrastructure of your hips, thighs, waist, abdomen, backside, and chest. But resistance training also gives your metabolism a long-term boost, prompting you to burn more calories even when you are at rest.

"Muscles require more energy per square inch per minute than fat," explains Dr. Mitchell. "So by doing things that increase your muscle mass, your body's caloric requirement goes up."

❏ Begin with exercises as simple as crunches (which tone the abdominals), lunges (which tone the thighs), and squats (which also tone the thighs)—basically any exercise that resists, or works against, your body, says Dr. Little.

❏ Add lightweight ankle weights and handheld weights to your routine. With dumbbells, start with three pounds and work your way up, says Nancy Karabaic, a certified conditioning specialist in Wheaton, Maryland. Or invest in some inexpensive resistance bands. All are available at sporting goods stores.

❏ Alternate between aerobic and resistance training, every other day.
For example, you might dedicate Monday, Wednesday, and Friday to aerobic exercise and Tuesday and Thursday to resistance training. Remember to spend a minimum of 30 minutes a day working out. As your body grows stronger, you can increase your exercise time, says Karabaic.

❏ If you are a beginner, set a goal of completing one set (8 to 12 repetitions) for each exercise you do. If you are using weights in your routine, you will know they are the right size for you if you feel comfortable doing the first 8 to 10 repetitions, but you really have to work hard to do the last few.

To work your trouble zones, Karabaic recommends the following exercises.

ABDOMEN: CRUNCH

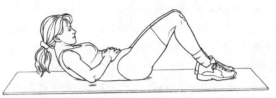

Lie on your back, with your knees bent and your feet flat on the floor. Rest your fingertips on your stomach, with your elbows out to the sides, as shown.

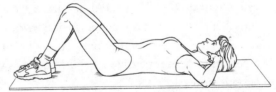

Tighten your abdominal muscles and lift your head and shoulders from the floor, exhaling as you rise. Hold the position for two to three seconds, then inhale as you lower and repeat for one set.

ABDOMEN: ROTATING OBLIQUE CRUNCH

Lie on your back, with your knees bent and your feet flat on the floor. Cup your fingertips behind your ears, as shown, with your elbows out to the sides.

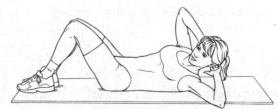

Leading with your right elbow, lift and curl your torso toward your left knee, as shown. Exhale as you come up and imagine touching your elbow to your knee. Hold for two to three seconds, then inhale as you lower. Do one set, then repeat on the opposite side.

HIPS: HIP ABDUCTION

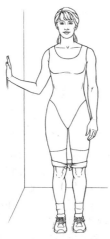
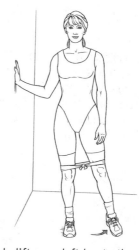

Stand sideways with the right side of your body about two feet from a wall. Place a resistance band around both legs, just above your knees. Place your right hand flat against the wall at chest height. Your feet should be flat on the floor, slightly apart.

Slowly lift your left leg to the side, as shown, and hold the position for two to three seconds. Return to the starting position, keeping your left foot just above the floor, and repeat. Complete one set with your left leg, then repeat with your right leg.

HIPS: LEG LIFT

▶ Lie on your left hip, with your left hand in front of you for support and your right hand on your hip. Bend your bottom (left) leg, keeping the top leg straight, as shown.

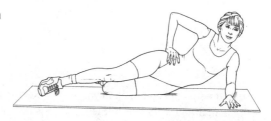

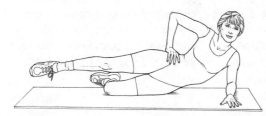

◀ Slowly raise your right leg six to eight inches from the floor, as shown. Hold the position for two to three seconds, then lower and repeat. Do one set, switch to your right side, and repeat the sequence.

TRICEPS (UPPER ARMS): TRICEPS EXTENSION

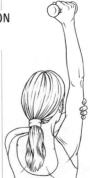

▶ Sit in a chair or stand with your feet shoulder-width apart. Hold a light (two- to three-pound) dumbbell in your right hand and raise it straight above your head while keeping your wrist straight, as shown. Do not lock your elbow. Use your left hand to hold the back of your upper right arm.

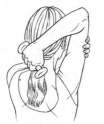

◀ Inhale and bend your right arm at the elbow and lower the weight behind your head toward the back of your neck, as shown. Your elbow should point almost straight to the ceiling. Exhale and slowly raise the weight over your head again by straightening your elbow. Repeat for one set, then work your left arm.

TRICEPS (UPPER ARMS): TRICEPS KICKBACK

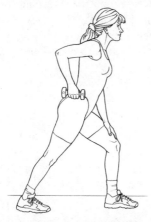 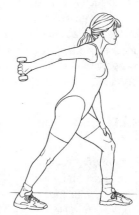

Hold a three-pound dumbbell in your right hand. Stand with your left leg about two feet ahead of your right leg, and your knees slightly bent. Lean forward, shifting your weight to your left leg. Tilt your upper body at a 30-degree angle, keeping your back straight. Bend your right elbow at a 90-degree angle. Swing your arm back so your right hand is at waist level, your palm facing in. Rest your left hand on your left leg for support.

Keeping your elbow stable at your side, slowly extend your right arm behind you until it is straight. Be sure to move only your forearm. Be careful not to lock your elbow. Repeat for one set, then repeat with your left arm. Remember to switch the position of your legs.

CHEST: CHEST CROSSOVER

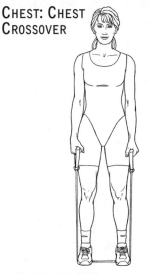 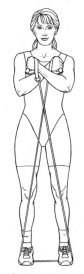

Stand in the middle of a resistance band. Hold the ends of the band in your hands at your sides, palms facing in, as shown. Your feet should be shoulder-width apart and your knees slightly bent.

Slowly raise your hands and cross your forearms so that they cover your chest. The resistance band will crisscross in front of you. Lower your arms to your sides and repeat for one set.

CHEST: CHEST PRESS

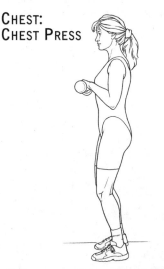 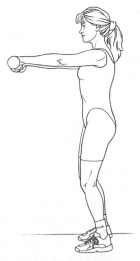

Stand with your feet shoulder-width apart and your knees slightly bent. Hold a pair of three-pound dumbbells at chest level. Your elbows should be at your sides, your forearms straight and your palms facing the floor.

Slowly push the weights straight in front of you until your arms are fully extended, as shown. Don't lock your elbows. Return to the starting position and repeat for one set.

BUTTOCKS: BACK LEG LIFT

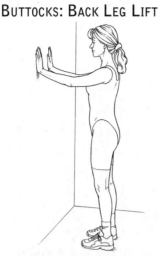 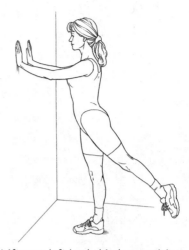

Stand facing a wall so that your toes are one to two feet from the base. Place both hands flat on the wall at shoulder height.

Lift your left leg behind you, raising it 6 to 12 inches. Keep your back straight. Lower your leg to the starting position, holding it just above the floor. Do one set, then repeat with the right leg. Once you are more comfortable with this exercise, you can put resistance bands around your ankles.

BUTTOCKS: LEG LIFT VARIATION

▶ Kneeling on a padded surface, lower yourself until your elbows and forearms rest on the floor and your weight is balanced on your knees and forearms. Lift your right leg about 12 inches from the floor, keeping your knee bent. The bottom of your right foot should be parallel to the ceiling, and your right thigh, from the top of your knee to your hipbone, should be parallel to the floor, as shown.

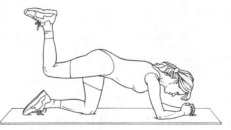

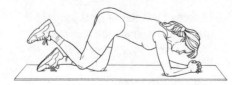

◀ Slowly lower your knee so that it hovers just above the floor, as shown. Repeat. Do one set with your right leg, then repeat with your left leg.

THIGHS: SQUAT

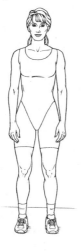

◄ Stand with your feet flat on the floor, shoulder-width apart. Bend your knees slightly and hold your arms down at your sides.

► Lower yourself slowly, as if you were going to sit in a chair. Extend your arms straight ahead as you squat. Stop when your thighs are almost parallel to the floor, as shown. Your back should be slightly arched, your knees should not extend beyond your toes, and your heels should remain on the floor. Pause, then rise and repeat for one set. If you want to try this exercise with weights, hold a pair of three-pound dumbbells in your hands and keep your arms at your sides.

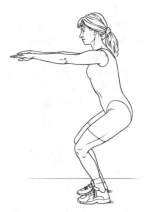

THIGHS: LUNGE

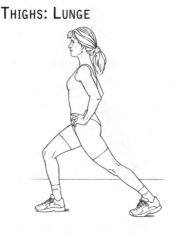

◄ Stand straight with your feet flat on the floor, shoulder-width apart. With your hands on your hips, step forward as far as comfortable with your right leg.

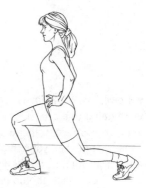

▶ Bend your right knee until your right thigh is parallel to the floor. The heel on your left leg will come up, as shown. (With time and practice, you should be able to extend the length of the lunge by increasing the distance between your legs.) Make sure that your right knee does not extend beyond your toes. Return to the starting position by shifting your weight to your front leg and straightening your back leg. Repeat with your left leg forward. (That's one rep.) To enhance the effectiveness of the lunge, hold a light (two- to three-pound) dumbbell in each hand or position your forward foot on a six-inch step, making sure that your whole foot is supported by the step.

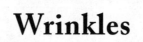

Wrinkles

When she was in her twenties, Debra Price, M.D., swore off the sun. Now a clinical assistant professor of dermatology at the University of Miami School of Medicine and a dermatologist in South Miami, she is glad that she did. The fortysomething doctor says that her skin is smoother and she looks less wrinkled than many of her contemporaries. "It always pays to protect yourself from the sun. The sooner you get out of the sun, the better."

Unprotected sun exposure is the leading cause of wrinkles. In fact, the sun's ultraviolet rays account for more than 90 percent of premature aging, Dr. Price says. Smoking, heredity, facial expressions, and the natural aging process explain most of the other lines that we see on our faces or hands. The sun wreaks havoc on the skin by breaking down collagen and elastin, two connective fibers. Collagen supports the skin and elastin gives it flexibility. Together, they give the skin its structure and tone.

You don't have to lounge in your bathing suit on a beach towel to add new wrinkles to your skin. Small but constant doses of ultraviolet rays from the sun can also lead to premature wrinkles, says Margaret A. Weiss, M.D., a dermatologist and assistant professor of dermatology at the Johns Hopkins Medical Institutions in Baltimore. "You can do just as much harm to your skin moving around as you can sitting still," she says. In fact, you can damage your skin just while walking to and from your car several times a day.

The good news for lifelong sun worshippers is that it's never too late to reverse some of the damage.

"Skin, like the rest of the body, has the capacity to repair itself," says Dr. Price. "Even if you do nothing else to combat wrinkles but use sunscreen and stay out of the sun, you will see improvement."

Prescription Rx
FOR IRONING OUT WRINKLES

Visit the cosmetics aisle at any drugstore or department store, and you will be overwhelmed by the choice of products promising younger, smoother, and hopefully wrinkle-free skin. While moisturizers help improve the appearance of wrinkles by smoothing and plumping up the skin, their effect is only temporary. Many newer skin-care products actually help diminish fine lines and wrinkles. It's as easy as A-B-C.

❒ Look for alpha hydroxy acids (AHAs). These naturally occurring acids—derived from plants, fruits, and other food products, such as sugarcane (glycolic acid) and sour milk (lactic acid)—can be found in over-the-counter creams, lotions, and gels. They improve sun-damaged skin by exfoliating dead skin cells on the skin's surface and uncovering the younger cells underneath. They also plump up the skin, in essence filling

MORNING

in the "dents" we know as wrinkles. Glycolic acid is the most widely used AHA.

Use an 8 percent AHA preparation on your face and neck twice a day—once in the morning and once at night, says Lorrie J. Klein, M.D., a dermatologist in private practice in Laguna Niguel, California. For the sensitive area around the eyes, use a fragrance-free 5 percent AHA eye cream.

❐ Consider beta hydroxy acids. Some women with sensitive skin find AHAs too irritating. If that's the case, try using a salicylic acid, known as beta hydroxy acid, instead. Available in moisturizers and cleansers such as Oil of Olay's Age-Defying Series, beta hydroxy acid exfoliates the skin and reduces the signs of lines and wrinkles as AHAs do, but with less irritation, says Dr. Price.

❐ Smooth on topical vitamin C. Unlike alpha and beta hydroxy acid products, which reverse skin damage by speeding up the exfoliation process, vitamin C might help prevent damage in the first place. As an antioxidant, vitamin C fights off free radicals, unstable molecules that form when the skin is exposed to sunlight and ultraviolet radiation. (Free radicals "steal" electrons from the body's healthy molecules, harming cells and leading to premature wrinkling and other forms of damage.) Vitamin C also helps the body produce new collagen, a protein that keeps skin smooth and firm. Unfortunately, the sun robs the skin of vitamin C right when it needs it most, according to Lorraine Meisner, Ph.D., professor of preventive medicine at the University of Wisconsin Medical School in Madison.

"One of the reasons that people get wrinkles is that they can't make new collagen because of inadequate vitamin C in the skin, and they can't make new vitamin C," explains Dr. Meisner. "Using a topical vitamin C feeds the skin from the outside."

MORNING

Because sun exposure depletes vitamin C levels in the skin, topical vitamin C should be applied daily—along with a sunscreen—before significant sun exposure. One topical vitamin C product is Cellex-C, a 10 percent vitamin C solution, available without a prescription from dermatologists and licensed aestheticians. Cellex-C also contains zinc (a trace mineral) and tyrosine (an amino acid), which help the vitamin penetrate the skin's surface, according to Dr. Meisner, who is co-inventor of the patented formulation in Cellex-C. The solution provides your skin with 20 times the vitamin C that you would get from your diet.

❐ Moisturize your skin in the morning. Dryness doesn't cause wrinkles, but it accentuates any you may already have, says Dr. Klein. "Wrinkles show up more when the skin is dry. You can hide wrinkles by plumping up the skin with moisturizer." If you have oily skin, you can skip the moisturizer, she adds.

MORNING

"People tend to apply moisturizer before they go to bed, so their appearance is improved for only four to six hours while they sleep," says William P. Coleman III, M.D., clinical professor of dermatology at Tulane University in New Orleans. "You may be better off moisturizing first thing in the morning."

Prescriptions
FOR STOPPING WRINKLES DEAD

Rx

Little can be done to stop the natural lines and sags that come with age, heredity, or facial expression. But most wrinkles can be prevented. Here's how.

❐ If you plan to spend most of your day indoors, going outdoors only occasionally, wear a moisturizer with sunscreen underneath your makeup, suggests Jonathan Weiss, M.D., assistant clinical professor of dermatology at Emory University in Atlanta and a dermatologist in Snellville, Georgia. Choose a moisturizer with a sun protection factor (SPF) of at least 15.

❐ If you anticipate being outside for any length of time, use a product with an SPF of 30 or higher. "Apply it 20 minutes prior to sun exposure, so that the sunscreen is well-absorbed," Dr. Jonathan Weiss says.

TIME IT RIGHT

❐ If you go swimming or perspire heavily, reapply the sunscreen after 80 minutes. If you stay cool and dry, you can wait up to three to four hours before reapplying, says Dr. Jonathan Weiss.

TIME IT RIGHT

❐ Cover up with lightweight, long-sleeved shirts and pants. And wear a broad-rimmed hat. But don't forget to use sunscreen on your face. "Sunscreen is still important when you wear a hat because water and pave-

WINTERTIME

ment reflect the sun's rays," says Dr. Jonathan Weiss. Don't forget to use sunscreen in the non-summer months, too. Winter's ice and snow reflect the sun's damaging rays.

DAYTIME

❏ Avoid sun exposure between 10:00 A.M. and 3:00 P.M., when the sun is most intense.

NIGHTTIME

❏ Sleep on your back. People who habitually sleep on one side develop a "sleep wrinkle," a vertical line that runs across the cheekbone, says Dr. Jonathan Weiss. It takes time, but you can teach yourself to sleep on your back.

❏ If you smoke, quit. Smokers are more likely to wrinkle prematurely than nonsmokers are. Among the possible reasons are that cigarette smoke damages the skin's connective tissue, and it constricts the blood vessels that supply oxygen to the skin. It also decreases vitamin A, which the body needs to protect against free radicals. Plus, smokers crinkle their eyes to avoid irritating smoke and purse their lips around the butt of the cigarette. These repetitive motions lead to wrinkles, says Dr. Margaret Weiss.

"If you don't quit for health reasons, do it for vanity," advises Dr. Price.

❏ Stay away from tanning beds. Don't be fooled by ads for tanning beds that promise a safe tan. Tanning beds use ultraviolet-A (UVA) rays, which penetrate the skin even deeper than ultraviolet-B (UVB) rays and lead to premature wrinkles.

❏ Avoid yo-yo dieting. Repeated weight gain and loss causes wrinkles by stretching then tightening the skin, says Dr. Margaret Weiss.

In particular, maintaining a steady weight helps to prevent crinkles and folds in the neck. "People who have always been athletic and stayed in shape usually don't have this problem," says Dr. Coleman.

Chapter 5

PRESCRIPTIONS
FOR EMOTIONAL HEALTH

A generation ago, the mainstream medical community largely dismissed the notion that emotions affect physical health. Reports of people overcoming serious illness through the power of positive thinking met with disbelief, even derision. According to the conventional wisdom of the time, only medicine—not the mind—could heal the human body.

That viewpoint began to change in the late 1960s with the pioneering work of Herbert Benson, M.D., associate professor of medicine at Harvard Medical School and founder and president of the Mind/Body Medical Institute at Deaconess Hospital in Boston. Dr. Benson discovered that meditation, a form of deep mental and physical relaxation, can slow breathing and heart rate and even reduce blood pressure. Subsequent research has suggested that daily meditation may also help correct irregular heartbeats and other cardiac problems.

These findings help substantiate the theory that emotional and physical health have a symbiotic relationship. Simply put, an upbeat mindset benefits your body. Unfortunately, the opposite also holds true: Persistent negative feelings can pave the way for physical disease.

You can see why it is so important to learn how to banish bad and blue moods as well as the emotions that accompany them—anger, depression, insecurity, and worry, to name a few. That's not to say that you should turn into a living, breathing smiley face. But instead of blowing up at the slightest provocation or withdrawing from family and friends, you can channel negative feelings in more positive, constructive, healthful ways.

This section offers dozens of simple, practical prescriptions for managing your emotions more effectively. For instance, you can defuse an angry outburst by sniffing the scent of rose. Banish the blues by eating smaller meals more often. Release nervous tension by practicing a technique called progressive muscle relaxation.

You will also discover innovative strategies for overcoming computer anxiety, coping with divorce, and curbing overeating. These and other lifestyle issues have strong emotional components that ever so stealthily undermine your energy, performance, and self-confidence.

Use this section as your guide to taking charge of your emotional health. Your body will thank you for it.

Anger

It's dinnertime. And in kitchens across America, the main course isn't the only thing stewing and boiling.

MEALTIME

"Dinnertime is tough for women, whether they work in or outside their homes," says Sandra P. Thomas, R.N., Ph.D., professor and director of the doctoral program in nursing at the University of Tennessee College of Nursing in Knoxville and author of *Use Your Anger*. "You're feeling all the stress that you have accumulated over the course of the day. You are tired and hungry, and you are trying to get dinner on the table. To top it off, your spouse and kids are probably just as tired and cranky as you." Together, these factors create a fertile forum for anger.

Anger—an emotion that can range from displeasure to rage—usually erupts when you feel rushed, tired, hungry, or sick, or you simply have too much to do. "Four of these five conditions frequently converge at dinnertime," observes Susan Heitler, Ph.D., a clinical psychologist in Denver and author of *The Power of Two: Secrets to a Strong and Loving Marriage.*

Other circumstances can provoke an angry outburst, too, says Dr. Thomas, who directed the first-ever large-scale, comprehensive study on women's anger. Even the most easygoing women often feel pushed to the brink when they aren't listened to or taken seriously, when they want to change a situation but can't, when they are lied to or deceived, or when they or their loved ones are hurt by an injustice. What peeves women most? Powerlessness—"when you want someone or something to change, and you can't make that happen," according to Dr. Thomas.

Of course, how you express that anger can have a significant impact on your health, according to Aron Siegman, Ph.D., professor of psychology and director of behavioral medicine in the department of psychology at the University of Maryland Baltimore County. "The repeated full-blown expression of anger—complete with screaming, clenched fists, and a raised voice—is among the primary risk factors for coronary heart disease in men," he notes. "Even though women are likely to express anger more subtly and indirectly, such behavior still places them at risk for coronary heart disease."

If you do forcefully blow off steam, your blood pressure will rise dramatically. "That's why chronic anger could literally kill you," says Dr. Siegman. In fact, research involving both women and men has shown that an episode of anger more than doubles the risk of having a heart attack within two hours after the outburst.

Admittedly, this may not mean much for healthy women between ages 30 and 45, for whom heart attacks are extremely rare, says Murray Mittleman, M.D., Dr.P.H., assistant professor and director of cardiovascular epidemiology at the Institute for Prevention of Cardiovascular Disease at the Beth Israel Deaconess Medical Center West and Harvard Medical School. Still, psychologists agree that regularly feeling and expressing anger isn't especially healthful—either for you or for those around you.

Prescriptions
FOR LETTING OFF STEAM

When you feel anger beginning to build, resist the urge to yell and scream. Anger vented this way won't get you anywhere—and in the long run, it could have serious physical and emotional consequences. Try these coping tactics instead.

❒ Breathe slowly and deeply. Only air—no words—should leave your mouth. Stay focused on your breath until you feel calm enough to deal with the situation rationally, says Dr. Thomas.

TIME IT RIGHT ❒ Put two drops of rose essential oil on a handkerchief, then inhale the scent for one to three minutes. Aromatherapists consider rose the classic remedy for anger, says Alan Hirsch, M.D., neurological director of the Smell and Taste Treatment and Research Foundation in Chicago. You can buy the essential oil in health food stores and some specialty bath-and-beauty shops.

❒ Count to 10. Counting is an old standby for coping with anger, but it works. It gives you time to frame an appropriate reaction to the situation, says Dr. Thomas.

TIME IT RIGHT ❒ Walk for 10 to 15 minutes. Walking releases the bodily tension that builds up when you are angry. If you are at work, take a quick trip around the block or up and down a flight of stairs. If you are at home, grab the mop or vacuum and clean up while you chill out, says Dr. Thomas.

❒ Create a buffer zone between yourself and the anger-provoking person or problem. For instance, if your kids are bickering while you are trying to prepare dinner, tell them that you need the kitchen to yourself for a certain amount of time, suggests Dr. Thomas.

❒ Allow yourself as much time as you need to cool off. "I tell women to hide under a rock until they are calmer and better able to identify the source of their anger," says Harriet Lerner, Ph.D., senior staff psychologist at the Menninger Clinic in Topeka, Kansas, and author of *The Dance of Anger.*

Rx ———

Prescriptions
FOR PRODUCTIVE PROBLEM-SOLVING

Once you have cooled off a bit, you are in a better frame of mind to contemplate what went wrong—and why you reacted so strongly. Here is how the experts suggest that you proceed.

❒ Accept your anger. "You have every right to feel the way you do when other people have treated you unjustly," notes Dr. Thomas. When

RETHINK Your Anger

If you are prone to angry outbursts, RETHINK can help you rein them in. RETHINK is an anger-management technique developed by a panel of educators and psychologists under the auspices of the Institute for Mental Health Initiatives, a nonprofit education foundation based in Washington, D.C. It was originally designed to teach parents not only how to manage their anger but also how to help their children manage *theirs*.

But experts say that anyone can benefit from using RETHINK. Women, in particular, stand to gain from learning how to deal with anger effectively. It can boost your self-esteem and give you a greater sense of control over your life, says Suzanne Stutman, a psychotherapist and president of the Institute for Mental Health Initiatives.

The next time you feel yourself becoming boiling mad, try the RETHINK-ing woman's approach to anger.

Recognize anger in yourself and others. Fatigue, shame, stress, or fear can trigger anger.

Empathize with the other person. If you were in her shoes, how would you feel?

Think about the situation differently. Can you find any humor in it? Is there another side?

Hear what is being said. What is the other person upset about? Where is she coming from?

Integrate love and respect with an honest expression of your anger.

Notice your body's reaction to anger. Breathe slowly and relax clenched muscles.

Keep your attention on the present problem. Don't let old grudges surface.

you are able to acknowledge your emotions, it actually diminishes your anger.

TIME IT RIGHT

❏ Schedule an appointment to discuss a problem. This works especially well in the workplace, where crises routinely erupt at day's end—just when everyone is feeling tired and cranky. Choose a date, time, and place to resume your discussion. And be sure to stick with it, says Dr. Thomas.

❏ If someone has made you angry, tell that person how you feel. You might say something like "I was just so upset with you that I had to take a walk. Now that I've calmed down, let's talk." This approach disarms the other person and makes her more willing to listen to you, according to Dr. Thomas.

❏ Speak softly and slowly. "Research has shown that during a confrontation, the person who argues loudly and rapidly experiences dramatic blood pressure fluctuations, while the person who argues softly and slowly does not," notes Dr. Siegman. Keeping your voice down has another advantage: It subtly persuades the other person to turn down her volume a couple of notches. Then the two of you can discuss the situation more rationally.

❏ Be specific about what you expect from the other person. Tell her not only what you want but also when you want it, advises Dr. Thomas. For example, if you are upset that your teenage daughter hasn't done her chores for the week, you might say to her, "I want you to clean your room by 5:00 P.M." The direct approach eliminates any ambiguity about your expectations. It also paves the way to discussion rather than confrontation.

❏ Walk away from a situation that you feel has gotten out of control. Simply tell the other person that you want to be left alone for a while, suggests Dr. Thomas. Then physically go someplace else until you have a chance to cool off.

MORNING

❏ Postpone your discussion until morning. That old saw about not going to bed angry doesn't necessarily apply to everyone. "When you feel tired, you can have a hard time resolving a problem," notes Dr. Thomas. Instead, use your usual pre-bedtime ritual to develop a plan of action. Tell yourself that you will talk to your husband in the morning or to your co-worker as soon as you arrive at work. This allows you to let go of your anger so that you get a good night's sleep. When you wake up the next morning, you will be at your well-rested best.

❒ Postpone your discussion for a couple of days. By playing the waiting game, you give yourself the opportunity to sort out what you need to address and what you can just let go, says Dr. Lerner. It also gives you time to think about the problem rather than reacting emotionally.

Medical **Alert**

Anger is a powerful emotion that at times can spin out of control. You should seek professional counseling if your anger is too frequent, too intense, or too prolonged, disrupting your personal or professional life or provoking you to hurt yourself or others, says Dr. Thomas.

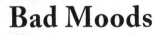

Bad Moods

When Holly Golightly had the *mean reds*—her term for a bad mood—she would just take herself out for breakfast at Tiffany's. Thank you, oh movie makers of Hollywood. For us real people, though, a visit to the world's classiest jewelry store is as impractical as it is unlikely to dispel a truly rotten mood.

Bad moods at breakfast are by no means relegated to the delightful likes of Miss Golightly. In fact, mornings are particularly tough times for lots of women (as well as men), says Robert Thayer, Ph.D., professor of psychology at California State University at Long Beach and author of *The Origin of Everyday Moods.*

"Though some people are morning people and others are night people, bad moods certainly occur at predictable danger times for many people," Dr. Thayer says. "Each of us has an internally controlled biological clock that governs our level of energetic arousal." According to Dr. Thayer, low energetic arousal leaves us vulnerable to anxiety, fatigue, and similar low-energy and high-tension states. High energetic arousal, on the other hand, can produce a combination of energy and tension, a state that may be mildly pleasant but that is associated with stress.

TIME IT RIGHT

We can actually wake up in a tense, tired state, which we perceive as a bad mood, says Dr. Thayer. By midmorning to early afternoon, though, most women are performing up to their energetic peaks.

Bad moods can flare up again in the late afternoon, says Dr. Thayer. "Problems that arise in the late afternoon can have the greatest impact on our moods because it's a time when our energy levels plummet," he adds.

Energy ramps up to a secondary peak in the early evening, and then drops steadily after dinner, until it reaches its lowest point of the day right before bedtime, notes Dr. Thayer.

Though the term *bad mood* is poorly defined in clinical psychology, most women know when they are having one, says Robert S. Brown Sr., M.D., Ph.D., clinical professor of psychiatric medicine at the University of Virginia in Charlottesville.

"A bad mood is different for every women, but generally, it is experiencing feelings ranging from sadness to anger," says Dr. Brown. "Bad moods have many triggers—they can be set off by everything from premenstrual syndrome (PMS) to irritating people."

Irritating people notwithstanding, psychologists frequently draw a connection between PMS and bad moods, though that connection might be more tenuous than many women believe.

A DAY IN THE LIFE OF YOUR MOODS

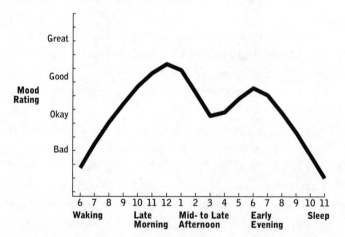

During the course of a day, you can expect your moods to fluctuate from good to bad to in-between, as shown in this graph.

Despite the fact that science doesn't absolutely connect that-time-of-the-month with bad moods, women generally believe in the link, according to Dr. Thayer. Semester after semester, virtually every one of his female advanced psychology students says that bad moods and PMS go hand in hand—even though the scientific research they study often indicates otherwise. Their convictions are based not on the uncertain science of PMS, but on their own experiences, he says.

MONTHLY

Prescriptions
FOR BANISHING A BAD MOOD

Rx

Just because occasional bad moods are inevitable doesn't mean that you can't limit their intensity and duration, says Mary Amanda Dew, Ph.D., associate professor of psychiatry, psychology, and epidemiology in the department of psychiatry at the University of Pittsburgh School of Medicine. "When you're in a bad mood, it is not always a good idea to simply hope it will go away," she says. "If it persists, you need to take action against the mood so that it won't engulf you and escalate into a more serious problem."

For a run-of-the-mill case of the mean reds, when utterly everything sets your teeth on edge—and when those around you run for cover—try these tips.

❏ Rate your moods. "Keep a mood diary for two months," says Ronald Podell, M.D., assistant clinical professor of psychiatry at the University of California, Los Angeles, director of the Center for Biobehavioral Psychiatry, and co-founder of the Westridge Psychiatric Medical Group, both also in Los Angeles. Rate normal moods as 0. Rate bad moods as -1 to -3 and good moods as +1 to +3. A -3 is a really bad mood and a +3 is a really good mood.

TIME IT RIGHT

Then, note your moods every few hours. "Keeping a mood diary enables you to see if your moods fall into patterns based on the time of day," says Dr. Podell.

❏ Steer clear of touchy topics—or touchy people. "A bad mood is as infectious as a bad cold," says Dr. Podell, who is also the author of *Contagious Emotions*. "When you are with someone who is in a bad mood, it is contagious—I call it mood fusion," he continues. Your bad mood infects your mate's mood and pretty soon, there is a lot of blaming, irritability, and anger. In a marriage, this vicious cycle can impede your sex life and create real marital discord. If both you and your partner are aware that you are prone to bad moods at certain times of the day, consider avoiding potentially provocative topics or activities at those times.

TIME IT RIGHT ❏ Walk briskly for 10 minutes. "Moderate exercise helps when bad moods occur during your low-energy periods," says Dr. Thayer. "Walk as if you were late for an appointment, but without the feeling of anxiety. Don't walk so fast that you become exhausted, but fast enough so that you become energized. Maintain an erect posture, relax your muscles, and let your arms swing naturally with your stride." The beauty of even a brief walk is that it not only raises your energy levels but it also helps reduce the muscle tension in your back, neck, and shoulders that contribute to a bad mood.

MEALTIME ❏ Don't skip meals. "Missed meals and dieting can affect your moods," says Dr. Thayer. "If you normally eat lunch, for example, and skip it, your mood will become negative because your blood sugar levels drop."

TIME IT RIGHT ❏ Sixty minutes after snacking—watch out. "We did one of the few published studies on the effects of sugar on mood," says Dr. Thayer. "We learned that after you eat a candy bar, for about 30 minutes, you will feel a burst of energy. But an hour after your snack, your energy will not only plummet but also sink lower than it was before you ate the candy bar. Worse, you are likely to feel edgy and tense for up to two hours." According to Dr. Thayer, the immediate sense of well-being right after noshing is what conditions most snackers to indulge. "If you could connect how bad you feel later to the candy bar you ate an hour ago, you would be less likely to go for the sugar load," he says.

❏ Do something to actively relax. Meditation and other relaxation exercises like visualization and slow, deep breathing can help you through a bad mood, says Dr. Dew. "Prayer can also be very useful. A strong belief that there is a force more powerful than you can be a major benefit in the midst of a bad mood," she says.

❏ Call an understanding friend. "Talking through your bad mood with a good friend can give you a fresh perspective on what's troubling you," says Dr. Dew.

❏ If you believe that your bad moods stem from PMS, take 25 to 50 milligrams of vitamin B$_6$ every day. According to Dr. Podell, the moods of two-thirds of the women who take it once a day seem to improve by their next menstrual cycle.

❏ Catch some rays. "Some people become lethargic and more snappish on dark, cloudy days," says Michael Cunningham, Ph.D., professor of psychology at the University of Louisville in Kentucky. "These people usually benefit from daily exposure to a light box—and I believe that everyone's mood improves by taking a nice trip to Florida."

Light boxes are available through mail-order catalogs and from commercial manufacturers. You will get the most benefit from the device if you consult your doctor first. She can show you how to use the box properly and create a treatment schedule for you.

Medical **Alert**

If you occasionally feel crabby for a day or two—or even a week—don't worry, says Dr. Dew. "But if you are in a bad mood for two weeks or longer, it could signal more serious problems. If you are also having trouble sleeping, if your eating habits change, or if you feel an overwhelming lack of interest in life, your bad mood could be depression, and you should seek guidance from a health professional."

Boredom

Boredom causes wrinkles. Don't laugh. It could be true, in a very convoluted way. You see, preliminary research suggests that boredom somehow contributes to the cellular breakdown that eventually sparks the aging process. What's more, chronically bored people may age faster than their more interested peers. And you thought boredom was just . . . well, boring.

Researchers believe that boredom has other health implications as well. For starters, it may play a part in the development of disease, according to Augustin De la Pena, Ph.D., a psychologist at the Clinical Monitoring Center in Los Gatos, California. In his book *The Psychobi-*

ology of Cancer, Dr. De la Pena reviews data from a broad range of scientific literature and concludes that chronic understimulation—or information underload stress, as he calls it—may be cancer-causing.

Chronic boredom and understimulation may have other health implications as well, says Dr. De la Pena. To assuage her boredom, a woman may respond by eating, smoking, or engaging in other unhealthy behaviors. These can put her at increased risk for obesity and other conditions.

Just what is boredom? "It's your body and mind telling you that you are understimulated, that you need more challenge and more activity in your life," says Susan Heitler, Ph.D., a clinical psychologist in Denver and author of *The Power of Two: Secrets to a Strong and Loving Marriage.*

Boredom can also signal that a particular area of your life is less fulfilling than it could be. "Maybe you have a fabulous relationship with your significant other, but you are bored to tears by your job," says Dr. Heitler. "Or maybe your job keeps you jumping, but you prefer the TV's company to your partner's at home."

Boredom can also mean that you are working too hard and not setting aside enough recuperative time. At its most serious, it may trigger depression or psychological withdrawal.

Fortunately, you can beat a hasty retreat from the state of boredom. And you don't have to scale Mount Everest to do it. (Although if that tickles your fancy, by all means go for it.)

Rx — *Prescriptions*
for a Stimulating Social Life

For women who are taking care of family and holding down full-time jobs, socializing doesn't stand much of a chance. Yet maintaining strong social ties is essential to a well-rounded, stimulating life.

To reestablish contact with the world around you, contemplate the kinds of people and activities that you enjoy. Brainstorm ideas about what would make your life more fun and satisfying. And consider these tips for reactivating your leisure time.

❏ Think of three community events or activities that have piqued your interest and commit to taking part in them. "People who are bored give themselves lots of reasons not to do X, Y, and Z," notes

Dr. Heitler. "You may have to make a deal with yourself to get involved—to do X, Y, and Z, no matter what." If you are stumped for ideas, check your local newspaper for announcements of events and volunteer opportunities.

❏ Try your hand at an activity that you perceive as completely out of character. "Getting 'unbored' may necessitate going beyond who you think you are and doing something other than what has traditionally been expected of you," explains Dr. Heitler. "If you think of yourself as very feminine and not very physical, consider trying inline skating or mountain biking or kickboxing."

❏ Enroll in a class that allows you to exercise your creative side. Choose any art form that intrigues you or that you think you would enjoy, even if you have never tried it before. "You don't have to be a great dancer to take adult ballet lessons or a great artist to sign up for pottery class," says Dr. Heitler. "The process of learning is in itself stimulating and fun, regardless of your skill level."

Prescriptions
for Engaging Employment

Rx

If your job bores you, you may need to discover ways to make it more challenging, suggests Dr. Heitler. Here are her suggestions for doing just that.

❏ Set professional goals for yourself. At times your job can pull you in all directions, scattering your attention and robbing you of your sense of purpose. Lack of focus can lead to boredom. Goals give you something to work toward. "Once you have a clear goal, your job may feel like it has more coherence and meaning," says Dr. Heitler.

"One of my clients was in this situation," she adds. "I asked her to sit quietly with her eyes closed and concentrate on what she really wanted professionally. An image came into her mind. She saw herself with a microphone in her hand, as though she was moderating a talk show. When she realized that she wanted a career in broadcasting, she began working more efficiently at her day job so that in the evenings she could take courses in preparation for a job at a local television station."

❏ Learn new skills that can enhance your job performance. "Boredom occurs when you perform the same tasks over and over again," says Dr. Heitler. "What seemed stimulating three years ago probably seems like the 'same-old same-old' now." She suggests attending management-training seminars, taking advanced computer courses, pursuing professional certification—anything relevant to your field of work. A bonus: The higher-ups will recognize your initiative and desire to improve. That may earn you a step up the career ladder.

❏ Consider changing your job. "Speak to your supervisor or personnel coordinator—someone you trust—about redefining your current position or moving into a new position within your company," advises Dr. Heitler. "If you have no opportunity for advancement where you work, you may want to consider updating your résumé and starting the search for another job."

Rx ——— *Prescriptions*
FOR ENHANCING YOUR HOME LIFE

Your after-five routine has begun to feel like an after-five rut: Make dinner, clean up, watch TV, go to bed. Your once-lively repartee with your partner has been reduced to a question-and-answer session. ("How was your day?" "Okay." "Did you pick up the dry cleaning?" "Yep.") Even sex has lost its sizzle.

If you think that your home life needs a little more oomph, it is up to you—not your partner—to initiate change. The following two tactics can help.

❏ Invite your mate to join you in trying something new. Give him a variety of appealing suggestions: working on a political campaign, volunteering in a soup kitchen, planting a garden, or just walking every night after dinner. "Put a positive spin on it and make sure that you tell him that you would prefer his company," says Dr. Heitler. "The important thing is that you make the offer.

"But don't let his reluctance dampen your enthusiasm," she adds. "If he isn't up to it, you can go ahead and make your life more meaningful."

❐ Take up a homemaking hobby, such as sewing, knitting, cro-
cheting, or quilting. Many women find these pastimes relaxing, rewarding,
and satisfying, says Dr. Heitler. "And they give you something worthwhile
to do if you can't pry your beloved husband out of his beloved recliner,"
she quips.

Computer Anxiety

Cartoons didn't do much to build our confidence in technology. Take
Wile E. Coyote. He designed brilliantly elaborate contraptions in his quest
to nab the Roadrunner. But inevitably, he ended up blowing himself—not
his quarry—to smithereens, often with the push of a button.

Come to think of it, maybe that's why so many of us grew up to
fear computers. We are absolutely convinced that somewhere on the keyboard is a "Destruct" button that, if pressed, could send us all to
kingdom come.

In fact, fear of destroying the computer or its contents is the number
one reason that many women suffer from computer anxiety, according to
Elliot Masie, president of the Masie Center, a computer training company
and international computer think tank in Saratoga Springs, New York.
"When I'm training a new computer user, the very first thing I tell her is
that she can do nothing to hurt the computer or damage its contents in
any way," he says. Many people also worry that they must learn incom-
prehensible lingo or master highly technical programming skills in order
to perform basic computer tasks. "But think about your VCR," says Masie.
"You may have trouble programming it to record four different shows over
the next three weeks, but you can certainly pop in a video and watch it.
The same principle applies to your computer—you don't have to be an expert to use it."

None of this is to say that women are more intimidated by com-
puters than men. While men are perceived as more mechanically inclined,
in reality both genders experience computer anxiety about equally, says
Herbert A. Simon, Ph.D., a Nobel laureate and the Richard King Mellon
University professor of computer science and psychology at Carnegie
Mellon University in Pittsburgh.

And when you take a look at the computer industry, you may notice that many companies have female executives in upper-management positions. What does this mean for you? Masie predicts that as women assume more leadership roles within the industry, computer products will become even more "female-friendly."

Rx — *Prescriptions* FOR GETTING YOUR FEET WET

The surest way for anyone to dispel computer anxiety is to jump in and experiment, says Dr. Simon. How long it takes for you to feel comfortable with the machine really depends on your own learning style. Use the following strategies to wade into the high-tech waters with confidence.

❏ Have someone show you the basics of computer operation, then explore your system on your own. "Well-intentioned family members and friends can destroy your bonding experience with your computer," says Masie. "Learning to use a computer is like learning to drive a car with a manual transmission. At first, you need someone to show you how to shift. But then you need to drive around alone for a while to get over your fear of grinding the gears."

❏ Ask a child rather than an adult for assistance. "Children have no fear of computers," according to Dr. Simon. "They can easily show you how to get around on one. And their freedom and willingness to experiment is contagious. A computer-savvy kid can make you computer-friendly fast."

❏ Read the most basic, simple instructions you can find. "Sometimes the manual that comes with the computer is just too complex and overwhelming for beginners," notes Masie. "Instead, you may want to try one of the many computer books in the . . . *for Dummies* series. They are informative, user-friendly, and very easy to follow—even for the most inexperienced computer user."

❏ Play the computerized version of solitaire. "With a familiar game like solitaire, you forget your computer angst and loosen up," says Rebecca

Pratt, director of the closing desk for *Newsweek* in New York City. "It's a great normalizing experience, especially if you are terrified that you could blow up your computer by pushing the wrong button."

Playing solitaire also helps beginning keyboarders become comfortable with the computer's mouse, the point-and-click device that accesses information, says Pratt, who has trained literally hundreds of *Newsweek* staffers about the intricacies of the magazine's computer system.

❐ Give yourself five hours to master your first task. "Concentrate on learning one basic program," suggests Masie. "Once you feel that you have a handle on that one program, you will have a much easier time progressing to more challenging tasks."

Prescriptions
TO BECOME BETTER EQUIPPED

Rx

You have mastered some basic skills and feel comfortable navigating the keyboard. These tips from the pros can ensure that your computer experience continues to be a positive one.

❐ Select software specifically designed for home use. Good choices include software bundles such as Claris Works and Microsoft Works. These products contain the basic programs that you will need at home, including word processing, database, and spreadsheet capabilities. They are good choices because each program within the bundle operates similarly; learn one and you can probably handle the rest, according to Masie.

❐ Subscribe to an all-purpose online service, such as America Online or Compuserve. These services have a number of advantages: They are easier to use than the Internet; they offer practical information (like food recipes and stock market quotes) as well as just-for-fun programs; and they provide simple electronic-mail (e-mail) service to anyone, anywhere in the world. Of course, they also provide access to the Internet, which you ultimately will want to master, says Masie.

❐ Explore the Internet world. "If you're new to computers, exploring the Internet is a great way to get a feel for your system," says Masie. "Have someone show you how to use the search function, then take it from there. If you run into a problem, you will probably find the solution on your own within a few minutes."

❐ Frequently save any document you have open and make a back-up copy of every file. These strategies safeguard your work in the event that your system "crashes," causing it to lose information.

❐ In the event of a problem, find someone who is familiar with computers or call the customer service department of the place where you purchased the computer. These people can explain to you what has happened and what you need to do in language you can understand. "If you call a help desk—which is something like a high-tech customer service department—you will probably end up speaking with someone who lives and breathes computerese," says Masie. "That can make you feel incompetent and inadequate."

Depression

The World Health Organization predicts that by the year 2020, depression will rank right behind heart disease as the world's second most disabling illness. And if the current trend continues, most of its victims will be female. Right now, women are three times more likely than men to develop depression.

LIFETIME

"Women do have times in their lives when they seem especially vulnerable to depression," says Laura Epstein Rosen, Ph.D., supervisor of family therapy training for the Special Needs Clinic at Columbia-Presbyterian Medical Center in New York City. Sometimes the risk is biologically driven, as when hormone levels fluctuate just after child-birth and just before menopause. Other times it is externally driven—perhaps by the death of a parent, divorce, job loss, or some other major life event.

Even everyday conflict can brew into mild depression, says Susan

Heitler, Ph.D., a clinical psychologist in Denver who wrote and recorded the audiotape *Depression: A Disorder of Power.* "When you want X and your partner wants Y, you have a problem," she explains. If you repeatedly give up what you want so that your partner gets what he wants, without seeking a mutually satisfying compromise, you may pay an emotional price in the long run.

Mild depression often manifests itself as deeply negative feelings of sorrow, guilt, discouragement, and powerlessness. More severe cases may be accompanied by symptoms such as loss of appetite, lack of sleep, and difficulty concentrating.

The good news about depression is that once you recognize that you have it, you can easily treat it. "By knowing when you are vulnerable to depression and by recognizing its signs and symptoms, you can get the help you need," says Dr. Rosen.

What's more, depression may draw your attention to some aspect of your life that needs evaluation and change, says Margaret Jensvold, M.D., director of the Institute for Research on Women's Health in Rockville, Maryland. "If you find yourself repeatedly getting upset or sad about the same situation, you need to come to terms with that situation, one way or another," she advises.

Prescriptions
FOR BEATING THE BLUES

Rx

For severe depression, you will need to see a doctor, who may recommend a combination of talk therapy and antidepressant drugs. Mild depression responds well to self-care measures like these.

❒ Drink one to two cups of St.-John's-wort tea every day. Research suggests that St.-John's-wort is just as effective as commonly prescribed antidepressant drugs, but with fewer side effects. Compounds in the yellow-flowered herb appear to stimulate brain cells.

To make the tea, pour one cup boiling water over one to two heaping teaspoons dried herb (available in health food stores). Allow the herb to steep for 10 minutes. Then strain the tea and set it aside to cool a bit before drinking it.

Because of its stimulant properties, St.-John's-wort should not be taken at bedtime, advises Varro Tyler, Ph.D., author of *Herbs of Choice*. The herb also increases your sensitivity to sunlight, making you burn more easily. So while you are using St.-John's-wort, limit the time you spend in the sun and use a sunscreen on all exposed areas.

❏ Eat six small meals, spaced three hours apart over the course of the day. Sticking with this schedule helps keep your blood sugar on a more even keel. "For some people, low blood sugar can trigger depression," says Dr. Jensvold. Of course, you should make sure that each of the six meals

---

A Visualization Prescription for Confronting Conflict

Depression often stems from an unresolved problem with another person—be it a spouse, a sibling, or a co-worker. The following exercise, recommended by Susan Heitler, Ph.D., a clinical psychologist in Denver who wrote and recorded the audiotape *Depression: A Disorder of Power*, can help you work through the situation so that both of you come out ahead—and happy.

❏ Recognize your negative feelings as depression.

❏ Look for the cause of your depression. Ask yourself what conflict or frustrating situation lies behind your sad feelings.

❏ Visualize your way out of the conflict with these simple steps.

1. Close your eyes. Ask yourself, "If I were mad at someone, who would it be?"

2. Allow the image of who you feel mad at to appear on your mental screen.

3. Pretend that you're Alice in Wonderland. You have just sipped the growth drops. See yourself grow bigger and

is well-balanced. Choose whole grains, fruits, vegetables, and nonfat or low-fat dairy products.

❐ Eliminate caffeine and sugar for two weeks and notice if you feel any better. "The more severe your depression, the more you will benefit from purging your diet of caffeine and sugar, though we're not sure why," says Larry Christensen, Ph.D., chairman of the department of psychology at the University of South Alabama in Mobile.

You probably already know the caffeine culprits: coffee, tea, cola, and chocolate. As for sugar, avoid candy, baked goods, and other treats. The

bigger until you tower over the person with whom you are in conflict.

4. From your new, powerful vantage point, reassess the other person and what each of you want.

5. Use what you can now see about that person to discover new possibilities for resolving your conflict in a mutually beneficial way.

To understand how this exercise supports conflict resolution, think of a woman who views herself as small and powerless in her relationship with her husband. Because of her self-image, she may be unable to assert herself effectively when a problem arises. Leaving the problem unresolved could cause her to become depressed.

If she visualizes herself as bigger and more powerful than her husband, she may notice things about him that she never did before. "For example, her husband's body language might tell her that he is actually scared or insecure," says Dr. Heitler. "Understanding him more fully can help her devise solutions to the problem that will benefit both of them."

sugars that naturally occur in fruits and other foods are okay, according to Dr. Christensen.

If your symptoms do improve during those two weeks of abstention, you could try reintroducing caffeine and sugar one at a time. You may find that you can tolerate one but not the other.

TIME IT RIGHT

❐ Do some aerobic exercise (the kind that pumps up your heart and respiration rates) for 20 to 30 minutes at least three days a week. "Any depressed woman who makes herself work out will experience a definite improvement in the way she feels about herself," says Robert S. Brown Sr., M.D., Ph.D., clinical professor of psychiatric medicine at the University of Virginia in Charlottesville. "The effort and vigor with which you work out is proportional to the physical and emotional benefits that you receive." In other words, the more you sweat, the less blue you will be.

❐ Write down how you feel. "Keeping a diary can help you work through your depression," notes Dr. Jensvold. It allows you to articulate, vent, and come to terms with your unhappiness.

❐ Create a human support system. "You need to have a friend or two to call upon when you are sad, someone who can give you the gift of listening," says Dr. Jensvold. But, she adds, make sure you share good times with that person, too.

Medical **Alert**

Read and respond to the following two questions.

1. Have you had a distinct period during which you felt down and unhappy or you lost your pleasure and interest in life?

2. Have you suffered from at least five of these eight symptoms for two weeks or longer?

✓ Appetite or weight changes
✓ Sleep problems
✓ Excessive fatigue
✓ Excessive agitation or lethargy
✓ Loss of interest or pleasure in usual activities
✓ Guilty feelings
✓ Slow thinking or indecisiveness
✓ Suicidal thoughts

If you answered yes to both questions—and especially if you have had suicidal thoughts—see your doctor. You may have severe depression, which requires professional care, says Gary Emery, Ph.D., director of the Los Angeles Center for Cognitive Therapy and author of *Rapid Relief from Emotional Distress*.

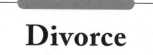

Divorce

Ask any woman who has weathered a divorce, and she will likely describe it as one of the most soul-searing experiences of her life. Even when a marriage has been difficult or impossible, ending it creates painful emotional fallout for everyone—particularly when children are involved. And that fallout can last, quite literally, for years.

"Getting over a divorce takes time," explains Constance Ahrons, Ph.D., professor of sociology at the University of Southern California in Los Angeles and author of *The Good Divorce*. "The only way to get past the pain and anger is to grieve the losses—perhaps for two to five years." The longer you were married, the longer your grieving process may be.

In many respects, coming to terms with divorce is like coping with the death of a loved one. "Divorce is the death of a dream—your vision of what your marriage and your future would be," notes Dr. Ahrons.

In addition to the initial grieving process, divorce can have even longer-term effects on your personal life. For instance, you may develop depression.

With all its baggage, emotional and otherwise, divorce marks a major transition in a woman's life. Yet sometimes starting over is the only real solution when a relationship is irreparably broken. If your marital ties are becoming undone, ask yourself these questions, suggests Diane Medved, Ph.D., a psychologist in Seattle and author of *The Case against Divorce*.

1. Are you unable to function because your relationship is punishing, distant, or unbearable?

2. Do you seek every possible opportunity to be apart from your spouse?

3. Would you rather be alone for the rest of your life than continue your marriage?

4. Are your values completely incompatible with your spouse's? (For example, you want monogamy, but he doesn't. Or you want children, but he doesn't.)

If you answer yes to any of these questions, your marriage is in some trouble. Two or three yeses mean that divorce is a real possibility, but you still have hope. If you answer yes to all four questions, divorce may be your only option. In any of these cases, you should find a good marriage counselor who views divorce as a regrettable last option, advises Dr. Medved.

Rx ——— *Prescriptions*
FOR PATCHING YOUR PARTNERSHIP

If you and your spouse take time to work out your problems at the first sign that the intimacy between you is gone, you just might save your marriage, says John R. Mondschein, a Fellow of the American Academy of Matrimonial Lawyers and an attorney in Allentown, Pennsylvania, who specializes in divorce law. "Couples who enter marriage counseling long after they have stopped communicating are in trouble," he notes. The person who initiates divorce may have been thinking about it for years and has already decided to go through with it. "You want to enter counseling before you reach this stage," advises Mondschein. "And you have to find a counselor who wants to support your marriage rather than help you ease out of it." These strategies can help you get the most from your counseling sessions.

❏ Ask people whom you respect and trust to recommend a marriage counselor. You may want to consult your closest friends, your doctor, your lawyer, or your clergyman. "Word of mouth is the best way to find an effective counselor since most states have no certification requirements and do not regulate the industry," according to Mondschein.

❏ Continue attending your counseling sessions, even when they become difficult or painful. Understand that repairing a marriage takes time, hard work, and commitment. During counseling, you may not always like what you hear, says Mondschein.

Know When to Call It Quits

Sometimes even the best counseling can't save a bad marriage. The following three factors make divorce virtually unavoidable, says Diane Medved, Ph.D., a psychologist in Seattle and author of *The Case against Divorce*.

Chronic addiction or substance abuse. If your spouse has a problem with alcohol or drugs but refuses to seek treatment, you may have little choice but to end your marriage, says Dr. Medved. The same holds true if your spouse has been in one treatment program after another without success, and nothing significant has happened to change his future prognosis.

Psychosis. The spectrum of mental illness can range from mild to severe and perpetually disturbing, according to Dr. Medved. The good news is that many conditions once thought to be incurable now are successfully managed with medication. If your spouse is undergoing treatment, you should try to hang in there until all medical options have been played out, she advises. But if your spouse has a psychosis—an inability to recognize reality and communicate with others—coupled with a prolonged lack of affection or desire to keep the marriage going, your only option may be to sever marital ties and move on.

Physical or emotional abuse. If you have been the victim of any kind of spousal abuse, seek help immediately. "No one should ever remain in a marriage in which her physical or mental well-being is in jeopardy," says Dr. Medved.

❐ Find another counselor if you are uncomfortable with the one you are seeing or if you have made little progress after several visits. Sometimes a counselor isn't the best match for you and your spouse. That doesn't mean that you should give up counseling altogether. Simply try someone else.

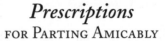

Prescriptions
FOR PARTING AMICABLY

Talking hasn't helped. Counseling hasn't either. You and your spouse argue constantly—or have stopped communicating altogether. Your children feel confused and hurt. Clearly, your marriage has suffered a meltdown.

How you initiate your divorce, and how you interact with your spouse as your marriage breaks up, helps determine how quickly you begin to heal emotionally. "Remember that time improves everything," says Dr. Ahrons. "There is life after divorce."

In the meantime, try these tactics to take some of the sting out of your split.

TIME IT RIGHT   ❐ Broach the subject of divorce with your spouse. "In most cases, the woman initiates the discussion of divorce," says Dr. Ahrons. "Simply mentioning the word *divorce* can be a turning point in a relationship." In fact, it's enough to prompt some couples to seek marriage counseling. "Call it shock therapy," adds Mondschein.

❐ Refrain from creating a marital crisis just so you have a reason to seek a divorce. "Even when you have endured a painful marriage, you may be unwilling to end it unless a crisis forces you to," explains Dr. Ahrons. And if no such crisis exists, you may subconsciously try to manufacture one.

Suppose one of you spends a lot of time away from home, either at the office or on business trips. This creates an emotional distance that can push the other person into an extramarital affair. The affair then becomes the reason for a divorce, even though the real problem is the demise of intimacy in your marriage.

❐ Prepare for the flood of emotions that begins once you and your partner formally agree to part. Read up on the subject of divorce. Talk to family members and friends who have experienced what you are about to go through. Consider joining a support group.

The initial separation is perhaps the most poignant and painful time of the entire process of divorce. You have to tell your children, decide who gets what, and deal with the reality that you will be on your own. "When one of you moves out, you begin to realize how much you are going to miss your partner. You may feel an overwhelming sense of loneliness and loss," notes Dr. Ahrons. But don't confuse these emotions with love, cautions Mondschein. Many couples reconcile at this time only to separate again because they misread the feelings they experienced.

"On the other hand," adds Dr. Ahrons, "many women experience a tremendous sense of freedom, release, and relief at the time of separation."

❏ Hire an experienced attorney who limits her practice to divorce and divorce-related matters such as property division, alimony, and child custody and support. Meet with each of your prospective choices to determine which one you feel will be most sensitive to your needs, suggests Mondschein. This means providing good client service as well as aggressive representation.

The American Academy of Matrimonial Lawyers can put you in touch with divorce lawyers practicing in your area. For more information, contact the organization at 150 North Michigan Avenue, Suite 2040, Chicago, IL 60601.

Prescriptions
FOR HIRING A MEDIATOR

Rx

If you and your spouse part less than peaceably, you may face a costly adversarial divorce, which can be time-consuming and emotionally draining. Mediation can help the two of you mutually work out everything from financial arrangements to custodial issues, says Mondschein. "It gives you the opportunity to ask yourself what you want your relationship with your spouse to be like once your marriage is over."

"Mediation usually doesn't produce more scars," agrees Dr. Ahrons. "It teaches you and your soon-to-be ex how to use negotiating and problem-solving skills. It also gives the two of you a chance to decide what kind of parenting partnership you will have with each other for the rest of your lives." In addition, mediation is likely to be far less expensive than a traditional divorce.

If you go the mediation route, you and your spouse will attend 5 to 10 sessions facilitated by an unbiased third party. "Most mediators have backgrounds in law, psychology, or social work," notes Mondschein. To make sure that you hire someone who is competent and qualified, he offers these tips.

❐ Choose a mediator with appropriate experiences and expertise. If your divorce involves complex financial issues—perhaps a large sum of money is involved or one of you is self-employed—you will want a mediator who has an accounting as well as a legal background. If your marital issues are more emotional than financial, or involve primarily children, you will more likely benefit from a mediator who has a background in psychology as well as in law.

The Academy of Family Mediators can refer you to a mediator with the appropriate training for your particular situation. Contact the organization at 4 Militia Drive, Lexington, MA 02173.

❐ Have a prospective mediator provide the names of some lawyers who have represented her clients. Then contact those lawyers and ask them specifically for their impressions of the mediator's negotiating skills, suggests Mondschein.

❐ Ask a prospective mediator how many complex divorces involving property and children she has negotiated, if those are issues for you. "You want someone who has plenty of experience handling situations that are similar to yours," notes Mondschein.

❐ Seek the advice of your attorney both before and between mediation sessions. While she won't directly participate in the sessions, your attorney plays a very meaningful role in the mediation process. She can help ensure that all of the property has been identified and properly valued. She is also responsible for drafting the agreement that you and your spouse reach.

Forgetfulness

Forget something? No big deal. It happens to every one of us—perhaps more often than we would care to admit. And while these synaptic slips may have something to do with the fact that we are getting older, they may just as well stem from stress or even boredom.

Certainly, age is a factor in forgetfulness. In fact, the quantity and quality of your memories began to deteriorate when you were just 18, says Glenn Smith, Ph.D., a psychologist at the Mayo Medical School in Rochester, Minnesota. "It's not that you remember less as you age," he explains. "It's that you need less time to acquire information at 18 than you do at 45—just as you need less time at 45 than you do at 75."

From your late teens to early thirties, you are under tremendous pressure to learn and recall information, observes Douglas Herrmann, Ph.D., a research psychologist in the department of psychology at Indiana State University in Terre Haute. "Older people may not actually have memory problems," he theorizes. "Rather, they may simply be under less pressure to remember and recall information. Different stages of life produce different levels of motivation and expectation."

Stress, not age, is responsible for most episodes of forgetfulness, believes Dr. Herrmann. "Emotionally charged events—childbirth, divorce, job loss, death of a loved one—can wreak havoc on anyone's memory at any age," he says.

Does gender play a role in how well we remember information? Quite possibly, yes. "The notion that women are better at remembering shopping lists and men are better at remembering directions is true," according to Dr. Herrmann. But as with age, gender-based differences in memory may be borne not of ability but of expectations.

"It's quite possible that women recall items on lists better simply because they are expected to," says Dr. Herrmann. "Likewise, men are expected to remember directions—and to never, ever stop and ask for them."

When you get right down to it, memory may be nothing more than a matter of experience, suggests Dr. Herrmann. "If a woman is good at remembering lists, it is because she has done most of the grocery shopping," he says. "And if a man is good at remembering directions, it is because he has done most of the driving." Reverse their experiences, and the woman will excel at remembering directions, while the man will shine at remembering lists.

Prescriptions
FOR MAXIMUM MEMORY

HERBAL
Rx

The search continues for the magic elixir that will boost brainpower and prevent memory loss. Some research hints at a possible link between blood sugar levels and memory. "Findings like these make me optimistic that there will someday be nutritional and drug aids to enhance cognitive functions such as the ability to remember," says Paul E. Gold, Ph.D., professor of psychology and member of the neuroscience program at the University of Virginia in Charlottesville.

In the meantime, if you want to remember better naturally, try these herbal remedies recommended by Kathi Keville, director of the American Herb Association in Nevada City, California, and author of *Herbs for Health and Healing*.

❒ Sniff the scent of rosemary essential oil. Aromatherapists have identified rosemary as a mental stimulant that enhances memory and concentration. You can buy the essential oil in health food stores and some specialty bath-and-beauty shops.

❒ Take ginkgo supplements according to the directions on the label. Numerous studies show that ginkgo not only improves blood flow to the brain but also enhances the brain's ability to use oxygen, says Keville. You can buy ginkgo supplements in health food stores. Be aware that you need to take the supplements for one to three months before you notice a difference in your mental performance.

Rx ———— *Prescriptions*
FOR TOTAL RECALL

You can sharpen your cognitive skills by learning a few tricks of the memory trade. The following techniques can help you remember anything with ease.

❒ Slow the rate at which you receive information. Studies have shown that people may experience memory lapses when information is presented to them at such a fast pace that they have little time to process it, says Dr. Smith. He recommends that you employ delay tactics to buy the time you need.

For instance, when you are introduced to someone at a party, engage that person in a brief conversation. Repeat her name, ask her where she works, compliment her on her outfit. This technique gives you time to commit her name to memory, plus it establishes associations that you can use to recall her name later on.

Just a Reminder . . .

Sometimes you may need more than mental tricks to keep track of everything on your schedule. You can have your pick of dozens of modern memory aids, from not-so-high-tech portable daily planners to state-of-the-art computer software.

Among the latest innovations catering to the fashionably forgetful is the specialized reminder service. For a small annual fee, a reminder service remembers important occasions such as birthdays and anniversaries for you. A week or so before the date, the service sends you a reminder postcard. It may even offer to buy your gift for the special occasion. To locate such a service, check the Internet under "Reminder Service."

❐ **Repeat information out loud.** For example, you could use this technique in the preceding party scenario. When you are introduced to someone, say the person's name: "Nice to meet you, Lynn." Later, say her name in conversation: "Have you tried that new restaurant on Elm Street, Lynn?" Then when you leave, say her name one last time: "Lynn, I really enjoyed our chat. I look forward to seeing you again soon."

❐ **Tune in to what you need to remember.** "Especially in stressful situations, you may not connect to the source that is presenting you with information," notes Dr. Smith. "Really attentive listening can go a long way toward helping you commit information to memory, whether it is a medical diagnosis from a doctor or directions to someone's home."

❐ **Use visualization to create associations** between what you want to remember and what is actually memorable. "When you meet someone for the first time, for example, pick out her most distinguishing feature and exaggerate it in your mind," suggests Dr. Smith. Then link it to their name, their job, or whatever else you want to remember.

❒ To memorize sequential information, visualize and rehearse it in the proper order. Dr. Smith refers to this as a memory path.

To create a memory path, first think of your usual routine when you arrive home from work. You unlock the door and walk in, hang up your coat, go upstairs to your bedroom to change your clothes, go downstairs to the kitchen for a snack, then sit down to read the newspaper. Associate the steps of this familiar sequence with the steps of the sequence that you need to remember.

For example, the night of the benefit dinner, you will want to remember to introduce yourself to the guest speaker (think of unlocking your door and entering your home). You will escort her to your table (hanging up your coat). You will introduce her to your associates (changing your clothes). After dinner, you escort her to the podium (getting a snack). Then you introduce her to the rest of the audience (reading the newspaper).

Medical **Alert**

Consult your doctor if you routinely (at least once a week) have trouble recalling important information, such as appointments or whether or not you have taken your medication, or if you routinely feel confused and lost in familiar situations, says Dr. Smith.

Guilt

What do women feel guilty about? Just about everything, it seems.

"Guilt is a ubiquitous emotion for women. Virtually all of us experience it from time to time," says June Price Tangey, Ph.D., associate professor at George Mason University in Fairfax, Virginia, and a clinical psychologist in Burke, Virginia.

Indeed, guilt can be an almost constant companion for some women because they feel compelled to fulfill so many expectations, adds Carole A. Rayburn, Ph.D., a clinical, consulting, and research psychologist in private practice in Silver Spring, Maryland.

What exactly is guilt? Generally, it is a troubling sense that you were responsible for something gone wrong or that you were unable to meet your or other people's expectations. Sometimes, it is a false perception—either the offense you perceive is imaginary or the cause is far deeper and widespread than you are admitting. Most any stressful situation or decision can trigger a backlash of guilt, deserved or not: arguing with your spouse ("I was unfair to him"); turning down a lunch date with a friend ("She needed to talk, and I wasn't there for her"); telling your boss that you can't take on another project because you already have too much to do ("I let the company down").

New moms are especially vulnerable to guilt, according to Dr. Rayburn. "Women who work outside the home often feel guilty about not spending enough time with their new babies," she points out. "Women who opt to stay home rather than returning to work often feel guilty, too, because they are depriving their families of a second paycheck or because they aren't currently pursuing their career." And deciding to place a child in day care has its own minefield of guilt-producing issues.

Shame, in most instances, can be more harmful than guilt, and psychologists stress the importance of knowing the difference between the two emotions.

"With guilt, you tell yourself, 'I feel bad for having done that,'" explains Dr. Tangey. "But shame makes you say, 'I'm worthless.'"

"Guilt motivates reparation," adds Richard Kolotkin, Ph.D., professor of psychology at Moorhead State University and a clinical psychologist in Moorhead, Minnesota. "It's a constructive emotion that pushes you to make amends for something that you have done or contemplate doing. Shame, on the other hand, is devastating and destructive since it motivates a desire to stay hidden. Shame implies a fundamental sense of being defective so that you may see yourself as a miserable failure when you have merely made a mistake."

Shame can be so deep-seated that it can lead to relationship and health problems, says Dr. Kolotkin. "Some women who have shameful feelings actually think of themselves as being concretely defective or deficient and undesirable," he explains. "They find ways to focus on these 'defects' to avoid confronting a much more fundamental sense of being flawed

Battling Day-Care Guilt

The issues surrounding child care generate a mother lode of guilt for many working moms. If you are concerned that day care may negatively affect your relationship with your child, one major study may help put your mind at ease.

In the study, a multi-million-dollar endeavor funded by the National Institute of Child Health and Human Development, researchers evaluated 1,300 families and their children. The researchers concluded that as long as a mother has a loving relationship with her child, the bond between them will not be eroded when the child enters day care. Only when a child has an insecure relationship with a troubled parent does day care create extra strain.

These findings are consistent with two decades of child development research. They support the premise that children who have secure relationships with their mothers show more emotional maturity and get along better with their peers and teachers than children who don't.

"The amount of time your child spends in day care or with a babysitter by no means diminishes her bond with you," says Carole A. Rayburn, Ph.D., a clinical, consulting, and research psychologist in private practice in Silver Spring, Maryland. "Just remind yourself that your child can't have too many people in her life who love her—and that includes babysitters, teachers, and other caregivers."

and unacceptable. This perception inhibits their desire for intimacy, because they believe no one could possibly be interested in them and they find reasons to support this notion. And we know that people who don't have close, supportive relationships with others tend to be less healthy than those who do."

Prescriptions
FOR CANCELING THE GUILT TRIP

While conquering shame may require professional help, getting over guilt may be more of a do-it-yourself job. For starters, give these tips a try.

❏ Set aside the notion that you can be all things to all people. The quest to be Superwoman is noble, but it is also highly unrealistic. It puts tremendous pressure on you and leaves you with an oppressive burden of guilt when you can't pull it off, says Dr. Rayburn.

❏ Ask yourself how you want to be as opposed to how others want you to be. "This is an important distinction because it changes your sense of where you find acceptance," explains Dr. Kolotkin. "The healthiest place to find acceptance is within yourself."

❏ Establish limits for yourself. "Become aware of what you can and can't accomplish in a day's time," advises Dr. Rayburn. "Don't let the expectations of others lead you to try to do more than you possibly can."

❏ Request help from family members and friends. If they balk, remind them that if you continue doing more than you can, you are going to burn out. Then you will be completely unavailable to them, says Dr. Rayburn.

❏ Monitor your self-talk (what you say to yourself in your mind) for "should" or "ought" statements. Telling yourself that you should have done this or ought to do that naturally fuels feelings of guilt and of behaving badly, according to Dr. Kolotkin. Do your best to edit these words from your vocabulary and to substitute more reasonable words and phrases like "it would be nice if I did . . ."

❏ Fix mistakes when you can, and when you can't, let go of them. TIME IT RIGHT
Guilt can be a useful tool if it makes you see that you have done something wrong, notes Dr. Tangey. If nothing can be done to change what has happened, at least you have the opportunity to avoid a repeat misstep in the future. "Women who realize this gain closure, move beyond guilt, and leave in their wake a better life," she says.

Rx ——— *Prescriptions*
FOR ESCAPING SHAME

While guilt may nag at you, shame is more subtle. It often hides behind feelings of unrealistic anger or even depression, notes Dr. Tangey. That is why you may need counseling to overcome shame. These strategies can help as well.

❐ Visualize yourself as you would most like to be (and not as you think others want you to be). Use visualization to identify your own ideals, values, and morality. This is important since it is much healthier to find acceptance from within yourself, and it can help you avoid confusing acceptance of self with acceptance by others. Having a clear mental picture of how you wish to conduct yourself in life gives you a healthy sense of pride. "And a healthy sense of pride is the antidote to feelings of shame," according to Dr. Kolotkin.

He suggests envisioning yourself in various challenging situations. Ask yourself how you, as the good person, would like to be—and not out of fear but out of desire. Then envision your response. For example, conjure a scenario that would make you really angry. Think the problem through, then picture yourself expressing your anger in a positive, constructive way. When you are done, pat yourself on the back to experience healthy pride. Say to yourself, "I really like the way I handled that."

❐ Enroll in an assertiveness training class at your local community college. Since shame is associated with an absence of power, assuming legitimate power through assertion can replace feelings of passivity with feelings of power and control, explains Dr. Kolotkin. This, in turn, helps dispel any sense of shame.

Medical **Alert**

If you are experiencing prolonged or intense guilt, it may best be handled by seeking professional counseling. Even in instances where it does not lead to serious depression, intense guilt is not healthy or productive, and it keeps a person from getting on with her life, explains Dr. Rayburn.

Hostility

Women aren't hostile. We may be upset, or irked, or downright ticked off. But hostile? Perish the thought.

Oh, we may *feel* hostile. But we would never describe ourselves that way. "Women view hostility differently than men do because it's not considered a socially acceptable female trait," says Margaret Chesney, Ph.D., professor of medicine and principal investigator for the prevention sciences group at the University of California, San Francisco, School of Medicine. "Labeling a woman as hostile may be perceived as belittling or insulting."

To be honest, psychologists and other experts in human behavior have a hard time defining just what hostility is. "Basically, a hostile person views others with cynicism and disdain, an attitude that has its roots in anger," explains Dr. Chesney. Still, she says, hostility is difficult to measure scientifically because it is such a fluid emotion. A person who is feeling hostile may be angry one moment and become passively aggressive the next.

Women, in particular, display hostility when they feel trapped in a particular situation or victimized by frequent frustrations, says Richard Carrera, Ph.D., a psychologist at the University of Miami in Coral Gables, Florida. Some women become verbally abusive and aggressive. But others turn inward rather than acting out.

"Women are more likely than men to exhibit hostility in passive ways," explains Dr. Carrera. "Rather than throwing things and resorting to violence, they tend to become quiet and withdrawn. They stop being nice to people. They start forgetting things, like appointments. And they stop showing signs of affection."

Clearly, hostility can have a negative effect on the people around you. It can have a negative effect on you, too, in terms of your health. Research has shown that compared with their more easygoing peers, women who are hostile run a greater risk of developing heart disease and other serious illnesses. They are also more prone to unhealthy behaviors such as overeating, smoking, and substance abuse.

Rx —— *Prescriptions*
TO KEEP YOUR COOL

Prone to hostile outbursts? Use the following strategies to mellow out in minutes.

☐ Take a 20-minute break from a provocative situation. You can go for a walk or water your plants or flip through a magazine. "Even though you have to come right back to the situation, getting some distance from it will lower your tendency to be hostile," explains Dr. Chesney.

☐ If you have more time, stroll around the local mall for two hours or so. "Women have a misconception that running away from a problem is wrong," says Dr. Chesney. "In fact, escaping for a short time may be what you need to rein in your hostility and deal with a situation more rationally."

☐ Recite a mantra. Dr. Chesney suggests saying to yourself, "In a month from now, this will be insignificant. I probably won't even remember this." Or, "Someday this will make a great story at a dinner party." This exercise enables you to reframe the situation and put it in its proper perspective.

Rx —— *Prescriptions*
FOR POSITIVE CHANGE

Because hostility does have serious health implications, you can do yourself a world of good by addressing its cause. These tactics can help.

☐ Identify the cause of your hostility. When you feel hostile, something has probably happened to provoke you, says Dr. Chesney. You need to ask yourself, "What's going on here? What's making me respond this way?" If you teach yourself to recognize your triggers, you can mentally prepare yourself to deal with them and minimize explosive reactions, she explains.

☐ Control stressors as much as possible. "I encourage women to enroll in stress-management courses," says Dr. Chesney. "You learn negotiating techniques and other coping skills that help prevent you from feeling overwhelmed and frustrated." Suppose you have a deadline at work that you know you can't possibly meet. Rather than responding hostilely, you can negotiate with your supervisor for a new deadline or for a helping hand to get the job done.

❑ If you can't change a situation, then change your perspective instead. You know how a new frame can make a picture look completely different? The same principle applies in life. "Suppose you dislike your job, and despite your best efforts, you can't find a better one," suggests Dr. Chesney. "Reframe your situation, putting it in a better light by focusing on what you are learning in this job that you will be able to use in the next one. Remind yourself that you won't have to stay forever, and redouble your efforts to find something more suitable."

❑ Find opportunity in adversity. Maybe you have to take time off from work because your child is sick and your husband is out of town. Rather than feeling hostile toward your mate because he is not there to help, relish the chance to spend some quality time alone with your child, says Dr. Chesney.

❑ Let your partner know what you expect when you share your feelings with him. Like most men, your husband may want to solve your problem for you. If all you want is a sounding board, tell him so. Dr. Chesney suggests this approach: "Do you have some time to hear about my day? It was wild. I don't need any advice right now, I'd just like to vent. Is that okay?"

Medical **Alert**

You should seek professional counseling from a psychologist, psychiatrist, or social worker if your hostility disrupts your personal or professional life or provokes you to hurt yourself or others, says Dr. Chesney. Ask your family physician for a referral.

Inhibited Sexual Desire

The average American woman is going places—like the office, the grocery store, the bank, the day care center, the dry cleaner, the PTA meeting. With a schedule like that, she barely has time to take a shower. So how can she possibly have time for regular, mutually satisfying sex?

"It's not necessarily that women aren't having sex because they don't want to," says Louise Merves-Okin, Ph.D., a licensed clinical psychologist and certified marriage and family therapist in private practice in Rydal, Pennsylvania. "Their problem is finding the time. I see lots of women in their thirties who are healthy, vibrant, and attractive. They love their husbands. They have successful careers, comfortable homes, attentive friends—and very young children. They tell me that they have no time or energy for pleasure."

Most of these women seek a quick fix for their waning passion, adds Dr. Merves-Okin. Ironically, the one thing that can solve the problem is the one thing they don't have. "Only time can help a woman get her sex life back on track," she notes. "She needs to work with her partner to revive romance and sexual desire. And if she doesn't take the time to communicate with her partner, her relationship could be headed for trouble."

Sometimes, though, inhibited sexual desire has nothing to do with lack of time, says Marilyn Volker, Ed.D., a sexologist in private practice in Coral Gables, Florida. "When a woman tells me that her desire is flagging, I look at three factors—what I call the three Ps," she explains. To find out if any of the three Ps might be affecting your sex drive, ask yourself the following questions.

Physical problems: Does something about your or your partner's body turn off either of you? Are you experiencing hormonal changes? Do either of you have an illness that takes a toll on your level of energy or physical comfort?

Psychological problems: Do you or your partner have concerns about sexual performance? Has your relationship been affected by job pressures, financial worries, or infidelity? Could an incident from your past, such as incest or rape, be hindering your trust of your partner?

Pharmaceutical problems: Do you or your partner abuse alcohol or recreational drugs? Are you taking a medication that could lower your sexual desire? (If you are not sure, ask your doctor or pharmacist.)

If you answered any of these questions affirmatively, you may have uncovered the cause of your stalled sex drive. You and your partner can try to work together to resolve the problem and get your sex lives back in sync.

Prescriptions
FOR AN ENTICING ATMOSPHERE

You can make any sexual encounter a more positive one simply by setting the right mood. To ensure that you and your partner are as relaxed and as comfortable as possible, take these tips to bed with you.

❐ Banish your parents' negative attitude toward sex from your bedroom. Bad messages from your formative years can sometimes intrude on good sex. "I tell some couples that they need to get their parents out of the bedroom, especially if those parents were abusive or raised them on unhelpful lessons like 'nice girls don't,'" says Gina Ogden, Ph.D., a sex therapist in Cambridge, Massachusetts, and author of *Women Who Love Sex*. She suggests making an event out of exorcising parental spirits. Tell them to leave, even if you have to make noise. Show them out the door and then shut it firmly. "This may seem simplistic, but it's an effective technique that allows you and your lover to enter into a sexual encounter as adults focused only on each other," she explains.

❐ Transform sex into a sacred ritual. "In my research, I have found that sex and spirituality have quite a connection," notes Dr. Ogden. "Some couples really take off on sex as a mystical experience. They make the bedroom a spiritual space by lighting candles and playing music that helps them feel open and safe. They practice deep breathing together. They honor and revere each other's bodies. And they look deeply into each other's eyes while they are making love."

Prescriptions
FOR MORE DESIRABLE SEX

Of course, good sex begins long before you even set foot in the bedroom. The following strategies can fill you with sweet anticipation.

❐ Recall pleasurable sensual experiences from your past. "Reconnecting to powerful feelings of sensuality—not necessarily *sexuality*—can go a long way toward helping you feel desire," explains Dr. Ogden. "Sometimes these playful, sensual memories predate adult sexual experience—like the time you went skinny-dipping when you were eight years old or you rolled around on the floor with your first puppy. Summoning the energy that infused your joy as a little girl can revitalize your sex life today."

❐ Exchange good deeds with your partner. "One woman told me that the most erotic words her husband can say to her are 'Honey, why don't you let me do the dishes?'" says Dr. Ogden. "Try to do nice things for each other. Good sex has a great deal to do with how you nurture each other."

❐ Give yourself permission to be sexual with your partner. "Sexuality isn't only about physical sensations. It is also about emotions," notes Dr. Ogden. She suggests taking time to play with each other before you

Four Days to Pure Passion

Remember how sexy you used to feel toward your mate? Remember how you planned for and fantasized about and anticipated your dates? Recapturing those emotions can help reawaken your sexual desire, says Lonnie Barbach, Ph.D., assistant clinical professor of medical psychology at the University of California, San Francisco, School of Medicine. If you want to rekindle romance and make sex sizzle, Dr. Barbach recommends the following four-day countdown to passion.

Day 4: Make a date with your mate. Write it in your calendar and his—in ink. And be sure to use the word *romance* in your invitation.

Day 3: Decide what you will do on your date. What will turn both of you on? A candlelit dinner? Dancing? A romantic movie? No matter what your dream date, you can help ensure that it happens by planning carefully. Make reservations, hire a sitter, or ask Grandma if the kids can spend the night.

Day 2: Start simmering. "This means thinking about your mate the way you did when you were dating," explains Dr.

have sex: Prepare food together and feed it to each other. Take showers or bubble baths together. Surprise each other in the intimate ways that only you know.

❒ Teach your partner to touch you in ways that you find pleasurable. "Women have told me that they can reach orgasm all over their bodies—for instance, when their partners massage their heads, nuzzle their earlobes, or suck their fingers," says Dr. Ogden.

❒ Encourage your partner to spend time stimulating you. "A lot of women say to me, 'My partner gets me just to the point where I'm about to explode, and then he moves on to something else,'" says Dr. Ogden. "Probably the most difficult part of a sexual relationship is learning how

---

Barbach. "Envision his body. Fantasize about his touch. Feel his lips on yours . . . you get the idea." Spend 10 to 20 minutes simply daydreaming about how romantic your date will be.

Date day: Prepare your body. Some women shave and perfume themselves, while others prefer to go *au naturel*, says Dr. Barbach. "Dress to impress your partner, in whatever turns him on. Invest in some sexy lingerie—or surprise him by not wearing any underwear at all."

Also, create an atmosphere that is conducive to romance. Turn off the phone, dim the lights, adjust the thermostat so that it is neither too warm nor too cold. Burn candles and play romantic music, if you wish.

Most important of all, make a sexy connection with your partner. "Talk to him. Tell him how happy you are to be with him. Tell him how important he is to you," suggests Dr. Barbach. "Strengthening your connection as a couple before you have sex will go a long way toward making your romantic evening a resounding success."

to cue your partner to continue doing what feels good to you. But asking for what you want is vital to your arousal."

❒ Avoid viewing intercourse as the be-all and end-all sexual experience. Mutual or solo masturbation can be very erotic, too, notes Dr. Ogden.

Rx —— *Prescriptions*
for a Passionate Partnership

Inevitably, there will be times when your partner is in the mood and you are not. And because you love him, you want to at least try to feel receptive to his advances. Here is how the experts suggest you do it.

TIME IT RIGHT

❒ Reset your sexual body clock. If you come alive well after 5:00 P.M., but he's raring to go at dawn, the two of you have some negotiating to do, says Dr. Ogden. You may want to try going to bed earlier so that you wake up earlier. Or arrange to "do lunch" with your partner, at least once in a while. "Or save sex for weekends, when the kids are staying with Grandma, the TV is unplugged, and the phone is off the hook," she suggests.

If morning stud/evening dud syndrome seems persistent, it is something that the two of you need to discuss. "Communicate openly and honestly with each other to be sure that other problems aren't interfering with your sex life," advises Dr. Ogden.

❒ Give yourself to your partner on occasion. "When you are not in the mood but your partner is, you may just want to say, 'This one's for you, kid,'" says Dr. Volker. "Giving yourself to the one you love can be a very sensual experience." What's more, seeing that your partner is satisfied may leave you feeling satisfied as well.

❒ Use a water-based lubricant such as K-Y Liquid or Astroglide. If you are not aroused, your vagina won't lubricate sufficiently for comfortable intercourse, explains Dr. Volker.

❒ If you and your partner are using a condom, avoid using oil-based products and petroleum jelly as lubricants. They can weaken latex condoms and render them ineffective, cautions Dr. Volker.

Medical **Alert**

See your gynecologist if your sexual desire continues to wane despite self-care measures such as those described above. You may have an underlying health problem such as chronic fatigue syndrome, depression, Lyme disease, or a thyroid disorder. And if you suspect that an emotional conflict is sapping your sexual desire, consider getting counseling from a psychotherapist or sex therapist, adds Lonnie Barbach, Ph.D., assistant clinical professor of medical psychology at the University of California, San Francisco, School of Medicine.

Insecurity and Low Self-Esteem

There are absolutely brilliant women who can do anything—except make a decision. They will analyze both sides of a problem, see all aspects of it, but they cannot bring themselves to decide what to do about it. "Such chronic indecisiveness stems from insecurity. And insecurity is a product of low self-esteem," says Carol Goldberg, Ph.D., a clinical psychologist and president of Getting Ahead Programs, a corporation based in New York City and Long Island, New York.

"When a woman has low self-esteem, she lacks the confidence to be assertive and decisive," explains Dr. Goldberg. "Low self-esteem holds you back and prevents you from reaching your full potential. When you can't take a risk or trust your own judgment, you have a hard time getting ahead—especially in the business world."

While low self-esteem can affect anyone, it is especially common among women who have endured some degree of physical or emotional mistreatment. "It may seem shocking, but it is true: Approximately one-third of all women have been abused by the age of 21," says Dr. Goldberg. "These women are at high risk for self-esteem problems, because being battered or berated by the important people in your life lowers your sense of self-worth and destroys your confidence."

Low self-esteem can breed other emotional troubles as well. But

LIFETIME

women often overlook this crucial connection, according to Eleta Greene, Ph.D., a psychologist and director of Creative Survival Systems in New York City.

"A woman may know that she is unhappy, but she may not know why," explains Dr. Greene. "She may tell herself, 'Nothing goes right for me. I'm depressed. I'm unhappy at work.' The problem may be that she does not realize her own self-worth. She doesn't realize her own intrinsic value. She may depend on other people's opinions for her self-validation rather than singing her own praises." Those people, however, may simply be reinforcing her low self-esteem.

In fact, how others respond to you may be a good indicator of your self-esteem status. "If your spouse, boss, or friends are constantly telling you to stop sitting on the fence and to make a decision already, you may want to consider the role that low self-esteem plays in your life," says Dr. Goldberg.

Rx ——— *Prescriptions*
FOR FEELING GOOD ABOUT YOURSELF

If your self-esteem could use a boost—or if you need a personal security blanket—consider these expert suggestions.

❐ Create a personal "bank book" for tracking your self-worth. This works much like an actual bank book—but instead of deposits and withdrawals, you are entering your assets and your perceived shortcomings.

You can use a blank journal for this exercise. On one side of a page, write down all of your good qualities. On the other side, write down your bad qualities. The catch: For every bad quality, you must flip the page and enter two good qualities. "This enables a woman to discover how she really sees herself," says Dr. Greene. "It also encourages her to give more weight to her 'credits' than to her 'debits.'"

❐ Replace negative self-talk with positive thoughts. "Sometimes a woman can be her own worst enemy by mentally replaying the harmful messages she heard back in childhood," says Dr. Greene. "The minute you catch yourself thinking, 'No wonder this went wrong. I can never do anything right. Things always end up badly for me,' stop yourself. Then think of at least five situations that have gone right for you and give them at least as much weight as you give your failures."

❏ Recall situations where you took charge. Women with low self-esteem often believe that they have no control over a particular situation. "Knowing that you were capable of taking charge in the past may convince you that you are just as capable now," says Dr. Goldberg.

Perhaps your child had a minor mishap. Think back to how you stopped her bleeding, called her doctor, and drove her to the hospital to get stitched up. You may have been shaking in your boots afterward, but you did what you had to do when you had to do it.

❏ Make a list of your abilities and accomplishments. Then review the list and circle those items that seem relevant to the current situation. This exercise can help you when you are having trouble making a decision, says Dr. Goldberg.

Suppose you are thinking of volunteering for a special project at work, but you can't make up your mind one way or the other. Decide what skills the project requires. Perhaps it needs a detail-oriented person who is dependable and always on time. When you scan your list, you may realize that you demonstrated those same talents when you successfully coordinated the PTA's bake sale last year. So you know that you are capable of handling the work project, too.

Mental Blocks

When confronted with the mountain, the Little Engine That Could might just as easily have slipped into reverse and rolled back home. Instead, he decided to accept the challenge. And eventually, he crested the peak, chanting, "I think I can. I think I can," all the way.

He had the right idea. Though the story may be coated with candy-cane sentimentality, experts say that even we grown-ups can learn a lesson from the Little Engine's "I think I can" mantra. It is the perfect remedy for overcoming a mental block.

When you have a mental block, you are unable to take action on a particular task or problem, explains Carol Goldberg, Ph.D., a clinical psychologist and president of Getting Ahead Programs, a corporation based in New York City and Long Island, New York. You may try to avoid making a major life decision or initiating a new project at work or even completing a menial chore.

A mental block can occur when you are faced with an unpleasant or difficult task—or with too many tasks at once. "When it came to a hard-to-start chore, such as filing a month's worth of old memos, men traditionally asked their wives or secretaries to handle it," notes Dr. Goldberg. "But if you are the wife or secretary who is always getting dumped on, you may reach a point where you feel that you are being treated unfairly. These chores, added to your own responsibilities, may make you feel so overwhelmed that you mentally stall out."

Rx ——— *Prescriptions*
TO GET THE JOB DONE

The workplace is littered with potential mental blocks. When you already have a full workload, taking on one more assignment can seem especially daunting. Use these strategies for success.

TIME IT RIGHT

❐ Create a timetable for completing a specific task. Suppose you have to clean up your office. Set aside 20 minutes every day for one week and use that time for organizing, putting away, and tossing out, suggests Dr. Goldberg.

❐ Break down a major project into smaller tasks. If you try to tackle the whole thing at once, you may quickly feel overwhelmed and frustrated, says Judith S. Beck, Ph.D., clinical associate professor of psychology in psychiatry at the University of Pennsylvania in Philadelphia and director of the Beck Institute for Cognitive Therapy and Research in Bala Cynwyd, Pennsylvania. That only tempts you to put it off. Instead, plan out the project in doable chunks. Allow yourself a reasonable amount of time to complete each chunk.

❐ Rethink what a project entails and eliminate any unnecessary tasks. If you are a perfectionist, you may put more into a project than you really need to, notes Dr. Beck. For instance, if your boss asks you to brief him on the Benson account, you don't necessarily have to walk into the meeting equipped with handouts, charts, and graphs. Some notes for your own reference should suffice.

Incidentally, the same rule applies on the home front. If you think that your kitchen is a mess, you can tidy up by doing the dishes and sweeping the floor. Reorganizing your cabinets, however, goes beyond the call of duty.

Prescriptions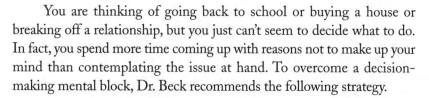
TO TACKLE HOUSEHOLD CHORES

These days, most women have two full-time occupations: the one they get paid for and the one they do gratis—otherwise known as housework. When you put in a full day at your "real" job, you don't necessarily feel like spending the evening wielding a vacuum cleaner or an iron. The following tactics can help you over the housecleaning hurdle.

❒ Use the "three-basket system" to clean out household clutter. Organizational experts recommend this technique as a means of simplifying housecleaning, says Dr. Beck. All you have to do is walk through your house with three baskets. In one basket, toss garbage, old magazines and newspapers, junk mail—everything that has outlived its usefulness. In another basket, put stuff that is out of place and belongs elsewhere. The third basket is for stuff that you are not sure about. "You can contain it now and deal with it later," she notes.

❒ Hire a professional to get the job done. "It is perfectly okay to hire someone to clean your house or wash your windows or mow your lawn," says Dr. Beck. "Where is it written that a household chore is done best only when it is done by you?"

Prescriptions
TO MAKE UP YOUR MIND

You are thinking of going back to school or buying a house or breaking off a relationship, but you just can't seem to decide what to do. In fact, you spend more time coming up with reasons not to make up your mind than contemplating the issue at hand. To overcome a decision-making mental block, Dr. Beck recommends the following strategy.

❐ Ask yourself what will happen if you do nothing. "Sometimes women have difficulty making decisions because they believe that they will be trapped forever by whatever they decide," explains Dr. Beck. "But doing something—even if it turns out to be the wrong thing—is better than doing nothing. Because when you do nothing, nothing changes."

Suppose, for example, you have received a job offer. You could accept the position and end up hating it. At worst, that means you would have to make another change down the road. But the chances may be equally good that you would end up loving it. The point is that if you are unhappy where you are now, you are probably better off trying something new than staying put.

Medical **Alert**

If you feel completely stuck in some aspect of your life, seek professional advice. "Part of being stuck is feeling that even discussing the problem with someone will trap you into a decision that you are not ready to make," explains Dr. Beck. "A good therapist can help you see all sides of the problem and approach it constructively."

Negative Thinking

Negative thinkers are human Eeyores. Much like the pessimism-personified gray donkey of Winnie the Pooh fame, they constantly put themselves down and think the absolute worst of themselves and the world around them.

"While the average person sees the glass as half-full, a negative thinker sees it as half-empty," says Carol Goldberg, Ph.D., a clinical psychologist and president of Getting Ahead Programs, a corporation based in New York City and Long Island, New York. "This pessimistic attitude can affect many aspects of a woman's life. It's as though a tape keeps playing the same message over and over in her mind: 'It's my fault. I'm a bad person. Everything I do turns out wrong.'"

Unlike male negative thinkers, who tend to take action to address whatever is bothering them, many female negative thinkers tend to dwell on their problems. "Women often allow their pessimism to overwhelm them," explains Judith S. Beck, Ph.D., clinical assistant professor of psychology in psychiatry at the University of Pennsylvania in Philadelphia and director of the Beck Institute for Cognitive Therapy and Research in Bala Cynwyd, Pennsylvania. "This prevents them from taking action to solve their problems."

Prescriptions Rx
FOR A NEW ATTITUDE

Like any other learned behavior, negative thinking can be unlearned, according to Susan Jeffers, Ph.D., an educator and author of *End the Struggle and Dance with Life*. "You can't change the world, but you can change the way you see the world," she says. "All you have to do is find the right tools." They include the following tactics.

❐ Look for the bright side of a bad situation. By slipping on a pair of those proverbial rose-colored glasses, you can face just about anything—even illness—with some degree of joy and hope, says Dr. Jeffers. And she knows what she is talking about. After years of teaching about the power of positive thinking, Dr. Jeffers found herself stricken with breast cancer. "I knew I had a choice," she recalls. "I could bemoan my fate, or I could use it to create something wonderful, even though on the surface there is nothing particularly wonderful about breast cancer."

In retrospect, says Dr. Jeffers, "Breast cancer was the richest, most empowering experience I ever had. And it made me know for certain that you can find the good in anything if you search hard enough."

❐ Before you turn in for the night, make a list of 50 positive things that happened that day. "When I give this assignment to women in my workshop, they say, 'Fifty? I can't even think of one!'" says Dr. Jeffers. "But the next day, they find themselves looking for goodness in their lives." Little things count just as much as big things, she adds. Like the sun shining. Or your child getting a good report card. Or your car starting on a frosty morning.

NIGHTTIME

❐ Encourage yourself with positive self-talk. "With positive self-talk, you remind yourself of your past accomplishments, and you persuade yourself that you have the ability to succeed again," explains Dr. Goldberg.

A Friend in Need

We all know someone whose personality hangs like a black cloud over those around her, just waiting to rain on their parade. If you find that spending time with a perennial party pooper brings you down, too, you may need to talk to her about it, says Judith S. Beck, Ph.D., clinical assistant professor of psychology in psychiatry at the University of Pennsylvania in Philadelphia and director of the Beck Institute for Cognitive Therapy and Research in Bala Cynwyd, Pennsylvania.

She suggests that you approach the person—whether she is a family member, friend, or co-worker—like this: "You have so much potential to be happy, yet I don't perceive you as a happy person. I wonder if you are seeing the positive and negative aspects of your life in a balanced way." Then you might take the opportunity to point out things in her life that she can feel good about.

If she doesn't take the hint, back off. "Don't take on the responsibility for changing her, and don't feel the burden of having to cheer her up all the time," advises Dr. Beck.

Suppose, for example, you want to ask your boss for a raise. Rather than convincing yourself that you don't stand a chance, focus on how hard you have worked over the past year, how others have praised your dedication and initiative, and how important you are to the company. Tell yourself that you are worth it.

❐ Recite affirmations. "Use a strong, uplifting statement to buoy your spirits when everything seems to go wrong," suggests Dr. Jeffers. "When I'm totally crazed, I keep repeating to myself, 'It's all happening perfectly. It's all happening perfectly. It's all happening perfectly.'"

❐ Cry when you need to. "Too many people believe that thinking positively means denying the pain we feel. To me, that's avoidance," says Dr. Jeffers. "The reality is that we have a lot of pain in our lives, just as we have a lot of joy. Crying healthy tears allows us to connect with and feel the pain." Only then can you begin healing emotionally.

❐ Relinquish your problem to a higher power. "I have a coffee cup on my desk that says, 'Let God worry about it,'" says Dr. Jeffers. "Once you've done all that you can to resolve a particular situation, you have to let go of it. You can't allow it to weigh down the rest of your life. That's when putting your problem in the hands of a higher power can be very comforting."

Nervous Tension

For the overscheduled, multitasked modern woman, nervous tension has become a persistent, unpleasant reality. It maintains an almost constant presence in our lives. In fact, on those rare occasions when we don't feel it, we tend to get suspicious and wonder why.

"Nervous tension is really just a sign that something is troubling you—something that you need to deal with as soon as possible," says Una McCann, M.D., chief of the Unit on Anxiety Disorders at the National Institute of Mental Health in Bethesda, Maryland. "At its most dramatic, it can provoke uncomfortable anxiety or even panic attacks. But even mild nervous tension on a day-in, day-out basis can cause a host of physical and mental symptoms."

Outwardly, nervous tension may display itself as a quivering voice, shaky hands, or profuse perspiration. But it can affect you internally as well, producing headaches, backaches, insomnia, stomach or gastrointestinal discomfort, and fatigue.

In women, hormonal fluctuations aggravate nervous tension, though scientists have yet to figure out how or why. They do know that women seem more prone to anxious feelings just prior to their periods as well as during puberty and menopause—times of life when hormone levels change dramatically.

LIFETIME

Rx —— *Prescriptions*
FOR EASING EDGINESS

When nervous tension seizes control of your body, use these strategies to regain the upper hand.

TIME IT RIGHT ❏ Practice progressive muscle relaxation. This technique, which involves systematically tensing and releasing your muscles, can help calm you down within just a few moments, says Dr. McCann. It's great for calming yourself before a meeting or social event.

To give progressive muscle relaxation a try, begin by clenching your hands into fists. Hold for 10 seconds, then release. Move on to your face, tensing and releasing the muscles there. Proceed to your neck, shoulders, arms, stomach, lower back, buttocks, thighs, calves, and feet. When you are done, you should feel completely relaxed.

TIME IT RIGHT ❏ Exercise for 30 minutes at least three times a week. "Nothing wallops nervous tension like a workout," notes Dr. McCann. "It stimulates the production of endorphins, your brain's own morphinelike chemicals. Endorphins fill your entire body with a sense of calm and well-being." Be sure to choose an activity that you enjoy and are comfortable with—perhaps walking, running, cycling, or swimming.

NUTRITION
Rx —— *Prescriptions*
FOR TENSE TIMES

When nervous tension hunkers down for the long haul, you need to pay special attention to your eating habits. The foods you choose—and the times of day you consume them—can influence your anxious feelings for better or worse. Here is what you can do to make your meals and snacks work for you.

❏ Eat a well-balanced diet that emphasizes whole grains, fruits, vegetables, and low-fat proteins. "Eating healthfully isn't a cliché," says Dr. McCann. "It's essential for reducing the angst of anxiety." Shoot for 6 to 11 servings of grains, 2 to 4 servings of fruits, 3 to 5 servings of vegetables, 2 to 3 servings of low-fat dairy products, and 2 to 3 servings of proteins (lean meats, poultry, fish, and beans) every day.

Handling Illness Head-On

Few circumstances make a woman more anxious than a potential medical problem. "Suppose you find a suspicious-looking mole or a lump in your breast," says Susan Heitler, Ph.D., a clinical psychologist in Denver and author of *From Conflict to Resolution*. "The very worst thing that you can do is try to wish it away. When you are dealing with a potentially life-threatening illness, remember that bad news is better than no news."

She suggests confronting the situation instead, using the following plan of action.

❒ List your symptoms in as much detail as possible—not "headache," for example, but "pounding pain on the upper right side of my forehead."

❒ As you review these specifics, write down any questions that come to mind.

❒ Find an appropriate doctor and get yourself examined. If your doctor confirms your suspicions, ask your questions about the condition.

❒ Learn all you can about your condition. Use bookstores, your community library, and the Internet.

❒ Seek a second opinion to get a more complete understanding of the problem as well as to verify the first doctor's diagnosis and suggested course of treatment.

❒ Eat smaller but more frequent meals instead of the standard three squares. Well-balanced mini-meals, spaced every three or four hours apart throughout the day, help keep your blood sugar level on an even keel so that you don't feel shaky and out of sorts. **TIME IT RIGHT**

❒ Curb your consumption of sweets such as candy, cookies, and ice cream. "Sugary treats may calm you at first," notes Dr. McCann. "But within an hour, you will feel even more drained and anxious." That's because sweets send your blood sugar level for a roller-coaster ride, and your mood rises and falls right along with it. "You should never eat solely to soothe tension," she advises.

❏ When you do feel hungry, choose turkey breast on whole-wheat bread over a candy bar. The protein in the turkey and the complex carbohydrates in the bread fill you up nicely so that you won't feel hungry again in an hour, according to Dr. McCann. What's more, the combination gives you a more steady supply of energy than either food alone. "Proteins and carbohydrates are broken down by different enzymes and have different time courses," she explains. "Therefore, unlike simple sugars that give you a rapid high, a combination of protein and complex carbs is like a slow-release energy capsule that lasts longer."

MEALTIME

❏ Eat your last meal or snack of the day at least two hours before bedtime. "Eating too close to bedtime can interfere with sleep, causing you to feel even more anxious and irritable in the morning," says Dr. McCann.

MORNING

❏ Limit your coffee consumption to two cups a day. While some women may tolerate caffeine better than others, it does contribute to the nervous jitters, says Dr. McCann. If you have difficulty getting by without coffee in the morning, try to stick with just one cup, saving the second cup for an afternoon break. You are less likely to get jittery if you space your servings throughout the day.

Rx

Prescriptions
TO BE PREPARED

Even the most laid-back, confident woman in the world can turn into human Jell-O under certain circumstances—like when she has to deliver a speech. Or ask the boss for a raise. Or go out on a date with someone for the first time.

Any of these events can evoke what is known as situational anxiety. But you can handle it like a pro—if you are prepared, says Susan Heitler, Ph.D., a clinical psychologist in Denver and author of *From Conflict to Resolution*. She suggests the following strategies for a tension-taming state of mind.

Podium Pointers

Some women have a love-hate relationship with public speaking. They rather enjoy making presentations to people, but they fear failure. What does it take to earn the audience's rapt attention for 15 minutes, 30 minutes, or longer?

Well, think about what makes a speech interesting to you. "New or surprising information, personal anecdotes, no more than three main points, a good story to illustrate each point, solid organization, clear but lively delivery—all are keys to memorable speeches," says Susan Heitler, Ph.D., a clinical psychologist in Denver and author of *From Conflict to Resolution*.

What if you are among the majority of women who would rather walk barefoot over hot coals than suffer the pain of public speaking? You may want to try cognitive therapy, says Una McCann, M.D., chief of the Unit on Anxiety Disorders at the National Institute of Mental Health in Bethesda, Maryland. Cognitive therapy is a counseling technique that can be used to help people examine how they look at problems and learn more constructive, accurate, and realistic ways to think and behave. Cognitive therapy can help you control the physical symptoms of anxiety—such as sweating and uncontrollable shaking—in as little as 12 weeks, notes Dr. McCann.

❏ Give yourself permission to feel anxious. "Anxiety is a yellow light, not a red stop sign," says Dr. Heitler. "Anxiety tells you to look at how you can deal more effectively with a potential problem. It doesn't tell you to give up on doing what you want to do."

❏ Create a plan of action. "Suppose it's your first day back at work following a vacation," says Dr. Heitler. "Rather than feeling tense, overwhelmed, and worried about the mountain of work piled on your desk, perform some triage. Get out your calendar. Set your priorities. Systematically attack each item and deal with it according to its importance."

❐ Gather information. "Information is often the best antidote to anxiety," notes Dr. Heitler, who wrote and recorded the audiotape *Anxiety: Friend or Foe*. No matter what awful situation confronts you, learn all you can about it. The knowledge you gain can help alleviate your distress.

Overcontrolling Tendencies

If there is ever a time to have an overcontroller around, it is during an emergency. She's the one who will take charge of the situation and see to it that everyone is safe and unharmed.

An overcontroller thrives on telling others what to do. She may think of herself as a born leader. She plans and micromanages not only every single aspect of her own life but also many aspects of everyone else's lives. And that's where she runs into problems.

In a way, overcontrolling tendencies seem like mothering instincts run amok. Women who are overcontrollers don't quite trust that adults are perfectly capable of making their own decisions, says Susan Heitler, Ph.D., a clinical psychologist in Denver and author of *The Power of Two: Secrets to a Strong and Loving Marriage*. "These women truly believe that things are not going to work out unless they tell people precisely what to do and when to do it," she explains.

That attitude evokes the ire of those subjected to overcontrolling tendencies. "If you're the overcontroller, your point of view is that you are simply trying to help, to make things work out right. But from the other person's point of view, her internal alarm is screaming, 'Help! I'm being invaded!'—and she takes action to resist the invasion. The result is tension and conflict," notes Dr. Heitler.

Are you an overcontroller? Take this quick quiz to find out.

✓ When working on a joint project with someone, do you look it over and tell your partner how to do his part differently?

✓ If your husband offers to vacuum, do you tell him exactly how you want it done?

✓ Do you supervise an experienced babysitter while she changes your child's diaper to make sure that she does it your way?

If you answered yes to these questions, you have at least a little over-controller in you. Changing your style may take some effort, but it can be done. Look at it this way: You can save yourself a whole lot of time and aggravation by letting others fend for themselves. "Once you return the focus to your own life, you can tune in to your own needs and take better care of yourself," says Dr. Heitler.

Prescriptions
TO OVERCOME OVERCONTROLLING

You have convinced yourself that the world would run better with you as benevolent dictator. Those around you would rather see you deposed. The following tactics can help you rein in your reign.

❏ **Speak up for your preferences, not for others'.** Suppose that you are going out for dinner with friends. When it comes time to choose a restaurant, some people in the group might want something quick and cheap, while others might prefer something more expensive and elegant. What do you do? If you are an overcontroller, you will most likely decide what everyone else wants.

"An overcontroller avoids conflict by making a plan that no one can challenge," says Dr. Heitler. "The problem is, the plan may not reflect what she herself or anyone else really wants." You are better off simply voicing your opinion, then trusting the group to make a shared, mutual decision.

❏ **If you have children, encourage them to take responsibility for** themselves as they get older. "Ceding the reins of power is essential to a child's development," says Dr. Heitler. "A new mom controls every aspect of her baby's life—and rightly so. But as the child grows up, Mom's role must shrink to allow for more autonomy." A child in elementary school may need a reminder about doing his homework, for instance. But a child in junior high should be allowed to be personally accountable. If he doesn't get his homework done, he will have to deal with the consequences.

LIFETIME

❏ **Discuss standards for household chores.** "You and your spouse need to agree on just how clean 'clean' is," advises Dr. Heitler. If your husband offers to clean up after dinner, for example, decide up front: Should the dishes be dried by hand or left to air-dry in the dish rack? Do the countertops need to sparkle? Must the floor be mopped or just swept? Once the two of you have agreed upon the job descriptions, leave your mate alone to follow through. "Then you can reserve your comments for thanks and appreciation," she says.

❐ Offer requests rather than criticism. Suppose you are going to a cocktail party at your boss's house, and your husband is wearing a tie and jacket that match only in his dreams. Broach the subject gently and tactfully: "This party means a lot to me, and I'm feeling quite nervous about it. I'm uncomfortable with the jacket and tie you're wearing. Would you be willing to change ties?" This approach is much more likely to produce the results you want than greeting your husband with "Omigod—are you gonna wear that?" says Dr. Heitler.

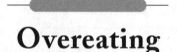

Overeating

Overeating has little to do with physical hunger. It has a lot to do with loneliness, sadness, boredom, restlessness—feelings that can send you searching for a quick food fix.

In emotionally turbulent times, eating can be soothing, satisfying, even rewarding. "You eat even though you aren't actually hungry because you have conditioned yourself to believe that food will comfort you," explains Peter M. Miller, Ph.D., director of the Hilton Head Health Institute in South Carolina.

LIFETIME

Women often begin overeating during transitional periods in their lives, notes Karen Eselson Belding, Psy.D., clinical director of the Renfew Center in Philadelphia, a women's mental health facility. She identifies four key periods when food can become a female's best friend.

✓ When a woman enters adolescence, as her body changes and is subject to scrutiny and judgment

✓ When a woman leaves home for college, career, or marriage

✔ When a woman experiences a reproductive event such as pregnancy, childbirth, or miscarriage

✔ When a woman passes through menopause

Stress can trigger overeating, too, according to Edward Abramson,
Ph.D., professor of psychology at California State University in Chico and
author of *Emotional Eating*. "Many women respond to 'background
stresses'—divorce, the death of a loved one, moving, a new job—by
bingeing on food."

Once you get in the habit of overeating, it can be hard to stop. "The
emotional prompts to overeat are often much stronger than the rational
thoughts not to," says Dr. Miller.

Still, experts emphasize that while overcoming overeating is difficult, it is by no means impossible. "The trick is to identify the emotion that
is troubling you and substitute a noncaloric way of dealing with it," explains Dr. Abramson.

Prescriptions Rx
FOR MINIMIZING THE MUNCHIES

If you are prone to overeating, you know how persuasive the urge to
binge can be. Here is how you can keep it in check.

❐ Eat three meals plus two or three snacks every day. For snacks, **DAYTIME**
choose fruits and other foods that supply no more than 100 calories each.
"The key to curbing overeating is to never allow yourself to become
hungry," according to Dr. Miller. Having a meal or snack every few hours
keeps your stomach satisfied.

❐ Keep yourself occupied in late afternoon and at bedtime. Women **NIGHTTIME**
seem most inclined to overeat at these hours of the day, notes Dr. Miller.
He suggests finding other activities that you can substitute for eating until
these danger times pass.

❐ When you feel the urge to eat, wait for 15 minutes. "You are not **TIME IT RIGHT**
saying no to your craving," says Dr. Miller. "You are just delaying it for a
little while." Women tend to believe that if they ignore their cravings, they
will become even hungrier. But the reality is that cravings come and go

in waves. If you give them time, they usually go away on their own within a matter of minutes, according to Dr. Miller.

TIME IT RIGHT

❒ Pass the time by doing something that you enjoy. Take a 15-minute walk, read a favorite magazine, plant a flower—anything to take your mind off your stomach, suggests Dr. Miller.

NIGHTTIME

❒ If you are battling the midnight munchies, first breathe deeply for a few minutes. Then write down or mentally review the reasons that you need to control your appetite, says Dr. Miller. Be sure to give those reasons a positive spin rather than a negative one. For instance, rather than telling yourself, "I need to control my appetite because I'm fat," try thinking, "I need to control my appetite so that I knock 'em dead at my class reunion next year."

TIME IT RIGHT

❒ If you still feel hungry after 15 minutes, choose a food and eat it slowly. "When emotions drive your eating, you tend to gobble the food so quickly that you don't even taste it," notes Dr. Miller. "The slower you eat, the more satisfying your treat, and the less likely you will be to overindulge."

So instead of grabbing the ice cream carton and digging right in, scoop out a one-half cup portion and put the rest back in the freezer. Then sit at the table to eat your ice cream, taking the time to savor each luscious spoonful.

Rx — *Prescriptions*
FOR BINGE-PROOFING YOUR HOME

Resisting the urge to overindulge becomes much easier when you keep temptation at arm's length. These strategies can help.

❒ Store food in the kitchen. "That means no peanuts in the living room and no chocolates in the family room," says Dr. Abramson. "Just seeing food triggers the urge to eat food."

MEALTIME

❒ At mealtimes, put a serving of food on your plate while you are in the kitchen. Then take only your plate—no pots, pans, or bowls—to the table. "Reaching for second and third helpings is much too easy when the food is sitting right there in front of you," notes Dr. Abramson.

Prescription for Mindful Munching

It is not what you eat but how you eat it that determines whether you win or lose the craving game. The following exercise can help you maintain a sense of calm, control, and choice throughout the eating process. It was developed by Jon Kabat-Zinn, Ph.D., founder and executive director of the Center for Mindfulness at the University of Massachusetts Medical Center in Worcester, and Elizabeth Wheeler, Ph.D., a clinic psychologist at the Center.

Two minutes before a meal: Sit quietly in your chair. Take five or six slow, deep breaths. Allow yourself to feel relaxed.

One minute before a meal: Honor your food. This is almost like saying grace, though it needn't be religious. If you are with other people, you might link hands around the table. Think about how your food is the product of sunlight, rain, earth, and other people's labor. Remember the work required to prepare and cook it. And appreciate the nourishment it offers your body.

Midway through a meal: Stop eating and take five slow, deep breaths. Sit quietly for just a moment. You might realize that you are no longer hungry.

Ten minutes after a meal: Take five slow, deep breaths. Focus on the physical sensations that the meal may be producing in your body. Most of these sensations should be pleasant. "But if a food makes you feel not so good afterward, you may decide to eat less of it in the future," says Dr. Wheeler.

❒ Buy foods in single-serving sizes. Instead of a half-gallon of ice cream, for instance, choose individually wrapped ice cream sandwiches. This strategy gives you built-in portion control, points out Dr. Abramson.

❐ For foods that you buy in bulk, create your own single-serving packages. You can divide, say, a bag of pretzels into single servings, then put each serving in a sandwich bag.

❐ Store tempting leftovers in your freezer. "In the time required to defrost and reheat a food, you are likely to lose your craving for it," says Dr. Abramson.

Rx ——— *Prescriptions*
TO FEEL GOOD ABOUT YOU

To truly change your attitude toward food, you may have to change your attitude toward you. "Unfortunately, we live in a culture with an insane standard of beauty—a 17-year-old waif who is 5 feet, 9 inches tall and weighs 110 pounds," says Dr. Belding. "The vast majority of us aren't fashion models. We are real women whose bodies normally gain about 10 pounds each decade." For most of us, trying to live up to the impossible ideal only leads to depression and low self-esteem—both of which can precipitate overeating.

Learning to love yourself as you are takes practice, but it is worth the effort. These tactics can make it a little easier.

❐ Cultivate a positive attitude toward exercise. "Realize that working out isn't about losing weight," says Dr. Belding. "It's about feeling good inside your body." If you are uncomfortable in a regular exercise class because of your weight, Dr. Belding suggests that you look for a class or a workout video designed especially for heavier women.

TIME IT RIGHT

❐ Exercise for as long as you comfortably can, then continue for one minute longer. Suppose you can walk for only five minutes. Do those five minutes, plus one minute extra. "Even very mild activity improves your mood, decreases your appetite, and takes you away from food cues. You don't have to puff and sweat," says Dr. Abramson. "Start at your own pace and gradually increase your time and effort."

❐ Substitute something fun for something fattening. Dip into a fragrant bubble bath instead of mint chocolate chip ice cream. Devour a romance novel instead of devil's food cake. Savor a play break with your daughter instead of a hot fudge sundae.

❏ Praise yourself for your successes. "Women tend to think in negative terms," says Dr. Abramson. "But patting yourself on the back when you pass up a doughnut is much more motivational than beating yourself up over eating one."

Poor Body Image

Every woman wants to look her best. Concern about personal appearance is normal and, in most cases, healthy. But for someone who has body dysmorphic disorder (BDD), concern becomes an obsession.

"Women who have BDD are perfectly normal-looking, even attractive," explains Katharine Phillips, M.D., associate professor of psychiatry and human behavior at Brown University School of Medicine and chief of outpatient services and director of the body dysmorphic disorder and body image program at Butler Hospital, both in Providence, Rhode Island. "Yet they worry incessantly that their hair is too curly, their nose is too big, their breasts are too small. They dwell on some perceived imperfection."

While its name is fairly new, BDD has been documented for more than a century. It currently affects an estimated five million Americans. This disorder is characterized by a fixation on a perceived physical flaw or defect—usually something that other people don't even notice.

When does meticulous grooming cross the line to BDD? "I start to worry when a woman spends more than an hour a day thinking about how she looks," says Dr. Phillips, who is also the author of *The Broken Mirror: Understanding and Treating Body Dysmorphic Disorder.* "And I consider the problem significant when it makes a woman anxious or takes her away from her day-to-day responsibilities or her enjoyment of life."

TIME IT RIGHT

Women who are diagnosed with BDD are often relieved just to find out that their problem is real. It is also highly treatable, responding well to psychological and medical therapies.

Rx

Prescriptions
FOR LIKING WHAT YOU SEE

To beat BDD, your best defense is to educate yourself about the condition. "BDD is easy to brush off because it is so under-recognized—even among mental health professionals," notes Dr. Phillips. Use these self-care strategies to help reshape your body image.

MORNING

❏ Allow just 20 minutes for grooming each morning. "This is all the time you should need to style your hair and put on your makeup," according to Dr. Phillips. "Some women with BDD literally take hours." She suggests setting a timer and forcing yourself to put down your brush when the bell goes off.

❏ Cover up or remove as many mirrors as possible in your home and office. This prevents you from constantly checking yourself in the mirror—and feeling worse each time you take a look, explains Dr. Phillips.

❏ Socialize with friends and co-workers. "Women with BDD are often tempted to hide themselves away," notes Dr. Phillips. "This only reinforces the problem." So accept invitations to parties, luncheons, and after-work gatherings, she advises. Remember that although your problem seems painfully apparent to you, it is likely to be invisible to others.

Medical **Alert**
Body dysmorphic disorder can be a serious condition, much like major depression, notes Dr. Phillips. Watch for these BBD warning signals.
  ✓ Obsessive worry about your looks for more than an hour a day
  ✓ Inability to perform daily activities as well as you could because you are preoccupied with your appearance—for example, you have difficulty concentrating at work
  ✓ Avoidance of social and professional functions
  ✓ A high degree of distress or anxiety
  ✓ A sense of hopelessness
  ✓ Feelings that you are worthless or that life isn't worth living
If you have any of these symptoms, you need to see a medical professional who is familiar with BDD and other obsessive-compulsive

behaviors, says Dr. Phillips. To locate a qualified practitioner or a BDD support group near you, write to the Obsessive-Compulsive Foundation at P.O. Box 70, Milford, CT 06460.

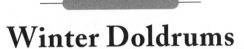

Winter Doldrums

For thousands of women, the worst day of the year is that Sunday in late October when daylight savings time ends. They know that for the next several months, the sun sets before dinnertime, leaving them with precious few hours of daylight to enjoy. Many of these women wish they could join the more sensible members of the animal kingdom who curl up in cozy hibernation until spring.

This dread of the dead of winter has become so common that the medical community has a name for it: seasonal affective disorder, or SAD. Since 1987, SAD has been recognized by the American Psychiatric Association as a distinct disorder.

WINTERTIME

After more than a decade of study, researchers believe that some 20 percent of the population—more women than men—experience blue moods as a result of seasonal changes in light, says Norman E. Rosenthal, M.D., chief of environmental psychiatry at the National Institute of Mental Health in Bethesda, Maryland. In fact, SAD symptoms often get worse at the end of daylight savings time.

LIFETIME

In women, SAD may have a hormonal link. You're more likely to develop the condition during your reproductive years than after menopause, according to Brenda Byrne, Ph.D., director of the seasonal affective disorder program affiliated with the light research program at Jefferson Medical College of Thomas Jefferson University in Philadelphia.

SAD affects women physically and emotionally, in varying degrees of intensity. How can you tell the difference between SAD and garden-variety winter blahs? "It is a question of severity of symptoms with SAD. You may experience a dramatic drop in your energy level," says Dr. Byrne. "You may also crave sweets and starches, sleep longer—even if that sleep is of poor quality—and desire sex less. Some women with SAD report difficulty concentrating and disinterest in social activities. Sadness and a depressed mood are also typical with SAD."

SUMMERTIME

Even though SAD is most common in the winter months, some women are affected by it in the summer months, too. "Three or four gray days in July leave some women feeling very low indeed," says Dr. Byrne.

Rx —— *Prescriptions*
TO BRIGHTEN DARK DAYS

If you have seasonal affective disorder—and only your doctor can tell you that for sure—light therapy can significantly improve your symptoms. In light therapy, you sit before a specially designed light box for a pre-scribed amount of time each day. Dr. Byrne stresses that you should use this treatment only in consultation with your doctor, who can show you how to use the box properly and set up a treatment schedule for you.

The following strategies can also help brighten your mood, whether you have SAD or a simple case of the winter blues.

❏ Install bright white lighting in your home and office. Fluorescent and incandescent bulbs work equally well, according to Dr. Byrne.

❏ Paint the walls inside your home in light, bright colors. Colors can make a big difference in the way you feel, explains Dr. Byrne. "Pay attention to how you personally respond to various hues," she suggests. "Notice which ones improve your mood and surround yourself with them."

❏ Try running an air purifier that generates negative ions in your home and office. (They are available at most home centers and health food stores.) Read the box label to ensure that it generates negative ions. "Very recent research suggests that some people who have SAD feel better when they use a negative-ion generator," says Dr. Byrne. "We don't yet know why, but it definitely appears to improve symptoms in some cases."

❏ Spend time outdoors. Yes, it's winter, and it's cold. But you get more mood-lifting light outside than inside. "I know one woman who bundles up and sits outdoors for 45 minutes every fair-weather day, reading her newspaper," says Dr. Byrne. "The newspaper reflects even more light into her eyes and maximizes the therapeutic benefits."

TIME IT RIGHT

❏ Engage in aerobic exercise for 30 minutes three days a week. *Aerobic* means any activity that elevates your heart and breathing rates, so running, bicycling, and brisk walking all qualify. "Women who remain active

Sweet Salvation

If you are among the women with seasonal affective disorder (SAD) who crave sweets, you should take care not to overindulge. In general, people eat more and exercise less in winter—the perfect formula for weight gain, notes Brenda Byrne, Ph.D., director of the seasonal affective disorder program affiliated with the light research program at Jefferson Medical College of Thomas Jefferson University in Philadelphia. Caving in to cravings can make you even more likely to put on the pounds. The solution? Eat less, exercise more, she says.

through the winter seem to have less-severe SAD symptoms than women who become sedentary," notes Dr. Byrne.

Medical **Alert**

Do not attempt to diagnose and treat SAD on your own, cautions Dr. Byrne. The reason is that SAD produces symptoms that are remarkably similar to other, potentially serious health problems, such as low blood sugar and thyroid disorders. If you suspect that you have SAD, see your doctor for a proper diagnosis. Also, seek professional counseling at once if you feel severely depressed or have suicidal thoughts.

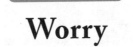

Worry

Mothers worry about their children. Wives worry about their husbands. Daughters worry about their parents. Women seem to worry their way through life. In fact, they seem to thrive on it.

"Many women may believe that time spent worrying is productive, but in reality, it isn't," says Rosemarie Schultz, Ph.D., a clinical psychologist and professor at the American Academy of Art in Chicago, where she teaches the psychology of creativity. "Worrying doesn't produce solutions to problems. Instead, worry fosters anxiety, saps your energy, and obscures your objectivity."

Worry can take one of two forms. An "if only" worry causes you to relive an unpleasant past event ("If only I hadn't said that"). A "what if" worry, on the other hand, takes you to some awful future event that may or may not happen ("What if I lose my job?"). Either way, you are contemplating a situation that is beyond your control. And that can lead to anxiety and depression, according to Thomas Borkovec, Ph.D., distinguished professor of psychology at Pennsylvania State University in University Park.

People tend to do most of their worrying during times of stress. "When you are under stress, your mind focuses on the source of danger," explains Dr. Borkovec. "But because stress reduces your ability to reason, you are more inclined to ruminate about a problem than to actually solve it."

When you get right down to it, though, you realize that worry is really nothing more than a bad habit. And, of course, bad habits are made to be broken.

Rx ——— *Prescriptions* TO WIND DOWN

Even if you are just thinking about bad things, they can make you feel absolutely awful, according to Dr. Borkovec. Your muscles tighten, your heart changes its normal rhythm, and your stomach does somersaults. To help you relax, he recommends that you find a quiet place and practice any or several of the following techniques once or twice a day for 10 minutes at a time.

TIME IT RIGHT   ❏ **Practice deep breathing.** In deep breathing, your stomach—not your chest—should rise and fall. Gradually slow your inhalations and exhalations as much as you can without becoming uncomfortable. As you become accustomed to this breathing pattern, you may want to whisper a word such as *relax* or *calm* as you exhale, says Dr. Borkovec. This helps deepen your sense of relaxation.

❑ Try progressive muscle relaxation. As its name suggests, this technique involves tensing and releasing each muscle group in turn until you feel completely relaxed. Begin with your hands, clenching them into fists and holding for about 5 seconds. Then release, and as you do, feel tension drain from your body for about 30 seconds. Repeat the tense and release sequence on all the major muscle groups in your body in the following order: arms, face, shoulders, stomach, buttocks, thighs, calves, and feet. By the time you finish with your feet, you should feel completely relaxed and free of tension, says Dr. Borkovec.

TIME IT RIGHT

❑ Conjure a relaxing mental image. Picture yourself lounging on a tropical beach or in a hammock under your favorite tree—anything that makes you feel calm and peaceful. Be sure to include all of your senses: smell the ocean, feel the heat of the sun, taste the pineapple. Really concentrate on this image, letting go of all other thoughts as you do, suggests Dr. Borkovec.

Prescriptions
TO WAYLAY WORRYING

Rx

Once you feel at ease, you can take steps to deal with your worry in a constructive way. Select from the strategies below when you feel a troubling thought taking hold.

❑ Tally the number of times you worry during the day. Dr. Borkovec suggests carrying a small notepad in your purse or pocket. Then each time you have a troubling thought, mark it down. Total the tallies at the day's end. This exercise should help put your worrying in perspective and give you the incentive to cut back.

DAYTIME

❑ Stay focused on the present. "The problem you are worried about doesn't exist in the here and now," says Dr. Borkovec. "By tuning in to the moment at hand, you learn to recognize the difference between thoughts of worry and what's really happening in your moment-to-moment life."

❑ Schedule 30 minutes each day as your official worry period. Choose a convenient, generally quiet time. You will want to avoid bedtime, though, since troubled thoughts could disrupt your sleep, advises Dr.

TIME IT RIGHT

Positive Pondering

A technique called cognitive restructuring can help you stop worrying about problems and start seeing them in more positive, productive ways. By pinpointing your worries, you can take steps toward solving them or dismiss them altogether.

The next time you catch yourself having a troubling thought, run it through the following sequence, recommended by Thomas Borkovec, Ph.D., distinguished professor of psychology at Pennsylvania State University in University Park.

1. What are you telling yourself that you find so troubling? Write down exactly what you are thinking.

2. Analyze what you have written down. Are your thoughts reasonable? What evidence do you have to support them? Has such an event ever happened?

3. If what you expect to happen does indeed happen, would you be able to handle it? What can you do to prepare for it? Have you ever handled a similar problem? A year after this "bad thing" happens, what difference will it have made in your life?

4. Think about your responses to these questions, and as you do, try to give them a positive spin. Write down these positive thoughts next to the original worry.

5. The next time this worry creeps into your head, counter it with the new, positive thoughts that you have written down. Remind yourself how carefully you examined the problem to come up with your good thoughts.

Borkovec. Choose a place as well—though not your favorite place, since you will come to associate it with worrying.

❏ Once you have established your worry period, put off worrying until the appointed half-hour. Whenever a troubling thought pops into your head, remind yourself that you can mull it over later. "You may even find that worry time becomes solution time because the problem gets your undivided attention," notes Dr. Borkovec.

❐ Distinguish between worries you can do something about and those you can't. Dr. Borkovec suggests evaluating each worry by asking yourself these questions.

✓ What actions can I take to reduce the possibility of the worry be-coming a reality?

✓ What information do I need to solve the problem?

✓ Who can help me solve the problem?

❐ Consider the worst-case scenario. If you are worried about losing your job, for example, ask yourself what the realistic consequences would be if that came to pass. Would you lose your home? Your family? Never work again? Decide what is most likely to happen, then think through ways to respond to those specific problems. "Pitting worry against reality puts everything in perspective," says Dr. Borkovec.

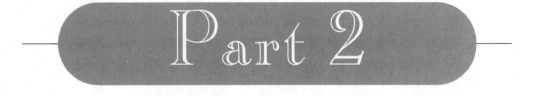

Part 2

PRESCRIPTIONS
FOR A HEALTHY LIFESTYLE

Chapter 6

Prescriptions
for Inactive Women

Some women view exercise the same way that they view sex. They think it is important, and they would like to do it more often, but they just can't seem to find time—or to make time.

That's too bad because exercise has a lot to offer health-wise. It helps you maintain a healthy weight. It lowers your cholesterol and blood pressure, which in turn slashes your risk for heart disease. It even bolsters your resistance to certain types of cancer.

"Exercise literally gives you more time," says Ralph Paffenbarger, M.D., professor emeritus at Stanford University School of Medicine. In his own studies, Dr. Paffenbarger has found that for every hour you work out, you gain an additional hour of life.

But if you are accustomed to an inactive lifestyle, even the promise of living healthier longer may not motivate you enough to get a move on.

You know that you are a certifiable sofa slug when:

✓ You haven't set foot in a gym since high school.

✓ You think resistance training is a psychological technique that involves learning to say no to everything—including exercise.

✓ You have never actually broken a sweat in your sweat suit.

✓ You watch a TV show that you dislike just because you have misplaced the remote and you don't want to get up to change the channel.

✓ You think that if God wanted people to walk, he wouldn't have given us cars.

You have no reason not to exercise—and every reason why you should. Here is what you can do to leave the sedentary lifestyle behind.

Rx — *Prescriptions*
FOR MODIFYING YOUR MINDSET

Getting in the exercise habit begins with your brain, not your body. You have to start thinking like an active person. That means finding ways to stay motivated. These tips can help.

❏ Make exercise a priority. "Tell yourself that exercise is important," says Ross Andersen, Ph.D., director of exercise science at the Johns Hopkins Weight Management Center in Baltimore. "Remind yourself every day—especially on those days when the rest of life seems to be conspiring to keep you from your workout."

As important as exercise is, it almost never has a deadline attached to it, explains Dr. Andersen. So it is easily bumped to the back burner—unless you make a mental commitment to it.

❏ Focus on how you feel rather than how you look. If you dream of achieving a supermodel-esque physique, you will probably be disappointed. "Most women simply can't look like Cher or Jamie Lee Curtis—it's not in their genetic makeup," notes Dr. Andersen. But you can feel good about yourself and your body. "Women tell me that exercise makes them stronger, helps them sleep better, gives them energy as well as a sense of accomplishment," he observes. "That's what I want them to home in on." These positive changes arrive within a few weeks after beginning an exercise program. They help keep people going.

❏ Substitute positive affirmations for negative self-talk. "People come up with horrible ways of describing themselves—fat, gross, disgustingly out of shape," says Michael Scholtz, director of fitness at the Duke

University Diet and Fitness Center in Durham, North Carolina. "All they are doing is beating up on themselves." When one of these critical messages floats through your brain, he suggests countering it with a positive statement, such as "I am a capable person who exercises every day and enjoys it." While this won't instantly change your self-image, it will make you aware of all the negative self-talk going on in your head and encourage you to think more positively.

❏ Sign up for beginner-level exercise classes. You will get the instruction you need to avoid injury, along with the support and encouragement you need to keep going. "Classes are especially helpful for women who have never exercised, who don't think they can exercise, or who feel embarrassed and self-conscious," says Christina Frederick, Ph.D., assistant professor of psychology at Southern Utah University in Cedar City. "For them, the right class and the right instructor can make all the difference in the world."

❏ Recruit an exercise partner. That way, on those days when you will use any excuse not to work out, knowing that someone is expecting you just might compel you to slip into your sweats and sneakers after all, according to Dr. Frederick.

❏ Consider hiring a personal trainer, if you can afford one. Particularly if you have a health problem that makes exercise difficult, a personal trainer can provide individualized guidance. "Find someone whose personality complements yours but who challenges you to improve," advises Dr. Frederick.

Prescriptions
FOR MAKING EXERCISE EASY

Rx

When it comes to customizing your fitness routine, keep in mind that you want to make your exercise sessions relatively hassle-free and as non-time-consuming as possible. Follow these guidelines to shape a routine that you can live with.

❏ Set aside at least 30 minutes every day for your workout. Mark it in your daily planner, just as you would any other appointment. This affirms the importance of exercise, explains Dr. Andersen. "You can say to

TIME IT RIGHT

yourself, 'I don't need to feel guilty. I'm doing exactly what I planned to be doing right now.' "

Your body actually appreciates this regularity, adds Scholtz. "Over time, your biological clock sets itself according to your workout schedule, so your body expects and wants an exercise fix at a certain time of day," he says. "If it doesn't get a workout, you end up feeling less energetic."

❑ Make sure that family members, especially children, understand that you are not available during your scheduled workouts. You may want

Prescriptions for Staying in the Swing

Maybe inactivity isn't your problem. Maybe you have been fairly active for years, but lately, your body doesn't seem to want to cooperate. You may have noticed that you are not running quite as fast, pedaling quite as far, or serving a tennis ball quite as hard as you used to. Especially if you are competitive by nature, the decline in your performance level may have you toying with the idea of giving up the sport you love.

This mindset—"If I can't do it the way I used to, I won't do it at all"—is quite common as people get older, says Michael Scholtz, director of fitness at the Duke University Diet and Fitness Center in Durham, North Carolina. "Some folks have a really hard time with it. I ask them to focus on the act of participating and the feeling they get from moving. This helps them to enjoy their sport in a different way."

If you simply can't do a sport anymore—say, knee pain prevents you from running—then find a suitable substitute. "Both biking and swimming can provide the same high level of cardiovascular fitness as running but without pounding on your joints," says Christina Frederick, Ph.D., assistant professor of psychology at Southern Utah University in Cedar City.

to write your workout times on a calendar and post the calendar in your kitchen. This can help you avoid last-minute requests for rides to soccer games and dance lessons.

❒ If you join a gym, choose one that is close to home or work. You are more likely to stop by the facility if you pass it on your daily commute, observes Scholtz.

❒ If you exercise at home, invest in some basic equipment such as a foam floor mat, a jump rope, an aerobic step, exercise tubing (for easy resistance training), and a pair of dumbbells.

True, it's not exactly the same. But consider the alternative. "Either you do what you can or you stop," observes Phil Mulkey, a former Olympic decathlete who continues to excel in his sport at the masters level. "And believe me, if you stop altogether, you go downhill real fast." He offers this advice.

❒ Exercise regularly. Being a weekend warrior is hard enough when you are 30. It is practically impossible as you get older.

❒ Give your body a chance to recover from your workout. You may need twice as much time as you did when you were younger. "Having access to a hot tub helps a lot," says Mulkey.

❒ Balance competitiveness with the potential for injury. Sure, you would love to beat the shorts off that cocky youngster on the other side of the tennis court, but you don't want to kill yourself doing it. "You need to know when to fold 'em," advises Mulkey. "I'm aware that people get a real thrill out of beating me, and I'm nice about it. I tell them that I have been beaten so many times in my life that all I'm trying to do now is even the score."

❒ Keep workout clothes and a pair of sneakers in your car. That way, you can exercise whenever the opportunity presents itself.

MORNING

❒ Exercise first thing in the morning. You are least likely to get outside interference at this time of day. "In my experience, even people who say that they are not morning exercisers adapt in a few weeks' time," notes Scholtz.

❒ Focus on consistency rather than intensity. When you are first starting out, your goal is to make exercise a habit, says Dr. Andersen. So don't worry too much about how fast or how far you walk, for example— as long as you are doing something for the amount of time you have allotted. You can worry about speed and distance later on, if you want.

Find the Beat That Moves Your Feet

When people walk in the great outdoors, they have a natural tendency to dawdle. You need to make sure that you maintain a faster-than-normal pace. Listening to music can help, says Maggie Spilner, walking editor for *Prevention* magazine. A song's beat quickens your steps so that you walk in rhythm. "Plus, music has a psychological effect that makes exercising seem easier," she notes. "Just be sure that you are alert to your surroundings. Keep one ear clear of the headphones or walk with a partner who is headphone-free. Stay on park trails where cars aren't allowed."

Following are some examples of popular songs and their miles-per-hour beat, based on the average stride length of a woman who is of average height (5 feet, 4 inches tall). You can simply hum the tunes you know to maintain a faster-than-normal pace while you walk. The list is provided by Metronome Jogger Pacing System in Shell Rock, IA.

3.8 miles per hour: "Mother and Child Reunion" and "Slip Slidin' Away," Paul Simon; "Don't Stop Believin'," Journey;

❐ Divide a 30-minute workout into 5- to 10-minute chunks. "Time is such a huge barrier to exercise that being active for a few minutes here and there throughout the day really excites people," explains Dr. Andersen. "They say, 'I can do that.'"

Time it right

❐ Look for opportunities to be active, even if it is only for five minutes. Despite your best efforts, things will occasionally intrude on your workout time. Rather than bag your workout altogether, do as much as you can wherever you can, recommends Scholtz. "Take the stairs rather than the elevator at work, or park farther away from the building rather than in the closest spot you can find," he suggests.

Time it right

"Feelin' Alright," Joe Cocker; "Wrapped around Your Finger," the Police; "After Midnight," Eric Clapton; "Legs," ZZ Top.

4 miles per hour: "Say You Love Me," Fleetwood Mac; "Don't Go Breaking My Heart," Elton John; "Maggie May," Rod Stewart; "Uptown Girl," Billy Joel; "Takin' Care of Business," Bachman Turner Overdrive; "Money for Nothing," Dire Straits; "Kodachrome" and "Loves Me Like a Rock," Paul Simon; "Cry Me a River," Joe Cocker.

4.2 miles per hour: "Mississippi Queen," Bachman Turner Overdrive; "It's Still Rock and Roll to Me" and "Moving Out," Billy Joel; "The Heart of Rock and Roll," Huey Lewis and the News.

4.4 miles per hour: "Big Shot" and "Only the Good Die Young," Billy Joel; "Message in a Bottle," the Police; "Sultans of Swing," Dire Straits.

5-plus miles per hour: "Stop, Stop, Stop," the Hollies; "Tell Her about It," Billy Joel; "Me and Julio Down by the Schoolyard," Paul Simon.

❐ Work through normal muscle soreness. What's normal? Well, you should expect a little tightness and discomfort in your muscles after you exercise, according to Scholtz. This type of soreness usually subsides over time, as your muscles adapt to your workout routine. If, on the other hand, you have pain that causes you to limp or leaves you unable to get out of bed in the morning, that's a sign that you are overdoing it and need to cut back.

Rx ———— *Prescriptions* FOR STICKING WITH FITNESS

You have penned your workouts into your daily planner. Now the big question: How, exactly, should you spend that time? The answer is entirely up to you—but just remember that the activity you choose can make or break your motivation. To keep exercise accessible and fun, heed this advice from the experts.

❐ Adjust your personal definition of exercise. "You can probably come up with at least one physical activity that you enjoy," says Scholtz. "You may not think of that activity as exercise, but it actually is."

❐ Try various activities until you find one that appeals to you. "Doing something pleasurable gives you the motivation to stick with it," according to Dr. Frederick. "Even though you may not engage in the activity every day, you will likely put in more hours per week than people who don't enjoy their workouts."

To find an activity you like, ask yourself these questions: What did you enjoy doing when you were younger? What sports were you good at? What activities have you always wanted to try? Perhaps ballroom dancing? Or inline skating? Or scuba diving?

DAYTIME

❐ Use your afternoon coffee break to walk the perimeter of your building—and see who has those nice corner offices.

❐ If you have a meeting with someone, ask her if she would like to walk and talk.

❐ Plan an active vacation. Take a walking tour of Paris or Rome, do a bed-and-breakfast bicycle tour of Vermont, or volunteer for a week with an environmental or community service organization.

Chapter 7

PRESCRIPTIONS

FOR EXERCISE FANATICS

Poll any group of health experts, and they will come up with at least two dozen reasons why women should exercise. Beyond trimming and toning your body, exercise boosts your energy, strengthens your bones, lowers your cholesterol and blood pressure readings, even prevents certain kinds of cancer.

But like overwatering a houseplant, overcooking fish, or overinflating a tire, overdoing exercise can cause problems of its own. According to the experts, you know that fitness has become an *un*healthy obsession when two or more of the following apply.

✓ You exercise for two or more hours a day most days of the week, even though you are not an athlete-in-training.

✓ You structure your personal and professional life around exercise.

✓ You are not competing, but you keep detailed records of your workouts.

✓ You become cranky, anxious, sluggish, or depressed if you miss your workout.

✓ You are obsessed with a single form of exercise, such as running, aerobic dance, or tennis.

✓ You base the intensity or duration of your workout on how fat you feel.

✓ You often feel tired, not energized, after your workouts.

✓ You need more and more exercise just to feel "normal."

✓ You are taking aspirin nearly every day to relieve exercise-related aches and pains.

✓ You repeatedly experience overuse injuries, such as tennis elbow, knee pain, shinsplints, or stress fractures.

✓ You continue to exercise despite an injury.

✓ You don't especially enjoy exercising anymore.

Most women who overdo exercise are chronic dieters obsessed with their weight, observes Joni Johnston, Psy.D., a clinical psychologist in Del Mar, California, and author of *Appearance Obsession*. "Overexercising can create a variation on the binge-purge of bulimia," she says. The "purge," in this case, is working out.

Other women start fitness programs to slim down and shape up, then end up becoming addicted. "This behavior is normal to some extent," acknowledges Christina Frederick, Ph.D., assistant professor of psychology at Southern Utah University in Cedar City. "But I believe that exercise can be a true addiction. It alters your brain chemistry to produce a feel-good high. Eventually, you crave that high, and when you don't get it, you become cranky and anxious. Your self-image evolves around exercise, and it crashes if you don't swim, bike, or whatever."

Some people get hooked by the sense of accomplishment that a good workout provides, adds Terri Manning, Ed.D., a health behavior specialist at the University of North Carolina at Charlotte. "They say that nothing makes them more fulfilled than a great day of training," she notes. "This holds true for both men and women, from ages 17 to 80."

With this skewed perspective, it's no wonder that overexercisers end up neglecting other, equally important aspects of a healthy lifestyle. "If you are driven to exercise for hours a day, you have little time for social activities and personal relationships," explains Dr. Frederick.

Rx ——— *Prescriptions*
TO WORK OUT WISELY

Of course, if you do have an addiction to exercise, you can't just kick the habit. Working out has far too many health benefits to give it up for

Prescriptions for Optimum Workouts

How much should you exercise? That depends on what you hope to gain from it. The following guidelines, recommended by Terri Manning, Ed.D., a health behavior specialist at the University of North Carolina at Charlotte, give you a general idea of what the optimum workouts would be for specific health goals.

❐ To achieve cardiovascular fitness, exercise at a moderate intensity (60 to 75 percent of your target heart rate) for about 30 to 45 minutes four or five days a week. (To determine your target heart rate, see "Aim for Your Target" on page 189.)

❐ Once you have achieved cardiovascular fitness, you can maintain it by exercising at a moderate intensity for about 30 minutes two or three days a week.

❐ To lose weight, exercise at a low to moderate intensity (50 to 65 percent of your target heart rate) for 45 to 60 minutes six days a week.

❐ To build extra strength and endurance, increase both the intensity and the time that you exercise so that you surpass the recommendations for cardiovascular fitness. "But why go beyond fitness?" asks Dr. Manning. "For most people, this has little to offer in the way of additional health benefits. It has more to do with a sense of accomplishment, with appearance, or, possibly, with addictive behavior."

good. To get fit without becoming fanatical, rebuild your exercise routine around these guiding principles.

❐ **Determine what level of fitness you want to achieve or maintain.** "In this case, you can use real numbers to help you set a goal," says Craig Morrison, Ed.D., associate professor of physical education at Southern Utah University. For instance, you may want to aim for a certain weight, body fat percentage, or blood pressure or cholesterol reading.

"People with exercise addictions often have trouble recognizing when they have achieved what they set out to do," explains Dr. Morrison. "They may initially have a goal, such as losing 10 pounds. But once they reach that goal, they feel so good and are getting so many compliments that they automatically up the ante—whether they realize it or not." Establishing a specific, measurable goal means that you can relax at some point, he adds. "You don't have to keep going. You can say, 'I'm here now. I can lay off a bit.'"

TIME IT RIGHT

❒ Decide how much exercise you need each day to reach your fitness goal, then hold yourself to that amount of time. If you need an hour, work out for an hour—but no longer than that. "Don't go for an extra half-hour run later in the day, and don't return to the gym for a second workout," advises Dr. Manning. If you consistently exceed your time limit, take it as a warning sign that your exercise habits may be spinning out of control.

MORNING

❒ Check your heart rate each morning to make sure that you are not pushing yourself too hard. "If your resting heart rate is at least 10 beats per minute above normal, it means that your body is busy recovering from the previous day's workout," explains Dr. Morrison. So take the day off from exercise—or at least take it easy.

TIME IT RIGHT

❒ Pay attention to how you feel before, during, and after your workout. Dr. Johnston suggests conducting quick self-assessments at the following intervals: as you warm up; 5 minutes, 10 minutes, and 30 minutes into your workout; and 1 hour, 5 hours, and even 24 hours afterward. Do any of your joints hurt? Do you have pain in your back or feet? Are you energized or tired? "Notice how the right amount of exercise makes you feel good, while overdoing it makes you feel bad," she says.

TIME IT RIGHT

❒ Substitute an hour of weight lifting for an hour of aerobic exercise two or three days each week. Women concerned about fat and flab may benefit from focusing more on adding muscle and less on losing pounds, says Dr. Frederick. That's because when you lift weights, body fat is replaced by muscle. And muscle gives you a trimmed, toned physique.

What's more, muscle burns calories constantly, which means that you can eat more. And when you eat more, you have a better chance of getting the nutrients you need, notes Dr. Frederick.

❐ Rotate among several activities that you enjoy instead of sticking with just one. This practice helps you avoid or overcome an obsession with one sport, when a need to go even faster or farther makes you push yourself too hard, says Dr. Johnston. Switching back and forth also helps prevent overuse injuries.

In fact, engaging in different activities may actually make you more fit than focusing on just one. For instance, both running and biking strengthen your legs and enhance your endurance. But by biking on alternate days, you give your knees and feet a break from the constant pounding of running.

❐ Engage in activities other than your regular workout that count as exercise. Play with your kids. Take your dog for a romp. Practice yoga. Plant a vegetable garden. "The idea is to have a component of your fitness routine that is relaxing," explains Dr. Johnston. "This reminds you that you don't have to go to a gym to exercise. You can just have fun."

❐ If you have to put in long hours to feel as though you had a good workout, reassess your routine. You may not be exercising efficiently, according to Dr. Morrison. Remember that quality, not quantity, counts.

If you run, you can intensify your workout by gradually adding sprints or hill work. If you usually walk on a treadmill or ride an exercise bike, switch to a stairclimbing machine on occasion. If you lift weights, add an extra set of repetitions. You may want to consult a personal trainer, who can show you how to make the most of your workout time.

❐ Change your fitness goals with the seasons. "Many athletes have one fitness goal for the summertime and another, slightly lower goal for the wintertime," explains Dr. Morrison. "They back off for the winter months to allow their bodies to recover, especially if they have been training hard." This downshift in activity also relieves the mental stress of maintaining a high level of fitness—and makes rebounding in spring even sweeter.

WINTERTIME

Prescriptions
TO SHAPE UP YOUR OUTLOOK

To overcome an obsession with exercise, you need to address it from an emotional angle as well as a physical one. In fact, emotional distress may have driven you to overexercise to begin with. The following strategies can help you adopt a more healthy, balanced attitude toward fitness.

❐ Stop counting calories. Chronic dieters play a kind of mind game with exercise, according to Dr. Johnston. "They tell themselves, 'Okay, I had 400 calories for breakfast, so I have to work out for an hour this afternoon.' It's a constant trade-off between tallying calories and figuring out how long to work out to burn off those calories."

This sort of compulsive thinking is a habit. To break the habit, you need to first become aware of it and then make a conscious decision not to act on your thoughts. "If it's too hard to stop counting calories altogether, then try to stop for at least one meal a day," suggests Dr. Johnston.

❐ Focus on the nurturing aspects of exercise. This gives your investment in fitness a brand-new bottom line. You want to work out because it makes you healthy, not because it burns calories and changes your appearance. "This subtle shift in mindset discourages addiction and encourages the sheer enjoyment of exercise," says Dr. Johnston.

❐ Skip your workout for one day. If anxiety sets in, write down what you are thinking and how you are feeling. Exercise fanatics, especially the previously plump, sometimes fear that if they miss even one workout, they may fall off the wagon completely, explains Edward Abramson, Ph.D., professor of psychology at California State University in Chico and author of *Emotional Eating*. "Even if this has happened to you in the past, it doesn't have to happen now. You can change your actions. Missing one day of exercise is not such a big deal if you know that you are going to be back at it the next day, or the day after that."

❐ Learn to manage emotional conflict without using exercise as a crutch. Overexercising is a way of escaping uncomfortable feelings such as fear, anger, and loss of control. "But working out never solves the problem that generated the feelings in the first place," explains Dr. Johnston. "It doesn't even allow you to work through those feelings. Like drugs or alcohol, exercise merely helps you avoid the problem temporarily."

You need to recognize, express, and work through emotional conflict without using exercise to blunt it. Learning how to do this takes time. "You need to stop long enough to get in touch with what is going on inside you," says Dr. Johnston. She suggests keeping a journal of your emotions, talking with friends, or setting aside time each day to sit quietly and monitor the thoughts that pop into your head.

❐ Engage in activities besides exercise that enrich your life and give it meaning. While exercise (and dieting) may be the center of your universe right now, it should never consume your very existence. "You lose out big if that happens," observes Dr. Abramson. Instead of becoming absorbed by solitary workouts, spend time with people you care about, volunteer for a good cause, or play. "You have people to see and things to accomplish that have nothing to do with your weight or fat grams or exercise," he notes. "You don't want to lose sight of that."

Medical **Alert**

Exercise fanaticism is often linked to an eating disorder such as anorexia or bulimia, says Dr. Johnston. Both can lead to serious health problems, including potentially fatal heart arrhythmia. If you are exercising a lot and severely restricting your calorie intake, you may be developing an eating disorder. See your doctor for help before you go overboard.

You should also see your doctor if your fitness routine leads to amenorrhea (cessation of menstrual periods), repeated stress fractures, or symptoms of depression and anxiety when you try to cut back or quit, advises Dr. Johnston.

Chapter 8

PRESCRIPTIONS

FOR CHRONIC DIETERS

When it comes to dieting, a fine line exists between self-discipline and obsession, between healthy moderation and joyless denial. A woman becomes a chronic dieter when, in her consuming quest for thinness, she crosses the line to the wrong side.

According to the experts, you know that you are edging toward chronic-dieter status when:

✓ You can recall every morsel of food that you have eaten in the past three days.

✓ You see a plate of food and automatically compute the number of calories or fat grams it contains.

✓ You often eat the same foods every day.

✓ Your day is ruined if you eat a "bad" food such as a nice, big chocolate bar.

✓ You eat only at certain times of the day.

✓ You prefer to eat alone.

✓ You ignore your body when it tells you that it is hungry or full.

✓ You can't pass a scale without hopping on for a quick weigh-in.

These traits may lead you to believe that all chronic dieters have weight problems. Surprisingly, this isn't the case. True, some chronic dieters are dangerously obese. Some are perhaps 10 to 15 pounds overweight. But some really don't need to slim down, says Edward Abramson, Ph.D., professor of psychology at California State University in Chico and author of *Emotional Eating*. "From a health standpoint, these women are at an appropriate weight," he explains. "But they don't meet their own idealized (and unrealistic) notion of how much they should weigh. As a result, they spend a tremendous amount of energy trying to shed those 'extra' pounds."

About half of all female dieters fall into this last category, estimates Joni Johnston, Psy.D., a clinical psychologist in Del Mar, California, and author of *Appearance Obsession*. "Whether they admit it or not, they are dieting for cosmetic reasons. They are trying to get their weight below their natural set points. And they have a hard time because their bodies resist."

The set point theory states that each person's body has a biologically determined weight, or set point, explains Dr. Johnston. The body is programmed to reach and maintain this weight. If you come from a family that has a large body type, you might have a higher set point than society dictates you should. If you go below your set point, however, either through dieting or illness, your body may go into starvation mode—even if you aren't actually starving—and begin to store fat.

Sometimes chronic dieting is driven not by a desire to look good but by a need to establish control. "By restricting her eating, a woman nourishes her sense of mastery and competence," explains Dr. Abramson. "Women who have eating disorders such as anorexia believe that if they ate normally, their lives would become chaotic and they would lose all control."

Admittedly, not everyone who fits the description of a chronic dieter experiences negative consequences from her behavior. Whether chronic dieting becomes a problem depends on a number of factors, including whether a woman needs to lose weight for health reasons, whether she is eating healthfully, and whether she allows her weight-loss efforts to drive other aspects of her life.

If, for example, a woman puts her life on hold until she loses weight (as many women do), she may miss out on a lot. "She may decide that she has to lose 10 pounds before she buys new clothes or goes dancing with her husband or takes a vacation," notes Dr. Abramson. "She's denying herself the opportunity to enjoy these things now."

More seriously, if a woman adheres to a nutritionally vacant diet, subsisting on lettuce and diet soda, she will develop nutrient deficiencies, says Terri Brownlee, R.D., a nutrition educator at Duke University Diet and Fitness Center in Durham, North Carolina. Worse still, if she routinely starves herself until her body rebels and sets off a binge, she runs the risk of developing a potentially life-threatening eating disorder such as anorexia or bulimia (binge-purge syndrome).

Rx — *Prescriptions*
TO NEVER SAY DIET

To correct a pattern of chronic dieting, you may actually need to stop trying to lose weight for a while, according to Dr. Johnston. "But that doesn't mean you're giving up—or that you're going to grow to gigantic proportions," she adds. "Over time, your body will find its natural weight. And you will learn to listen to your body, feeding it when it's hungry and stopping when it's satisfied." If you are ready to leap off the weight-loss bandwagon, these tips can help you do it.

❏ Get rid of your scale.

MONTHLY

❏ If you must keep your scale, gradually cut back your weigh-ins to just one a month. And when you do step on the scale each month, make sure that it is on the same date at the same time and that you are wearing the same clothes. "This gets you off the roller coaster of minor weight fluctuations that occur from day to day," explains Dr. Johnston. "You'll see that your weight actually stays pretty much the same."

❏ Use the fit of your clothes to assess how you are doing. Even if you need to shed pounds for health reasons, you will know whether you are succeeding by how loose (or tight) your clothes feel, says Dr. Johnston.

❏ Aim for a healthy weight range rather than one magic number. For instance, if your ideal weight is 125 pounds, then try to stay between 120 and 130 pounds. "Your weight can fluctuate within the range," according to Dr. Johnston. "This gives you permission to go a little over—

or under—your ideal weight. You won't feel a need to overcorrect a small, temporary gain by restricting calories. As a result, you will eat more normally."

❏ Focus on getting fit rather than losing fat. "Some people may be genetically programmed for overweight, at least as it's defined by contemporary standards," says Dr. Abramson. "If that's the case, you may be better off simply trying to shape up, even if you don't slim down." Regular exercise—30 minutes a day, every day—is the best way to accomplish this, he adds.

Prescriptions
TO DITCH THE DIET MENTALITY

Rx

Chronic dieting is as much an emotional issue as a physical one. In fact, how you feel about yourself pretty much determines whether you go on a diet in the first place. The following strategies can help you resolve underlying emotional conflict and develop a healthier self-image—one that is not so wrapped up in what you weigh.

❏ Identify which aspects of your life you can control and which you can't. Imposing rigid eating rules on yourself may be a way of compensating for a situation that you feel powerless to do anything about.

Begin by asking yourself what in your life has made you feel out of control, suggests Dr. Abramson. Is your job overwhelming you? Has a rift developed between you and your husband? Do you feel as though you have no time to yourself?

Then look at what you can control. "I ask women to keep track of the decisions they make," says Dr. Johnston. "This opens their eyes to the fact that they do have choices. It empowers them to say, 'Yes, I do control my life.'"

❏ Praise yourself once a day for all of the things that you do well. This helps put your weight in proper perspective, according to Dr. Johnston. Maybe you can't wear a teeny-weeny bikini. But are you a loving parent? A caring friend? Have you done a good deed for a stranger? These things speak volumes about your character—and they are much more important than an extra 5 or 10 pounds.

❐ Treat yourself twice a week to non-food-related activities that give you pleasure. "This helps a woman address a sense of emotional deprivation, which often manifests itself as severe dieting, overeating, or both," explains Dr. Johnston. "It encourages her to explore what she really wants and needs in life."

Of course, your sense of pleasure is entirely individual, adds Dr. Johnston. If soaking in a candlelit bubble bath doesn't appeal to you, then perhaps sleeping out under the stars, calling your best friend, or taking a long walk by yourself does.

Rx ———

Prescriptions
FOR SENSIBLE WEIGHT LOSS

So what if you really need to slim down? Don't even think "diet," suggests Dr. Johnston. Instead, think "healthy eating"—and feed yourself only when your body tells you that it's hungry. As you revamp your weight-loss plan with this new view in mind, heed this advice from the experts.

DAYTIME

❐ Consume three small meals plus two healthful snacks each day. This eating plan prevents you from becoming so hungry that you lose control and gobble everything in sight. "Chronic dieters tend to starve themselves all day, then overeat at night, when excess calories are most likely to be stored as fat," notes Brownlee.

❐ Learn to visually assess serving sizes. A serving of meat, for instance, weighs in at three ounces—roughly the size of a deck of playing cards. A serving of pasta is a mere half-cup, a clump about the size of a tennis ball.

❐ Determine a healthy calorie intake for a woman your size. Most women consume between 1,500 and 1,800 calories a day—more if they exercise regularly. So cutting your calorie intake to 1,200 a day gives you an appreciable deficit and may leave you feeling hungry, according to Brownlee. Generally, women should not go below 1,200 calories a day. Many active women can lose weight at 1,500 calories a day.

There's a simple formula for calculating your healthy calorie intake. Consider that you need 10 calories per pound to maintain your weight.

Nutrition Prescriptions to Supplement Your Diet

If you are restricting your calorie intake in order to lose weight, you may not be getting all the nutrients you need from foods. Vitamin and mineral supplements can help make up for any shortfall. Here is what the experts recommend.

❒ Take a multivitamin that supplies the Daily Values of all the essential vitamins and minerals. "A multivitamin can cover those nutritional 'gray areas' where you might be coming up short," says Terri Brownlee, R.D., a nutrition educator at Duke University Diet and Fitness Center in Durham, North Carolina.

❒ Take a calcium supplement, if necessary, to meet the recommended daily intake of 1,000 milligrams for women between ages 25 and 50. You will need to get a rough idea of how much calcium you are consuming from foods, according to Brownlee. For instance, one cup of milk and 1½ ounces of cheese each supply about 300 milligrams of the mineral. Three ounces of tofu provides more than 580 milligrams (but read the label to make sure your tofu was prepared with calcium sulfate). And one cup of dark leafy greens such as chopped kale contains more than 90 milligrams.

(This figure accounts for basic daily activity but excludes exercise.) To lose a pound a week, you should cut your calorie intake by 500 calories a day. For example, a person who weighs 180 pounds could consume 1,800 calories a day to maintain her weight (that's 180 pounds times 10 calories per pound). To lose a pound a week, she would have to cut back to 1,300 calories a day (that's 1,800 minus 500).

❒ Consume between 20 and 30 percent of your daily calories as fat. If you are following a 1,500-calorie-a-day eating plan, for example, 300 to

450 of those calories should come from fat. That translates to roughly 30 to 45 grams of fat a day.

Chronic dieters often try to avoid fat altogether, when in fact they may benefit from having at least a little bit of the nutrient in their diets. Fat is necessary for some basic body functions such as temperature regulation and absorption of fat-soluble vitamins. "And, if you don't consume at least some fat, you get hungrier more often, because fat helps to prolong the sensation of satiety," explains Brownlee. "Plus, fat carries the flavor of foods. So if you eat a fat-free meal and you don't like the taste of it, chances are that you will eat something else to satisfy you, which adds calories."

 TIME IT RIGHT

❏ Assess your overall eating pattern rather than your daily diet. "The truth is, most people have days when they eat nothing but junk, days when they eat only healthful foods, and days when they eat next to nothing," says Linda Smolak, Ph.D., professor of psychology at Kenyon College in Gambier, Ohio, and co-author of *Developmental Psychopathology of Eating Disorders*. "Your body can self-correct for overeating or undereating if you pay attention to its hunger and satiety cues."

Medical **Alert**

Chronic dieters run the risk of developing an eating disorder, especially bulimia, advises Dr. Smolak. "Some people can deny hunger better than others," she says. "But eventually, a feedback mechanism kicks in that compels you to eat—often to seriously overeat."

If you find yourself bingeing frequently, using purges such as laxatives, vomiting, or even overexercising, or if you have lost so much body fat that your menstrual cycle has stopped, you need professional help. Your doctor can direct you to the nearest eating disorders clinic or to a psychologist who specializes in eating disorders.

Chapter 9

PRESCRIPTIONS

FOR THE MARRIED

AND HARRIED

Time. Everyone would like more of it. No one seems to have enough.

For the typical working wife and mom, the time bind seems especially acute. She spends 8 or more hours at her "real" job, then arrives home to a second shift of cooking, cleaning, schlepping the kids around, and supervising homework. She may be blessed with a husband who pitches in—but he seldom has a second to spare himself. By the time she collapses into bed, she has put in about an 18-hour day. And, lucky her, she gets to do it all again tomorrow.

You know that you're officially "married and harried" when:

✓ You are so busy that you have to schedule "snuggle time" with your spouse.

✓ You have been getting 6 hours of sleep a night, tops, since your second child was born 10 years ago.

✓ You are putting in more hours on the job than you want to, but you are afraid that you'll be fired if you ask to cut back. And besides, you need the money.

✓ You would like to spend more time with your children, but other obligations always seem to interfere.

✓ You are fed up with waiting in lines, getting stuck in traffic jams, playing phone tag, picking up everyone else's clutter, and wading through junk mail.

If you feel that you can't keep up your current frenzied, unforgiving pace, know that you are not alone. Many women are struggling to strike a balance between their personal and professional lives. "They are concerned that they don't have enough time to enjoy life or to be with their children as they grow up," explains Pamela Kristan, founder of the Practical Matters, a family-management business in Dorchester, Massachusetts.

Some women have the option of giving up their jobs, or at least cutting back their hours, so they can spend more time with their families. Others have no choice but to work. "Their salaries go for basic needs, not luxury items," explains Nancy Marshall, Ed.D., senior research scientist with the Center for Research on Women at Wellesley College in Wellesley, Massachusetts.

What's more, women seem to be working harder than ever. Figures released by the Bureau of Labor Statistics indicate that compared with women in the mid-1970s, women today are putting in even more hours on the job—about 2 more hours a week, or 104 more hours a year. Why the increase? "It could be that more women are working, that more women are working full-time, or that some women are working more than 40 hours a week," suggests Dr. Marshall.

To make the move from harried to happy, you need both practical and soul-searching solutions. You can apply professional time-management techniques to your personal life or take advantage of the latest in timesaving technology. And you must examine your values and your attitude toward time, says Kerry Daly, Ph.D., associate professor in the department of family studies at the University of Guelph in Ontario and author of *Families and Time: Keeping Pace in a Hurried Culture.*

Prescriptions
FOR FINDING LOST TIME

Rx

Okay: You know that you are busy, but do you really know where all your time goes? Chances are that you have a couple of minutes, or a couple of hours, tucked away in your schedule somewhere. Here is how to go about finding them.

❒ Keep a time diary for one week, writing down what you are TIME IT RIGHT doing every 15 minutes. This is the most accurate way to see exactly how you spend your time, according to Karen Goebel, Ph.D., professor of consumer science and extension specialist at the University of Wisconsin in Madison. "At the end of the week, you can look over your notes and see if your activities reflect what is important to you," she says. You may notice that you run a lot of errands with your car, for example, and decide that you don't want to spend your time that way.

❒ Once you have identified potential time-wasters, brainstorm alternatives for handling them. If you want to reduce the amount of time you spend running errands, for instance, you might want to consolidate trips or share carpooling with someone else, suggests Kristan.

Prescriptions
FOR PARING DOWN

Rx

Simplifying your life in other ways can help slow your hectic pace and free up time for the things that matter most to you. Take advantage of the following suggestions, and you are guaranteed to find seconds to spare.

❒ Designate a space in your home for doing paperwork, and keep it organized. Paper clutter does more than steal time by making you look for things in a shuffled mess. It also creates mental clutter—a sense of overload and lack of control, according to Nancy McGahey, a franchise owner in Rochester, New York, for Priority Management, an international corporate-training company.

❒ Create a "bill book," which can be as simple as a three-ring binder with pocket inserts. When a bill arrives in the mail, write the amount and due date on the front of the envelope, then put it in your bill book. "The biggest advantage of this system is that I know where my bills are," says McGahey. "They're all in one place, not lying on the kitchen counter or wherever else I may have opened the mail."

❒ Use direct deposit and automatic bill payment. Most banks offer these services, which save you the time you would normally spend writing checks, waiting in line at the bank, and running to the post office.

❒ Make a list of the items that you usually buy at the grocery store, then have the list photocopied. This way, you can simply circle items as they run out. It saves you the hassle of writing a new list each week, and it helps you shop more efficiently.

TIME IT RIGHT

❒ Take a late lunch and do your grocery shopping between 2:00 and 3:00 in the afternoon. Or if you live near a 24-hour supermarket, shop after 10:00 at night. Either way, you avoid the noontime and after-work crowds.

❒ If you are looking for a particular item, call various stores to check its price and availability. You will save yourself a bundle of time and energy by not having to chase the item all over town.

❒ Request your husband's assistance with chores and errands. You may think that what needs doing around the house is all too obvious. Your spouse, however, seems to remain oblivious. "So it's up to you to ask for help," says Ruth Klein, author of *Where Did the Time Go?: The Working Woman's Guide to Creative Time Management.*

"Meet your husband on neutral turf outside your home, at a time when you are not ready to blow your stack," suggests Klein. "Tell him that you are overwhelmed and need help. Negotiate what you will do, what he will do, and what your children can do."

❒ Consider hiring one person or service to lend a helping hand around your home. For this to work, of course, you must first accept the fact that you simply don't have time to handle everything yourself, says Jeff Davidson, director of the Breathing Space Institute in Chapel Hill, North Carolina, and author of *The Complete Idiot's Guide to Managing Your Time.* You may opt for a cleaning person or a nanny, a grocery store that delivers or a dry cleaner that picks up at your home.

Prescriptions
FOR FOCUSING ON FAMILY

As you spend less time dealing with life's little details, you will have more time to devote to your family. Here's how to make the most of every minute.

❐ Work with your spouse to develop goals and priorities for your family. If you have children, you may want to ask for their input, too—but it is essential that your and your husband's family values align, says Kristan. Together, you can plan time for what matters and let the unimportant stuff slip by. For instance, you and your spouse may agree that a clean house or a manicured lawn means less than spending time each day with your kids or with an aging parent who needs your help.

❐ Write down your family goals and priorities, then review them regularly. "Realize that your family values are dynamic and may change over time," advises Dr. Goebel.

MONTHLY

❐ Maintain a master monthly calendar that shows every family member's schedule and activities. This allows you to see the big picture so that you can avoid situations in which someone is supposed to be in two places at once, explains McGahey.

❐ Have children ages 10 and older prioritize their own activities. And if their plans conflict with yours, you don't necessarily have to be the one to change. "You should feel comfortable telling your child that a certain event won't work for you and that she has to reschedule it," advises McGahey.

TIME IT RIGHT

❐ Schedule a family meeting for 10 to 15 minutes each Sunday afternoon or evening. This gives everyone an opportunity to hear who is doing what during the upcoming week, says McGahey. You can update your calendar, hash out conflicting appointments, and let the kids know in advance when Mom is going to be away on a business trip or when Dad won't be home for supper.

❐ Make sure that your family time includes free time. People tend to plan their family time around specific, structured activities. But you need to leave the schedule open on occasion. "This is especially good for

(continued on page 482)

Beat the Clock on Household Chores

Rather than stockpiling household chores for the weekend, why not do what you can during the week? Just a few minutes here and there can keep your home neat and clean—without taxing your free time.

The following "to do" list gives you a general idea of how long you need to complete specific tasks, says Jeff Campbell, owner of the Clean Team, a San Francisco–based cleaning service, and author of *Clutter Control* and *Speed Cleaning*. Use the list to make the most of your available time—or to assign chores to your spouse and kids.

5 MINUTES

- ❑ Load or empty the dishwasher
- ❑ Put a load of laundry in the washer
- ❑ Remove a load of clothes from the dryer and fold them
- ❑ Clean the litter box
- ❑ Clean the kitchen counters or table
- ❑ Shake out the tablecloth or place mats
- ❑ Make one bed
- ❑ Strip the sheets off one bed and take them to the laundry basket
- ❑ Clean under one bed
- ❑ Clear the clutter off one bureau
- ❑ Clean a toilet
- ❑ Go through the mail and throw out the junk mail
- ❑ Put out the trash for pickup
- ❑ Shake out or vacuum the doormats

15 MINUTES

- ❑ Water the houseplants
- ❑ Wash the dishes by hand
- ❑ Clean the stove top
- ❑ Sweep the kitchen floor
- ❑ Scrub out that badly burned pot that has been sitting in your sink for two weeks
- ❑ Clean either the bathroom sink and toilet or the tub

❏ Pick up in the living room or family room
❏ Vacuum the cat hair off the couch
❏ Vacuum high-traffic areas around your home
❏ Dust a shelf of books
❏ Wash four windows (hint: use a squeegee)
❏ Sweep the porch or garage
❏ Clean the crud off the barbecue grill
❏ Pull weeds

30 MINUTES

❏ Spot-clean the carpet
❏ Pick up, vacuum, and dust the living room, dining room, or bedroom
❏ Thoroughly clean the bathroom
❏ Clean up and reorganize the mess in the medicine cabinet (discard old or unused items)
❏ Clean up and reorganize the mess under the kitchen sink (discard old or unused items)
❏ Plan a week's worth of menus and use them to make up your shopping list
❏ Clean the oven
❏ Pay a month's worth of bills
❏ Balance your checkbook
❏ Wash all of the windows in one room
❏ Give the dog a bath

60 MINUTES

❏ Thoroughly clean the kitchen
❏ Scrub and wax the kitchen floor
❏ Wash the walls and ceiling in the bathroom
❏ Clean and reorganize the linen closet
❏ Mow the lawn
❏ Clean the patio and outdoor furniture
❏ Wash and vacuum the car
❏ Wax half of the car

kids, because they learn to take care of themselves and to pursue their own interests," explains Kristan.

❏ Recognize moments of spontaneous quality time. "Many of life's most important interactions occur out of the blue, at odd moments—like when you and your spouse are sharing the bathroom sink or you are driving your child to soccer practice," says Dr. Daly. These events, however brief, are just as important to the fabric of your family life as a Saturday afternoon of planned quality time.

TIME IT RIGHT
❏ Reserve at least 20 minutes every day just for yourself. Walk, meditate, breathe deeply—do whatever it takes to restore your equilibrium and energy. "If you don't regenerate yourself somehow, you won't have anything left to give at home or at work," notes Klein. "So allowing this time for yourself is very important."

Rx —— *Prescriptions*
FOR WORKING SMARTER

Maybe you love your job—you just wish it didn't take so much time away from your private life. It doesn't have to. Consider these tactics to manage your workload more effectively.

TIME IT RIGHT
❏ Allow your answering machine or your secretary to screen your calls, then make your callbacks within 24 hours. "Answering phone calls when they come in is one of the biggest time-wasters around," says Klein. It's not that you spend a lot of time talking but that your concentration is disrupted. When you hang up the phone, you may have a hard time refocusing on your work.

TIME IT RIGHT
❏ Cluster your phone calls between 11:00 A.M. and noon or between 4:15 and 5:00 P.M. "At these times of day, your calls are likely to be brief and to the point, since people are likely to be watching the clock," explains Klein.

❏ Ask your boss to help you prioritize your workload. "Tell her, 'I can do this or that, but not both. So which do you need now, and which can wait?'" suggests McGahey. Of course, if you try this tactic, be prepared to explain why each task will take a certain amount of time to complete.

❒ Avoid committing to a project that you know you don't have time for. "It's better to underpromise and overdeliver than to overpromise and underdeliver," says Davidson.

❒ Take 5 to 15 minutes at the end of each workday to plan what you must do the next day. "If you map out your day first thing in the morning, you might be overly optimistic about what you can accomplish," explains McGahey. "But by 4:30 in the afternoon, you're harried, you're bloodied, you're beat. In that frame of mind, you are going to be a lot more realistic about what you can and can't do the next day."

In addition, try planning for Monday on Sunday evening rather than Friday afternoon, when you have already checked out mentally, suggests McGahey.

❒ Create a boundary between your professional and personal lives that you are comfortable with. Some people have to draw a sharp line between work and home so that their thoughts aren't one place while their bodies are another, says Dr. Marshall. This may mean not taking work home or not checking the office voice mail on vacation days.

Other people, though, do better with a more permeable boundary. "When they are at work, they like to phone home to check on the kids. And when they are at home, they like to be available to handle a crisis call from the office," explains Dr. Marshall. "They don't like things to stack up on them."

Chapter 10

Prescriptions

for Single Mothers

Women follow a variety of paths to single motherhood. Some choose the role via adoption or insemination—artificial or otherwise. Other women find themselves parenting alone when they are divorced or widowed.

Entering the ranks of solo "momdom" changes your perspective. You know your outlook has changed when:

✓ Your idea of fine dining is any place without a drive-up window.

✓ You would rather lose your best friend than your best babysitter.

✓ Even your back-up plans have back-up plans.

While every single mom has a unique parenting situation, she likely shares with other single moms a deep sense of isolation. "Most single mothers feel alone and cut off when they don't have another adult to help out—whether in an emergency or in the day-to-day business of raising a child," says Sirgay Sanger, M.D., founder of the Parent/Child Interactive Program at St. Luke's/Roosevelt Hospital and the Early Child Care Center, both in New York City, and author of *The Woman Who Works, The Parent Who Cares.*

When isolation persists, it can cause problems for both mother and child. Dr. Sanger identifies three of the most common hazards.

Overintensity. The absence of other adults to lend support and perspective seriously strains the bond between mother and child. And that situation may leave both parties feeling misunderstood and alienated from each other, particularly when a conflict arises between them.

Overinvestment. Studies have shown that single working mothers are more likely than married working mothers to project their own ambitions and goals onto their children.

Overprotection. Single mothers tend to be more restrictive with their children about normal activities such as exploration.

If any of these problems surfaces, it needs to be addressed right away. Otherwise, the child may experience emotional troubles later on, says Dr. Sanger.

Prescriptions
TO MAINTAIN BALANCE

Rx

"When I was in medical school, I always felt that I left my job too early, then arrived home too late for my children," remembers Barbara Majeroni, M.D., assistant professor of family medicine at the State University of New York at Buffalo. "Single mothers often feel torn by the need to be in two places at once."

And because they focus on the needs of others, single moms often ignore their own physical and emotional welfare. And that can jeopardize their health.

Is it even possible to satisfy other people while maintaining your own sanity? Absolutely—if you employ these expert-recommended strategies.

❏ Pay attention to what your body tells you. "Headaches, muscle tension, and exhaustion are warning signs that you are under too much stress," advises David Edelberg, M.D., clinical instructor at Northwestern University in Evanston, Illinois, and founder of the American Whole Health Centers in Chicago, Denver, and Bethesda, Maryland. "If you don't alleviate the stress that is causing your symptoms, your symptoms can become chronic health problems."

❏ Pamper yourself on occasion. "When was the last time you did something just for yourself?" asks Dr. Edelberg. He suggests arranging a sleep-over for the kids at Grandma's or a friend's so that you can have an entire weekend to yourself. If you can afford it, retreat to a spa or hotel. If not, simply enjoy some well-deserved quiet time at home—soak in an aromatic bath, read a book, watch a movie.

❏ Establish a social support network for yourself, especially if you have no family members or friends to turn to. "Find out if your area has a single mothers' club," suggests Andrea Engber, founder and director of the National Organization of Single Mothers and co-author of *The Complete Single Mother*.

"If not, you may want to start one by posting notices at your kids' schools and on community bulletin boards," Engber says. Also, consider joining the PTA, the YM/YWCA, and other family-oriented organizations. (For more information about the National Organization of Single Mothers, write to P.O. Box 68, Midland, NC 28107.)

❏ Turn to your church, synagogue, or other religious organization for spiritual support. "Spirituality offers a host of emotional benefits to both single mothers and their children," notes Ronald G. Nathan, Ph.D., clinical psychologist and professor of family practice and psychiatry at Albany Medical College in New York. "Prayer is a relaxing antidote to the stress that accompanies single motherhood. Also, many churches and synagogues have single mothers' groups."

NUTRITION Rx

Prescriptions
TO FEED THE FAMILY

"The challenge for the busy single mom is to get a good-tasting, well-balanced meal on the table without resorting to canned ravioli," says Dr. Majeroni. Fear not: It can be done. Here's how.

MORNING

❏ Abandon the notion that only hot, homemade meals are wholesome. "If you are pressed for time, you should feel comfortable serving your kids a bowl of cold cereal and a glass of juice for breakfast or wholewheat crackers, cheese, and fruit for lunch," says Barbara Whedon, R.D., nutrition counselor and outpatient dietitian at Thomas Jefferson University Hospital in Philadelphia.

Prescriptions to Care for Sick Kids

Three words a single mom dreads: "Mom, I'm sick."

"When your child becomes ill, you may feel overwhelmed and powerless," says Ronald G. Nathan, Ph.D., a clinical psychologist and professor of family practice and psychiatry in the department of family practice at Albany Medical College in New York and co-author of *Their Stress Is Your Stress.* "It can challenge your sense of control, and that can be highly stressful."

Though you can't anticipate everything, you can evaluate all of your sick-child options well before you need them. Here is what experts recommend.

❒ Prearrange your child's care in the event that she becomes ill. "A sick child needs nurturing," explains Dr. Nathan. "Ask your boss if you can work at home on days when your child is under the weather. If that doesn't work out, then check whether your community has a sick-child day care center. Or find out from the school nurse what other single moms do when their children become sick."

❒ Think twice about letting your child stay home alone. "Whether a child can stay home by herself when she has a mild cold, for example, depends so much on her level of maturity," says Barbara Majeroni, M.D., assistant professor of family medicine at the State University of New York at Buffalo. "I've seen 11-year-olds who can care for themselves competently, as well as older children who are completely unreliable. Certainly, any child under age 10 needs an adult nearby who can check in on her periodically."

❒ Evaluate whether your child really needs to stay home from school. "You should keep your child at home if she has a temperature, taken orally, of more than 100°F," advises Dr. Majeroni. "If she has strep throat or another infectious condition, she should stay home for at least 24 hours after beginning antibiotics."

❒ Prepare your meals on the weekend. "Roast a turkey or cook a delicious soup or stew that you can serve a few times during the week," suggests Whedon. And don't forget to recruit your children to help out in the kitchen—it's a special, loving way to spend some time together as a family.

MEALTIME

❒ Make sure that you are eating healthfully, too. Single moms instinctively prepare wholesome meals for their children, but they seldom do the same for themselves. "I ask single mothers to recall everything that they have eaten within the past 48 hours," says Dr. Edelberg. "Then I ask them, 'Is this the meal plan of a woman who loves herself?' "

Rx ———— *Prescriptions*
FOR FOOLPROOF PARENTING

In your role as a single mom, you will find that the three Ds—discipline, dating, and Daddy—occasionally conspire to disarm you. But you can outmaneuver them in ways that are beneficial to both you and your children. These tactics can help.

❒ Teach your children by setting a good example for them. "Your children model your behavior," explains Dr. Sanger. "So if you expect them to help clean up after a meal, you need to initiate the task. Then they will pitch in."

❒ Keep chores fun and appealing. "Never make your kids feel sorry for themselves with statements like 'I wish you didn't have so many chores, Jack, but you're the man of the house now,' " advises Dr. Sanger.

❒ Take dating slowly. "Make sure that your kids understand that no man can affect your relationship with them," suggests Dr. Sanger. "Avoid asking them, 'What do you think of so and so?' every time you go out with someone new." And if you are inclined to have a beau stay overnight, wait until you have established a steady, committed relationship with him, and think about the influence this will have on your children's emerging behavior.

❒ Refrain from competing with your former spouse for your children's affections. "When your ex buys your kids the entire toy store and takes them on exotic vacations, your self-esteem—and your control of anger—can suffer," notes Dr. Sanger. "What's worse, kids tend to temporarily go for the glitter and attraction of the latest gimmick." Your best defense is to instill in your kids a bulwark of core values. Take them to museums and parks, bake cookies with them, work on arts and crafts with them. Help them to decide for themselves which accomplishments are most satisfying. "If you make creative, inexpensive activities seem fun, your kids will get in the spirit, too—and you will enrich their values," says Dr. Sanger.

Chapter 11

Prescriptions
for Workaholics

Once her job was her passion. Now it's an addiction.

Like the alcoholic who craves her next drink, the workaholic needs to work to feel good about herself. So she spends long hours at the office and takes projects home with her, disrupting the delicate balance between her professional and personal lives. Family and friends chide her for working so much. They may even call her a workaholic, which she soundly denies.

"Like any addiction, workaholism is very persuasive and convincing," according to Len Felder, Ph.D., a psychologist based in Los Angeles and author of *The 10 Challenges*. "Your brain always comes up with a non-negotiable reason why you should work even harder."

You know that your job has taken over your life when:

✓ You think about work all the time—weekends, holidays, and vacations included.

✓ You are often tired, irritable, and short-tempered.

✓ You have trouble delegating tasks.

✓ You can't say no to new assignments, even when you are already overwhelmed.

✓ The laptop computer spends more time in your lap than your children do.

✓ The last time you took a vacation, stamps were a quarter and George Bush was president of the United States.

Some workaholics alienate themselves from family and friends. They become insensitive and self-centered. They try to bully the people around them to compensate for their inability to control the chaos of their internal world. Other workaholics try so hard to please everyone that they not only overextend themselves at the office but also do everything for their kids, spouses, parents, and friends, says Dr. Felder. In both cases, the work that used to bring satisfaction becomes a source of burnout and resentment.

"Ultimately, the workaholic reaches a point where she says, 'Is this it? Is this what my life is all about?' This wake-up call can be devastating," says Renee Magid, Ph.D., president of Initiatives, a company based in Fort Washington, Pennsylvania, that is committed to helping organizations enhance the quality of work life and personal life, and author of *Work and Personal Life: Managing the Issues.* "You have to remind yourself that life is not a dress rehearsal. You get just one chance to do it right."

Prescriptions
TO PINPOINT THE PROBLEM

Rx

To overcome workaholism, you first have to acknowledge that you have a problem. Heed the early warning signs, says Dr. Felder. Here's how to recognize them.

❏ Pay attention to physical warning signs such as stomach, back, and neck pain. "These are clues that something is wrong," notes Dr. Felder. "Don't dismiss them or cover them up with aspirin."

❏ Listen to your family, friends, and co-workers. "If your spouse tells you that you seem stressed-out, if your friends complain that you are never available, or if your co-workers say that they can never sit down and have a discussion with you, consider these important clues that you may have a problem with workaholism," says Dr. Felder.

❐ Consider your own feelings. If the work you previously enjoyed now seems burdensome, irritating, or boring, you might be edging toward workaholism.

Rx —— *Prescriptions*
TO WEAN YOURSELF OFF WORK

If you suspect that you have workaholic tendencies, you need to regain balance between your professional and personal lives. These measures can help.

❐ Schedule daily 15-minute appointments with an imaginary client named Liz. Then use those 15 minutes to briefly escape the pressures of the workplace. You may want to take a short walk, water your plants, read an inspiring book, or just sit quietly—whatever you need to do to break a pattern of workaholism, says Dr. Felder. Just be sure to take your appointment with Liz as seriously as you would any other appointment on your calendar. That means no cancellations.

❐ If you have your own office, turn off the lights, put up your feet, and sit quietly for 10 minutes. You may want to play some classical music—"or any music that makes you feel great," suggests Dr. Magid. "Those 10 minutes of rest will give you two hours of energy."

❐ Learn to say no to assignments that are absolutely not your responsibility. "Don't agree to take on extra work just because you are trying to be nice or to prove that you can handle it," advises Dr. Felder.

❐ Delegate projects to others who have lighter workloads than you do. If you don't have the authority to delegate, then at least ask your supervisor for assistance. You need to decide which projects you want to keep for yourself and which you can off-load to co-workers, says Dr. Felder.

❐ Let others know when they request the impossible from you, then offer them alternative solutions. For example, suppose your supervisor hands you a lengthy or complicated project at noon and wants it completed by 5:00 P.M. the same day. Explain to her that you could have the work done on time, but that it may be of lesser quality than if you had a more realistic deadline such as noon the next day. With this approach, you are neither a complainer nor a victim, explains Dr. Felder. You are a professional who gives people choices.

❒ Explain to others how they can help lighten your load. Don't wait for family members and co-workers to offer help. "Many workaholics believe that they will be rescued once someone notices how burned-out they are," says Dr. Felder. "The trouble is, that someone is usually focused on her own life and obligations."

Prescriptions
TO STRENGTHEN FAMILY TIES

Rx

Once you have reined in the demands of your job, you can reclaim your relationships with your loved ones. Use these strategies to get your private life back on track.

❒ Learn from others' mistakes. Look at the people in your life who burned out, suffered ill health, ruined their marriages, or became estranged from their kids—all because they put the professional ahead of the personal. "Sometimes a negative role model can motivate a person to make positive changes," notes Dr. Felder.

❒ Put your job in perspective. Your life includes so much more than just work. "If you define yourself by your job and then lose that job, you will be devastated," says Dr. Magid.

❒ Resist the temptation to contact the office outside regular business hours. From voice mail and e-mail to laptop computers and cellular phones, modern technology makes keeping in touch with work easy. The question is, do you really have to? It is something to ask yourself before you check in at the office after hours.

❒ Set aside one hour every day—before or after work—to exercise. Consider this your private time, when you won't be distracted by professional or personal responsibilities, says Dr. Magid. You can join a fitness center or simply make space in your home to work out.

TIME IT RIGHT

❒ Schedule time alone with your mate, and protect that time against any interruptions, advises Dr. Felder.

❑ When you make plans with your spouse, children, or friends, treat those plans not as sacrifices but as a lifeline for keeping yourself sane and balanced. "In your mind, you have to value these people just as much as your most important project or client," explains Dr. Felder.

❑ Refrain from overscheduling your leisure time. Putting too much on your plate will make you—and those around you—anxious, says Dr. Magid.

❑ If you haven't taken a vacation for years, begin with a four-day weekend. Anything longer than that may prove too stressful for you, according to Dr. Felder. If you enjoy your extended weekend, plan for a week next time.

Chapter 12

PRESCRIPTIONS

FOR FREQUENT TRAVELERS

Well, the ad in the newspaper did say "travel required." But when you accepted your job, you had no idea that you would be away from home this much.

You know that you're a too-frequent traveler when:

✓ You live out of your suitcase—even when you are at home.

✓ You own four watches, each one set to a different time zone in the United States.

✓ The porters at the airport greet you by your first name.

✓ You call your landlord to request room service.

✓ You have put 25,000 miles on your company car in just six months.

While a travel-filled career may seem glamorous, it also has its downside. The grueling pace takes its toll on your body. And it jeopardizes your efforts to maintain the regular schedule that helps you eat right, exercise regularly, and sleep soundly.

But you can make even a business trip a pleasure. You just have to follow some basic rules of the road—or rails or air.

Rx ——— *Prescriptions*
FOR A SMOOTH FLIGHT

From the moment you pack your suitcase to the moment you pick it off the airport luggage carousel, airplane travel can be an exhausting—even unnerving—experience. To make your air time as comfortable and stress-free as possible, experts recommend the following strategies.

TIME IT RIGHT

❐ Drink eight ounces of water or fruit juice every hour during your flight. These fluids prevent dehydration, says Edith Hogan, R.D., a consulting nutritionist in Washington, D.C., and a spokesperson for the American Dietetic Association. Dehydration is a common problem among those traveling by air. The humidity in a typical airplane cabin ranges from 2 to 20 percent. By comparison, normal humidity ranges from 60 to 65 percent.

❐ Take bottled water on the plane with you. That way, you are covered in case you become thirsty but you can't get the attention of a flight attendant, according to Diana Fairechild, a former flight attendant, an airline passenger advocate, and author of *Jet Smart*.

❐ Refrain from drinking alcohol, which may actually contribute to dehydration.

❐ Use a portable air filter. Such a filter hangs around your neck, drawing in air to purify it before noiselessly venting it out and up toward your face, explains Martha H. Howard, M.D., medical director for Wellness Associates in Chicago. The device is especially useful for frequent flyers, who often are confined to small, enclosed areas with little fresh air for long periods of time. These folks tend to get sick more often than the general population. You can order portable air filters from specialty catalogs that cater to people with chemical sensitivities or environmental illnesses.

❐ Pack your own pillow. Buy one that you can scrunch up and store in your carry-on bag, suggests Karen Goodwin, editor in chief of *Frequent Flyer* magazine. Neck pillows are designed for travel and come in a variety of styles, including inflatable, water-based, and filled with buckwheat hulls. They are sold in specialty catalogs that cater to travelers.

❑ Take a sweater or shawl on board with you. You can use it to protect yourself against the plane's cool and fluctuating temperatures, says Fairechild.

❑ Carry an eye mask with the words *Do Not Disturb* written across it. It can come in handy if you decide to do some in-flight snoozing, says Fairechild.

❑ Also carry your own earplugs. Some airlines supply earplugs to first-class passengers on certain international flights, according to Fairechild. Otherwise, you are on your own.

❑ During takeoff, swallow frequently, chew gum, sip water, or nibble on fruit. This helps prevent the painful ear blockage that often accompanies a rapid change in altitude, says Quentin Regestein, M.D., director of the sleep clinic at Brigham and Women's Hospital in Boston.

❑ During landing, pinch your nose and push your tongue against the back part of the roof of your mouth. Make sure to breathe through your mouth. This technique, called the Frenzel maneuver, also protects against pain by keeping the ears open, says Dr. Howard.

Prescriptions
TO ELUDE JET LAG

Rx

For many people, airplane travel presents no problems until after the plane lands. That's when jet lag can set in. To get your body clock in sync with your new time zone, try these strategies.

NIGHTTIME

❑ If you are heading east, go to bed 15 minutes earlier each night and get up 15 minutes earlier each morning for 2 days for every hour you gain as you cross time zones. For instance, if you are going to gain six hours as you travel eastward, follow a revised sleep/wake schedule for 12 days before your departure. This tactic won't prevent jet lag, but it can help ease its aftereffects, says Dr. Regestein.

MORNING

❑ If you are heading west, says Dr. Regestein, go to bed 15 minutes later each night and get up 15 minutes later each morning for one week before your flight. Generally, people recover from westbound flights more quickly than from eastbound flights.

TIME IT RIGHT

❏ Set your watch to your destination time zone as soon as you board the airplane. Then coordinate your usual activities with the new time, advises Kenneth Groh, Ph.D., assistant biologist in the biological and medical research division of the Argonne National Laboratory in Argonne, Illinois.

For instance, when your watch says that it is daytime in your destination city, do what you can to stay awake in-flight—turn on your overhead light, talk to your neighbors, walk up and down the aisle. If possible, eat your dinner when it is dinnertime in your destination city. "Your goal is to get your body clock running on destination time," explains Dr. Groh.

TIME IT RIGHT

❏ If you are traveling to Europe, book a flight that leaves an East Coast airport after 9:00 A.M. and arrives at your destination before 9:00 P.M. Flying during daylight hours helps to minimize jet lag.

Melatonin: A Remedy for Jet Lag?

If you spend much of your travel time jetting between the coasts, you are probably well-acquainted with the exasperating symptoms of jet lag: difficulty falling or staying asleep, daytime fatigue, and gastrointestinal distress.

For every time zone you cross, your body needs about one day to recover, says Quentin Regestein, M.D., director of the sleep clinic at Brigham and Women's Hospital in Boston. That means your internal body clock takes about three days to reset after a trip from New York to Los Angeles—and even longer after a trip to Europe.

Some researchers believe that they have found relief for jet lag in the form of the hormone melatonin. Melatonin is released within your body only during nighttime hours. It is believed to help reset your internal clock by informing your body that it is becoming dark outside. Melatonin may play a role in making you feel tired at bedtime and alert in the morning in part by helping to lower your body temperature, which normally peaks

❐ The first morning in your destination city, go outside and soak up some sunshine. Bright light can help reset your internal body clock naturally, explains Dr. Regestein.

Prescriptions
FOR WOMEN ON THE GO

NUTRITION
Rx

No matter what your mode of travel, eating nutritiously away from home can present a challenge. A fast-food burger here, a pack of "plane nuts" there, and soon you have consumed twice your usual number of fat calories in one day—and with few vitamins and minerals to show for it.

The trick to sticking with your healthful eating habits is to plan

---

in the late afternoon and then gradually drops until early morning.

Although widely available as a supplement, melatonin has not been approved by the Food and Drug Administration for any purpose, cautions Margaret Moline, Ph.D., director of the Sleep/Wake Disorders Center at the New York Hospital–Cornell Medical Center in White Plains, New York. "Melatonin looks promising," she says. "But it's very important to understand that research has not yet proven its safety or effectiveness."

The actual content and purity of melatonin pills is generally unknown, adds Dr. Regestein.

If you want to try melatonin as a remedy for jet lag, consult your doctor for the proper dosage before you buy anything. Melatonin is available in relatively huge doses, so taking a pill raises your blood level of the hormone far above normal, says Dr. Regestein. When this happens, you may experience some hangover-type grogginess the next morning, he explains.

ahead, says Hogan. "You'll save yourself time and money, and you'll get the foods you like," she notes. Here is what she and other experts advise.

TIME IT RIGHT

❐ Request a special meal at least 72 hours before your flight. These days, many airlines offer their passengers low-fat, vegetarian, and kosher meals, says Hogan. To get one, though, you most likely have to notify the airline in advance.

❐ Pack pretzels, mini-bagels, and dried fruit in your carry-on bag. You will have something to munch on in the event that your flight gets delayed, according to Hogan.

❐ If you are traveling by car, stock a mini-cooler with individually wrapped cheeses and crackers, fresh fruits and vegetables, and other nutritious snacks. Individually wrapped items provide automatic portion control, notes Hogan. For foods that you can't buy this way, simply place single servings in resealable plastic bags.

❐ Also stock your mini-cooler with leftovers from the previous day's meals. If any of the food requires reheating, Hogan suggests using the microwave oven in a convenience store.

❐ If fast food is your only option, order a plain burger and a side salad with low-calorie dressing.

❐ Refrain from opening the mini-refrigerator in your hotel room. You may even want to throw a towel over it so that you can't see that it's there, says Hogan. Unlocking the fridge invariably reveals a Pandora's box of fat-filled (not to mention expensive) treats.

EXERCISE Rx

Prescriptions
TO TAKE ON THE ROAD

Traveling may tempt you to break from your exercise routine. Ironically, this is when you can least afford to slack off, says Joe Ogilvie, a certified personal trainer at Chelsea Piers in New York City and Canyon Ranch in Lenox, Massachusetts.

These days, most hotels offer fitness equipment. If your hotel doesn't, you can still take advantage of other forms of exercise—walking,

An Herbal Prescription for Rapid Recovery

When you travel, be sure to pack your bags—tea bags, that is. A cup of chamomile tea can help you relax after a long and stressful journey, says Martha H. Howard, M.D., medical director for Wellness Associates in Chicago. Plus, you can dunk the tea bags in cool water and apply them under your eyes to combat the puffiness that comes with being tired.

jogging, even aerobic workouts in your room, suggests Ogilvie. To break a sweat in any city, try these tips.

❏ If you have a layover, walk the various concourses of the airport while you wait for your connecting flight. "It's much too easy to just sit there like a blob," says Ogilvie. "Use the time to squeeze in a good workout." You may want to stow your carry-on luggage in a locker rather than toting it with you.

❏ Pack a jump rope and resistance bands. They take little room in your suitcase, and you can use them in your hotel room, notes Ogilvie.

❏ Diversify your exercise routine to include more than one type of activity. If you limit yourself to one type of exercise machine or one type of class, you are setting yourself up for trouble, says Ogilvie. You may not have access to that particular activity when you travel.

❏ Book a fitness session or massage in your destination city. The Fitness Connection offers free referrals to personal trainers and massage therapists. The fees that these professionals charge vary by location. You should schedule their services at least 24 hours in advance, if possible, says Lori Schoenhaus, a certified personal trainer and founder of the Fitness Connection. They can be contacted by writing to P.O. Box 108, Fair Lawn, NJ 07410.

TIME IT RIGHT

❐ Find a fitness facility near where you are staying. *The Fitness Guide* by Kyle Merker tells you where you can work out while you are on the road. It lists health clubs, exercise classes, and hotels with gyms in about 45 U.S. cities. If you can't find a copy in your bookstore, ask the salesclerk if one can be ordered for you.

Rx — *Prescriptions*
FOR A SAFE, COMFORTABLE STAY

Where you stay when you are traveling can make all the difference in the success of your trip. While you probably don't need anything over the top in extravagance, you at least want your accommodations to be . . . well, accommodating. To make your hotel room feel more like home, consider these pointers from the pros.

❐ Select a hotel with 24-hour room service. Whether you arrive early or late, it is important to know that you can still get food if you are hungry, says Fairechild. Travel across time zones may require you to eat at irregular hours for a couple of days until your body adjusts.

❐ When you make your reservations, request a nonsmoking room. Leftover smoke in the drapes, bedding, and carpet is allergenic. Plus the sprays used by the cleaning crew to cover up the smell can sometimes irritate the respiratory system.

❐ When you check in, request a room near the elevator. These are among the safest rooms, because you don't have to walk through a number of empty corridors to get to them, notes Goodwin.

❐ If you have any concerns about the safety of the hotel parking lot, arrange with hotel security to have someone escort you to and from your car, advises Goodwin.

❐ If someone knocks on your door and identifies himself as hotel staff, call the front desk to confirm who he is before you open the door.

Chapter 13

PRESCRIPTIONS

FOR SHIFT WORKERS

The shift worker may as well live on the other side of the world. She goes to bed when everyone else is getting up. She eats breakfast when everyone else is having dinner. She punches in when everyone else is heading home.

Approximately one-fifth to one-quarter of the population has a nontraditional work schedule. For these folks, the conventional nine-to-five routine doesn't exist. They may work every day from 11:00 P.M. to 7:00 A.M. Or they may be on a rotating shift, meaning that each week they work a different 8-hour segment of the 24-hour cycle.

If you are a shift worker, you can probably vouch for the fact that adjusting to a new sleep/wake schedule is no easy task. "If the human body came with an owner's manual, it would say, 'Do not operate at night,'" says Jack Connolly, Ph.D., president of ShiftWork Consultants in Springfield, Missouri. "We are not biologically programmed to be awake and alert at night. We evolved as daytime movers and nighttime sleepers. So when we try to alter this powerful pattern of behavior, we are bound to have problems."

Certainly, shift work takes a toll on your physical and mental health. Shift workers are prone to weight gain, depression, chronic fatigue syndrome, gastrointestinal disorders, ulcers, heart disease, irregular menstrual cycles, and infertility. They are more likely than the general population to have accidents at work and on the road. And they have a harder time maintaining their topsy-turvy schedules as they get older. Clearly, shift work is not for everyone.

You know that shift work has begun to get the best of you when:

✓ You always feel tired.

✓ You easily become frustrated and irritable.

✓ You feel isolated from your family and friends.

✓ You believe that no one else understands the situation you are in.

✓ You have developed a low tolerance for people and situations that bother you.

Why is shift work so hard on the body and spirit? Primarily because it interferes with your body's biological clock, which gets reset every day by the rising and setting of the sun. This creates a natural cycle called a circadian rhythm, explains Harold Thomas Jr., M.D., chief of emergency medicine at Portland Veteran's Hospital in Oregon. Many bodily functions have circadian rhythms, from the sleep/wake cycle to the vital signs (heart rate, respiratory rate, temperature, and blood pressure).

Circadian rhythms do not readily reverse themselves, which explains why shift workers have trouble staying alert at night and sleeping during the day. To make matters worse, external cues such as bright sunlight filtering through window blinds and aromatic coffee brewing in the kitchen conspire to tip off your body clock that it is time to get up when, in fact, it is time to sleep.

Rx ——— *Prescriptions*
FOR GETTING A GOOD DAY'S SLEEP

Shift work robs you of sleep in more ways than one. Not only are you going against your body's circadian rhythms, but you are also getting less shut-eye overall. Research has shown that people sleep 1½ to 2 hours less during the day than at night.

You can improve your chances for an afternoon of sound, satisfying slumber by heeding this advice from the experts.

DAYTIME

❐ Wear a sleep mask to block out light.

❐ Cover your bedroom windows with room-darkening drapes or shades.

❐ Wear foam earplugs to block out noise. Even if it doesn't wake you, noise disrupts your sleep cycle and compromises your sleep quality, explains Dr. Thomas.

❐ Run a small fan or a white-noise machine while you sleep. Either gadget produces a low, steady tone that helps block out other sounds, says Janie O'Connor, a shift-work consultant and trainer for Interface: Work/Family in St. Paul, Minnesota. You can find white-noise machines in large department stores and specialty catalogs.

❐ Disconnect the phone, or at least turn down the ringer.

❐ Set your bedroom thermostat between 65° and 70°F. A cooler temperature makes sleeping easier, says Ronald Novak, Ph.D., assistant professor in the school of medicine at Case Western Reserve University in Cleveland.

TIME IT RIGHT

❐ Exercise before you go to work rather than before you go to bed, especially if you have trouble winding down. Working out within three hours of bedtime may keep you awake because your body has not had a chance to shift gears. On the other hand, regularly exercising before or during your work hours can actually improve your sleep quality, according to Quentin Regestein, M.D., director of the sleep clinic at Brigham and Women's Hospital in Boston.

If you have trouble fitting a workout into your schedule, try to reserve at least one of your break times for a fast walk, suggests Dr. Regestein.

❐ Ask your employer to install brighter lights. Exposure to bright lights helps your body's internal clock reset more quickly to keep you awake and alert at night, says Dr. Thomas.

TIME IT RIGHT

❐ For more personalized light therapy, use a high-intensity light box before going to work. Light boxes improve adaptation to an irregular work schedule. They are the treatment of choice for those who have seasonal affective disorder (SAD), a form of wintertime depression caused by shortened periods of daylight, says Dr. Thomas. A typical daily session with a light box can range from 30 minutes to two hours. You should ask your doctor to prescribe an appropriate amount of time for you. Light boxes are available through commercial manufacturers. For a listing of manufacturers in your area, write to the Society for Light Treatment and Biological Rhythms, 10200 West 44th Avenue, Suite 304, Wheat Ridge, CO 80033.

DAYTIME

❐ Invest in a pair of really dark wraparound sunglasses. Put them on before you step out into daylight for your commute home, advises Dr. Regestein. The glasses reduce the morning light signal that tells your body clock that it is "awake time" rather than sleep time.

❐ Carpool to and from work. If you have at least one other person in the car with you, you can help each other stay awake and alert. And that may save you from a sleep-related accident. In focus groups conducted by Dr. Novak and his wife, Susan E. Auvil-Novak, professor in the Frances Payne Bolton School of Nursing at Case Western Reserve University, 43 of 45 night-shift nurses had been involved in at least one accident or near-accident in the previous year.

❐ Ask your doctor about melatonin supplements. In its natural form, melatonin is produced by your brain and released during the hours of darkness to make you fall asleep. Research has shown that the synthetic form of melatonin, taken as a supplement, may help your body adjust during the first few days of shift work.

Be aware that melatonin has yet to receive approval from the Food and Drug Administration for any purpose, advises Margaret Moline, Ph.D., director of the Sleep/Wake Disorders Center at the New York Hospital–Cornell Medical Center in White Plains, New York. The supplement looks promising, she says, but not enough research exists to substantiate its safety or effectiveness.

NUTRITION
Rx

Prescriptions
FOR NIGHTTIME NOSHING

While shift workers may lose sleep, they apparently gain weight. In a study conducted by Allan Geliebter, Ph.D., a research psychologist in the Obesity Research Center at St. Luke's/Roosevelt Hospital in New York

City, night-shift workers gained an average of nine pounds over nine years. Day-shift workers gained less than one pound over the same time span.

Why the difference? For starters, the night-shift workers reported eating more and exercising less than their daytime counterparts. Plus, they ate a sizable "dinner" closer to bedtime, which may have slowed their metabolism (the body's calorie-burning mechanism).

To maintain a healthy weight and to avoid the gastrointestinal distress common among night-shift workers, try the following dietary strategies.

❒ Eat half of your meal (the one you take to or buy at work) now and save half for later. To guard against weight gain and postmeal drowsiness, several nurses in the Novak/Auvil-Novak focus groups used a technique called meal-splitting. They ate just half of a normal portion of food during the first break on their shifts, then ate the rest during a subsequent break.

❒ Keep healthful snacks—fresh fruit, low-fat yogurt, whole-grain crackers—on hand. And ask your employer to stock equally nutritious items in the company vending machines.

❒ Eliminate, or at least cut back on, spicy foods. Sure, they taste good going down. But your body has a hard time digesting fiery fare, explains Dr. Novak. And a churning stomach can keep you awake when you should be sleeping.

❒ Limit your consumption of coffee and other caffeinated beverages to the first two to four hours of your shift. After that, stick with water and fruit juices. Caffeine consumed too close to bedtime can disrupt your ability to sleep, says Dr. Novak.

❒ Refrain from drinking a pre-bedtime nightcap. Alcohol, like caffeine, impairs sleep, advises Dr. Connolly.

Prescriptions
FOR MAINTAINING FAMILY TIES

The women who fare best with shift work respect the fact that they are on different schedules than many of their family members and friends. They don't try to live in both worlds at once. "The women who struggle

Prescriptions for Togetherness

It's tough for any working couple to spend quality time together during the week. It's nearly impossible if either spouse is a shift worker. Different schedules mean different times for eating, sleeping, and just hanging out. The challenge is to find that hour or so each day when you are both free—and to use it wisely.

When the two of you finally find some time alone, any of the following activities can help you reconnect on an emotional level, suggests Susan Heitler, Ph.D., a clinical psychologist in Denver and author of *The Power of Two: Secrets to a Strong and Loving Marriage*.

❑ Lounge in comfortable chairs or get rockers for your living room. Rocking creates an especially calm and comfortable mood, even for people with fast-paced, frenzied lives.

❑ Take a hike. Walking is especially helpful when you and your spouse need to discuss a difficult or sensitive issue. Research has shown that people feel less threatened and defensive when they are side by side than when they are face-to-face.

❑ Exercise. Choose an activity that you both enjoy—perhaps cycling, running, or strength training. Whether you work out in a health club or at home, build a routine that you can rely on for healthful together time.

❑ Prepare a meal, even though the two of you may eat it separately later on.

❑ Grab sketch pads or watercolors and explore your creative talents.

❑ Get intimate. Sex offers communication, fun, exercise, and creativity all rolled up in one. It is the ultimate activity for strengthening the bond between the two of you.

try to maintain their daytime orientation and 'incidentally' work at night," says O'Connor. "For instance, they respond to phone calls during the day, even though that's when they should be sleeping."

The following tactics can help ensure that your personal life is in sync with your professional life.

❐ Post a big calendar where everyone in your family will see it. Then write everyone's schedule on it, including your own work and sleep times, suggests O'Connor.

❐ If your schedules allow, ask your partner to drive you to and from work. This gives the two of you an opportunity to spend some time alone together, notes O'Connor.

❐ Adopt a pet. A furry, four-legged companion helps to ease the loneliness of shift work, according to Neal Voron, founder of the Night Shift Initiative, a Web site devoted to shift-work issues. "When you get home at three o'clock in the morning, a greeting from your pet feels really good," he says.

Chapter 14

PRESCRIPTIONS FOR CAREGIVERS

Once, she fed you, diapered you, clothed you, nursed you, loved you, and protected you from harm. Now, decades later, it's your turn.

"Caregiving is largely about women caring for women," says Thomas Humphrey, executive director of Children of Aging Parents (CAPS), a not-for-profit foundation based in Levittown, Pennsylvania. "Today's caregiver is typically a 34- to 49-year-old woman who is likely to spend more years taking care of an aging relative than she did raising her children."

You know you have become a caregiver when:

✓ A little old lady who looks a lot like your mom is permanently ensconced in your guest room.

✓ You've had to childproof your home—though your kids are long past puberty.

✓ Instead of buying Pampers for your infant, you're buying Depend incontinence garments for your father.

✓ You consider it a good day when your live-in mother-in-law remembers your name.

✓ You can't remember the last time you went to a movie, read a book, or took a bubble bath.

"It's good to be needed, to give love, and to perform worthwhile tasks," says Barbara Wich, M.D., a fellow in women's health at the William F. Middleton Veterans Administration Hospital at the University of Wisconsin in Madison. "But caregivers can suffer from severe burnout—it's a relentless, 24-hour-a-day occupation."

Burnout isn't the only problem that can bedevil caregivers, says Dale A. Lund, Ph.D., professor of gerontology and director of the gerontology center at the University of Utah College of Nursing in Salt Lake City. "We call them heroes, these women who unselfishly care for their elderly loved ones," he says. "But heroic caregiving can lead to depression, marital troubles, health problems, and lots of guilt, anger, and resentment."

Caregivers must realistically balance their own needs with the needs of the person they are caring for, says Dr. Wich. If that sounds nearly impossible, read on.

Prescriptions ——— Rx
FOR FACING THE FUTURE

If you have parents or other beloved elders, it is likely that at some point in time you will become their caregiver. You could become a long-distance caregiver, a full-time caregiver, a part-time caregiver, or just an occasional caregiver. No matter which caregiving hat the future holds for you, start planning now to make sure that the hat fits comfortably when your time comes to wear it.

❏ Tackle the tough issues. The time to talk to your beloved elders about the future is now, before your care is needed, says Dr. Wich. "Make a date to discuss values and other hard issues so that you know what your elder would want in the event she is unable to speak for herself," she advises. "Discuss the what-ifs of illness, incapacity, and death. Have your elder make her wishes clear. Suggest that she prepare an advance directive, either a medical power of attorney or a living will, to outline her wishes legally. These forms can be obtained from your medical doctor and can be implemented through your attorney."

❐ Make changes now. If an elder is becoming frail but is still capable of caring for herself, consider modifying her living situation now, even if it seems premature, suggests Dr. Wich. "Suggest a move from a too-large home to something more manageable. Think about putting her name on an assisted-care housing list. It can take years for a name to get to the top of some housing lists, and there is no harm in saying no if your name comes up before you are ready."

❐ Accident-proof the home. "Don't wait till your elder becomes frail to install safety devices in her home," cautions Dr. Wich. "Install grab bars in the bathroom and handrails in the stairwells. Make sure that lighting is bright and adequate, especially in the kitchen, bathroom, stairwells, and outside of the home. Remove slippery throw rugs and install nonskid carpet on hard floors. Eliminate clutter and uneven surfaces so that walking paths are clear. Set the hot water heater at 120°F or less. Install smoke alarms and make sure that they are operational."

❐ Keep up social activities. "Encourage your elder to maintain her support systems, such as the bridge club, church activities, or whatever she likes doing," says Dr. Wich. "Scout out recreational activities that your community has for seniors and encourage her to attend. Check with your local agency on aging for information and referrals. Also, newspapers, senior centers, and churches may have information on resources in your area that provide social support and enjoyable activities geared toward older persons."

❐ Think twice before moving an elder into your home. "Try to maintain your elder in her own home or assisted facility," says Dr. Wich. Before moving an elder anywhere, consider options that are acceptable to both you and her. Know that if you and your elder have a difficult relationship now, it is unlikely to improve once she is under your roof. "In fact, it will be far worse," she says. "Once an elder becomes dependent upon you, all kinds of hostility and resentment can surface for you both. Control issues make getting along with each other difficult and can make life miserable for your entire family. If you are dealing with someone who was a miserable parent, subconsciously you may see this as a time of payback, which is a prescription for disaster."

Don't even think about moving your elder into your home if she needs a more structured and supervised setting. If she has violent outbursts, has substance abuse problems, smokes in bed, or is given to wandering or other dangerous behavior, then she requires continuous supervision, suggests Dr. Wich. "Taking such an individual into your home may create divided and stressful demands. You'll crash very quickly, and you stand the chance of destroying your relationship with yourself, your elder, your children, and your spouse," says Dr. Wich.

You should also consider alternatives to home care if your elder has round-the-clock nursing needs or is uncontrollably incontinent, recommends Dr. Wich. Such services are expensive, so you will need to plan ahead to finance them. Inquire about community resources, Medicare funding, medical assistance, sliding-scale payment options, and Veterans Administration assistance, if eligible.

❏ **Seek out support.** For help with any caregiving need, contact Children of Aging Parents at 1609 Woodbourne Road, Suite 302A, Levittown, PA 19057. If your elder lives far away, contact the National Association of Professional Geriatric Care Managers at 1604 North Country Club Road, Tucson, AZ 85716. Two other organizations that can offer assistance are the Alzheimer's Association (also known as the Alzheimer's Disease and Related Disorder Association), 919 North Michigan Avenue, Suite 1000, Chicago, IL 60611; and the National Stroke Association, 96 Inverness Drive East, Suite I, Englewood, CO 80112.

Prescriptions
FOR GETTING RESTFUL SLEEP

A caregiver needs seven to eight hours of efficient, restful sleep every night to function effectively, says Michael Janson, M.D., director of the Center for Preventive Medicine in Barnstable, Massachusetts. To get the shut-eye you need, he recommends trying these tips.

❏ **Do nothing too stimulating,** emotionally or physically, for 30 minutes before bedtime.

NIGHTTIME

❏ **At bedtime, lie in bed** and breathe slowly, regularly, and deeply for a few minutes.

Dispense a 30-Minute Vacation

A half-hour break. It's the impossible dream when you care for someone with Alzheimer's disease. "What caregivers need most is just a little time to themselves," says Dale A. Lund, Ph.D., professor of gerontology and director of the gerontology center at the University of Utah College of Nursing in Salt Lake City. So Dr. Lund and his team, who have been studying caregivers for more than a decade, developed "Video Respite," a series of videotapes that simulates a visit by a warm, caring person. Each tape offers simple, interactive experiences—familiar old songs, holiday memories, a trip to the good old days. Some even feature friendly dogs and gentle hand exercises. "The videos can calm people who are in the moderate or advanced stages of Alzheimer's disease," says Dr. Lund.

"If someone can watch TV, they are likely to enjoy these tapes—over and over again," Dr. Lund says. That can give you, the caregiver, the chance to slip into a hot bath, read a book, or do absolutely nothing. The tapes range in length from about 25 to 55 minutes, and cost from $35 to $58 each.

For more information, write to Innovative Caregiving Resources at P.O. Box 17332, Salt Lake City, UT 84117.

❐ When you feel very calm, close your eyes and visualize yourself somewhere peaceful—the beach, for example. Examine the scenery in detail. Hear the waves, see the grains of sand, feel the breeze on your skin, watch the waves lap onto the shore, listen to the gulls. Immerse yourself in the details, focusing for a brief moment on each one before moving on to the next.

Prescriptions
FOR CAREGIVERS

NUTRITION
Rx

As a caregiver, you need 10 times more energy than most women. Here is a life plan designed to boost your energy, increase endurance, and enhance your vitality, specifically designed for caregivers by Dr. Janson.

❒ Skip the coffee. "For some women, even one cup of coffee in the morning can disturb their sleep at night," says Dr. Janson.

MORNING

❒ Moderate your alcohol intake. "A glass of wine (5 ounces) or a beer (12 ounces) at dinner, one to three times a week, may have healthful benefits. But more than that can affect your performance—even the next day," Dr. Janson continues.

❒ Avoid soda altogether. "The sugar, phosphoric acid, and caffeine in soda leach calcium from your system," Dr. Janson says.

❒ Lighten up on sweets. "Too much sugar can be devastating to a woman who is stressed-out," says Dr. Janson. "It causes blood sugar fluctuations, which in turn can cause mood swings." Sugar that occurs naturally in fruits is fine, but avoid candy, cookies, cakes, and ice cream. "And be careful about 'naturally sweetened' foods," he says. "They often use highly concentrated fruit juice or other sweeteners that have similar effects to refined sugar. Even natural sweets like honey and maple syrup are easy to overdo, so be sure to read food labels and avoid products with ingredients like fructose and glucose."

❒ Graze on plant foods. "A diet high in fiber foods—natural whole grains, oatmeal, fruits and vegetables—keeps your bowels functioning regularly," says Dr. Janson. In addition, eating a broad variety of fruits, vegetables, grains, and beans will ensure that you get a good supply of bioflavonoids, which are chemical pigments found in plants. According to Dr. Janson, bioflavonoids enhance the protective benefits of vitamin C and improve the strength of blood vessels, in addition to having a host of other physiological benefits.

❒ Take a divided dose multivitamin/mineral supplement. "I tell caregivers to take a good high-potency multivitamin every day," says Dr.

Janson. "Look for the kind found in health food stores that are divided into four to six pills daily."

❏ Take 400 to 500 milligrams of magnesium a day. "It's an important supplement for women who are under stress because it helps mitigate nervousness and irritability," says Dr. Janson.

Note: The recommended dosage of 500 milligrams exceeds the Daily Value for magnesium, which is 400 milligrams. If you decide to give supplements a try, and particularly if you have heart or kidney problems, you should be working with a doctor who is willing to monitor your progress. Also, if you experience diarrhea when taking these supplements, cut back your dosage until your symptoms subside.

EXERCISE Rx

Prescriptions
FOR THE OVEREXTENDED

Biking, jogging, or brisk walking are excellent for defusing stress. Even housework and gardening may qualify, as does any activity that gets your heart pumping and makes you sweat.

TIME IT RIGHT

❏ Exercise four or five times a week and work up at least a mild sweat for a half-hour or so. "The sweatier you get, the better," says Dr. Janson, "but don't get too out of breath."

❏ Get out of the house. "Though you could use an at-home exercise bike, it's important that caregivers take breaks away from the home. If you can't get out on the bicycle or track, make a commitment to join a gym and to use it regularly," advises Dr. Janson.

Medical **Alert**

Being a caregiver could lead to depression. If you have trouble sleeping or your eating habits change or you develop a lack of interest in life, you could be headed for a more serious problem, says Mary Amanda Dew, Ph.D., associate professor of psychiatry, psychology, and epidemiology in the department of psychiatry at the University of Pittsburgh School of Medicine. If these symptoms continue for two weeks or longer, seek out professional help.

Chapter 15

PRESCRIPTIONS

FOR LIFE ON THE GO

What's not to love about technology? These days, we have computers, modems, fax machines, pagers, cellular phones, and high-tech messaging services. We have microwave ovens. We have VCRs, virtual reality, and online shopping. In short, we have everything we need to make life faster, easier, and better.

Everything, that is, except time. There simply isn't enough time to go around. And as a result, you probably feel as though there isn't enough *you* to go around.

"Years ago, trend watchers predicted that by the year 2000, we would be a nation of leisure," says Martin Goldberg, M.D., clinical professor of psychiatry at the University of Pennsylvania School of Medicine in Philadelphia. "Although we have all of the modern contraptions that were supposed to free up our time, the opposite has happened. Technology has complicated our lives even further. We have more responsibilities, and we expect more of each other as individuals."

Society, in general, expects a lot more of women. "We have this notion that if Martha Stewart can bake brioches, stencil a floor, preside over a staff meeting, and make dried floral arrangements for every room in her house all before lunch, then every woman can do the same," notes Dr. Goldberg.

You know that your life has gotten too hectic when:

✓ Your daily planner is thicker than the Manhattan phone book.

✓ Your car phone has a fax.

✓ Your beeper has changeable cases and doubles as a fashion accessory.

✓ You dream in "to do" lists.

✓ Post-it notes cover your computer, your fridge, your bathroom mirror, and occasionally your clothes.

While some women thrive on this not-a-second-to-spare lifestyle, others quietly bend to its pressures. They may skip healthful meals, ignore their exercise routines, and come up short on restful sleep. Their marriages and other personal relationships may suffer. So may their health.

If any of these ring a bell with you, slow down long enough to read the following prescriptions for leading a full and happy—if hectic—life.

NUTRITION Rx

Prescriptions
for Fast Food

When you are on the go, your healthful eating habits can be the first thing to fall by the wayside, says Georgia Hodgkin, R.D., Ed.D., associate professor in the department of nutrition and dietetics in the School of Allied Health Professions at Loma Linda University in California. Following are some tips for maintaining dietary sanity when the rest of your world has gone haywire.

❐ Plan meals one week in advance, then shop ahead for quickly prepared, healthful foods. "Make purposeful food choices so that you don't get stuck eating meals that aren't nutritious," suggests Dr. Hodgkin.

❐ Substitute five or six healthful snacks for the standard three meals a day. When your schedule is full, you may benefit from small but nutritious "snack-meals," says Michael Janson, M.D., director of the Center for Preventive Medicine in Barnstable, Massachusetts. This style of eating, called grazing, not only keeps you energized and alert but also helps you to lose weight and lower your cholesterol, if you make the right selections.

Choose low-fat, low-sugar foods such as fresh fruits, unsweetened applesauce, raw vegetables, prepackaged lentil soup, whole-wheat bread, air-popped popcorn, rice cakes, and broiled salmon, suggests Dr. Janson. "Grazing is a good eating plan in general, and you can do it forever. Just make sure that you eat a variety of foods in reasonable portions."

❐ Rely on kitchen equipment that makes meal preparation easy. "Between your microwave, your toaster oven, your slow cooker, and your freezer, you can prepare ahead and get a good meal on the table quickly, no matter how pressed for time you may be," according to Dr. Hodgkin.

❐ Consume enough fiber-rich foods each day to meet the Daily Value of 25 grams. "A high-fiber diet keeps the bowels regular," notes Dr. Janson. He suggests eating plenty of whole grains, especially oatmeal, brown rice, and whole wheat, as well as starchy vegetables such as potatoes, yams, squash, and corn. Avoid white flour and other foods made from refined wheat, which has had its fiber removed.

❐ Make healthful fast-food choices. "These days, you can find baked potatoes with toppings, burritos, and side salads on the menus of most fast-food restaurants," says Dr. Hodgkin. Even pizza can be nutritious if you're careful when you make your choice: Order a pie that goes heavy on veggies and light on cheese—and ask whether you can get a whole-wheat crust.

You can make your fast-food meal even healthier by adding a vegetable, a fruit, or a glass of skim milk, advises Dr. Hodgkin.

❐ Curb your consumption of caffeinated coffee. "If your life is already hectic, the caffeine in coffee can jangle your nerves even more," notes Dr. Janson. "For many women, even one cup in the morning can disturb sleep at night. Losing sleep is the last thing you need when you lead a hectic life."

Prescriptions
FOR FITTING IN FITNESS

No matter how busy your schedule is, you can find time to exercise, says Larry A. Tucker, Ph.D., professor of health promotion at Brigham

Timeout for Instant Relaxation

If your daily routine has you on the go every moment, you owe it to yourself to slow down and smell the roses—at least for an instant, as often as you can each day.

"Even a very busy woman can invest 20 minutes a day for a couple of weeks to learn how to relax rapidly," says Ronald G. Nathan, Ph.D., a clinical psychologist and professor of family practice and psychiatry at Albany Medical College in New York and co-author of *The Doctors' Guide to Instant Stress Relief*. "Once you learn how to relax, you can do it anytime, anywhere. Even very short sessions can produce long-term benefits."

To ensure that you are using the proper technique, you should consider investing in a relaxation tape or getting trained by a professional, advises Dr. Nathan. But to get you started, he offers this very basic form of relaxation.

1. Find a place where you will not be disturbed for 20 minutes. Sit there comfortably in a well-supported position.

2. Close your eyes. Gently let go of any unwanted thoughts, and gradually breathe slower and deeper until you feel completely relaxed.

3. Continuously repeat to yourself a word that sounds pleasing and has positive meaning for you. *Beach, vacation,* and *honeymoon* are good choices, says Dr. Nathan.

By practicing this technique regularly, you will soon be able to quickly trigger an optimal state of relaxation that can counter the negative effects of stress, explains Dr. Nathan.

What about those days when you don't have a 20-minute time slot to spare? "The average American spends 40 minutes a day just waiting—often in a state of anger or anxiety," says Dr. Nathan. "So make waiting work for you by giving yourself a healthy stress break." Simply close your eyes; take a slow, deep, satisfying breath; and repeat your cue word. "I call it an instant relaxant," he notes.

Young University in Provo, Utah. And if you intend to stay healthy while maintaining that hectic pace of yours, exercise is absolutely essential.

"Virtually all humans function best when they work out regularly," explains Dr. Tucker. "Exercise offers literally over a thousand different physical benefits. For the woman on the go, in particular, exercise defuses stress and increases strength and stamina."

The following suggestions can help you make exercise part of your daily routine.

❐ Exercise in the morning. "Women who successfully fit their **Morning** workouts into their schedules often start their days by exercising," says Dr. Tucker. This may mean that you have to get up an hour earlier than usual. "The advantage is that you can get your workout over with and start your day with a feeling of achievement." He suggests working up to at least 30 minutes of exercise a day, seven days a week.

❐ If morning workouts simply don't suit you, then exercise at **Daytime** lunchtime. "Take a brisk 30- to 40-minute walk, stopping to pick up a healthy sandwich or salad on your way back to the office," suggests Dr. Tucker.

❐ Combine exercise with another activity. "Busy women often juggle a couple of tasks at once. You can do the same with exercise," says Dr. Tucker. "Read your company's annual report or catch up on the news while you are on a stationary bike or a treadmill."

Prescriptions
for Strengthening Your Union

Rx

A life on the go often means precious little time with your mate. And that can fuel any stress that you are already feeling. "Each of you starts doing your own thing, so you are spending more and more time apart," explains Dr. Goldberg.

Just being aware of this problem can propel you to its solution. Here is what Dr. Goldberg suggests you do.

❐ Schedule one or two 45-minute appointments with your spouse **Time it right** each week. Write the appointments in your and your spouse's calendars. Then use this time to chat with each other. "You have 45 minutes to warm up and start talking," notes Dr. Goldberg. "If you find you have nothing to say to each other, then discuss that. Don't abandon the conversation until 45 minutes has passed."

❏ If you can, plan your chat times with your spouse for the weekend. "Sundays after church and Sunday evenings are very popular because people tend to be most relaxed then," says Dr. Goldberg. "The worst time is right after work, when people feel exhausted and overextended.

"Avoid other outside interference during your chat, such as television, music, even knitting," advises Dr. Goldberg.

❏ Take a walk with your spouse. Getting out of the house makes for a productive chat, and walking while you talk is quite relaxing.

Chapter 16

PRESCRIPTIONS
FOR PARTY GIRLS

At the risk of sounding spiritless, there is such a problem as having too much fun. It's not a problem most of us have, mind you. Some of us even fantasize about it. But every now and then, a woman comes along who is so focused on experiencing pleasure, seeking adventure and constant social interaction, that it is detrimental to other aspects of her life—health, family, work, and community.

You know that you have officially earned party girl status when:

✓ You spend your workday thinking about where you can go for happy hour.

✓ You seriously considered venturing out during the decade's worst blizzard.

✓ You are so seldom at home that your dog thinks you are an intruder.

The question is when does the pursuit of a good time become excessive?

"On the one hand, a lifestyle focused on socializing may reveal a person as a true extrovert," says Rebecca MacNair-Semands, Ph.D., a psychologist in the student counseling center at the University of North Carolina at Charlotte. This means that you are at your best when you are in the company of other people—which, incidentally, may make you a natural for a job that requires lots of networking.

On the other hand, too much socializing may be a way of putting deeper problems out of sight, out of mind. "A person might be using socializing or partying to avoid dealing with a difficult or troubling situation," suggests Dr. MacNair-Semands.

Perpetual partying can have health implications as well, especially if you routinely engage in the risky, addictive behaviors that are so closely linked to a life of fun—things like drinking and taking drugs and smoking. In addition, casual and unprotected sex poses health dangers, since it makes you a prime candidate for sexually transmitted diseases, including AIDS.

Younger women, in particular, tend to cultivate the party girl role, primarily because they have a social network to support it, explains Bela Chopp, Ph.D., clinical director in the student counseling center at Oakland University in Rochester, Michigan. Plus, they are still making the transition to adulthood. "Once your schooling ends, you are expected to assume adult responsibilities. That can seem terribly frightening," notes Dr. Chopp. "So you delay the process by seeking refuge in your social life. It's as though you are in denial: 'If I don't think about what I have to do, then I don't have to do it. I can pretend that it doesn't exist.'"

Rx —— *Prescriptions*
FOR FINDING DIRECTION

The term *party girl* makes it sound as though only young women can be addicted to socializing. But the term extends to any woman who still feels a compulsion to go out as much as humanly possible, even at the sacrifice of her job or family. Such women often lack a firm sense of who they are and where they are going—they struggle with so-called identity issues. "They tend to have problems with self-esteem, they rely on others to give them direction, and, out of fear, they may avoid tackling the question 'What do I want to do with my life?'" says Dr. Chopp. "This question is tough to deal with, especially when you are in your twenties or thirties and you have most of your life ahead of you."

Understand that the road to self-discovery takes a lifetime to travel. You can make the journey a little easier for yourself by heeding this advice from the experts.

❐ Establish personal and professional goals for yourself. What sorts of things do you want to accomplish in life? Do you want to further your education? Climb the career ladder? Focus on children?

LIFETIME

By giving your life direction, goals create and sustain interest, energy, and focus, explains Dr. MacNair-Semands. And they help prevent boredom, which can get you into trouble.

❐ Break down long-term goals into manageable short-term goals. "People freeze up when faced with the question 'What am I going to do with my life?' " says Dr. Chopp. "It's just too overwhelming and frightening." So instead, ask yourself where you want to be five weeks, five months, five years from now. This baby-step approach helps whether you are planning out your life, remodeling your home, or coordinating a project at work.

❐ Determine what you must do to reach your goals. "In career counseling, we suggest that people conduct informational interviews," says Dr. MacNair-Semands. "This involves talking to successful professionals about what they do in a typical day, what they like and dislike about their jobs, and what level of education and training they needed to advance to their current positions. This exercise helps people recognize what they need to do to achieve their goals."

❐ Before you go to bed each night, spend 10 minutes quietly reflecting on your day. Think about how it has been meaningful to you, whether you have advanced toward your goals, whether you feel lost or off-track. "This sort of quiet time can be especially balancing if you are normally moving nonstop," notes Dr. MacNair-Semands. "It allows you to focus more on the consequences of your behavior when you are acting in a way that doesn't feel healthy to you." It may also prompt you to take greater responsibility for your actions and where they lead you.

NIGHTTIME

❐ Write down your thoughts. "You might want to ponder some of the same questions that a college counselor would pose to a student," suggests Dr. MacNair-Semands. "What do you enjoy? When you feel your best, what is it that you are doing? What are your values now, and what did you grow up believing? Of the values you grew up with, what do you no longer find important or want to replace?"

❏ Find someone to be your sounding board. Sometimes extroverts do better talking with others than spending time alone, says Dr. MacNair-Semands. If this describes you, enlist a family member, a friend, or a psychologist to help you hash things out.

Rx — *Prescriptions* FOR SMART SOCIALIZING

As you determine where you are headed in life, your perspective on partying may change. The following strategies can help you let the good times roll—responsibly.

❏ Stop engaging in behavior that puts your health at risk. Let's face it: Your body has to last you a lifetime. You are not doing it any favors if your socializing includes heavy drinking, smoking, drugs, or casual and un-protected sex. "Unfortunately, most people have a hard time recognizing and admitting that their behavior has spun out of control," according to Dr. Chopp. "For instance, young people who drink excessively often de-lude themselves into believing that they can stop any time they want. But they never actually put themselves to the test."

❏ Look for healthy alternatives to partying. If you sense that your desire to socialize is driven by some underlying impulse, try to identify what that impulse might be. "For example, perhaps you have a need for risk-taking or excitement," observes Dr. MacNair-Semands. If that's the case, you may want to try an activity such as scuba diving, mountain biking, or rock climbing.

TIME IT RIGHT ❏ Exercise for at least 30 minutes each day. "Working out is an ex-cellent alternative to risky behavior," notes Dr. MacNair-Semands. It also helps to dispel built-up anger and anxiety.

❏ Join a group whose interests match your own. Watch your local newspaper for meeting and event announcements from hiking clubs, reading groups, and church organizations, among others.

❐ Stay socially active. You can find ways to reduce risky behavior without decreasing or limiting your fun, says Lori A. Lefcourt, Ph.D., a licensed psychologist in the university counseling center at George Washington University in Washington, D.C. "The wisest older people never forget to have fun, even though *how* they have fun may change," she explains. "I believe that the older you get, the more you understand and appreciate the value and need for longtime friends, celebrations of hard-earned success, and time spent just relaxing."

When you are young, you have more time and less focus, so you don't realize how valuable such social occasions are. But when you are in your forties, fifties, sixties, or beyond, that occasional night of total debauchery really is much more fun—simply because it is so rare.

Medical **Alert**

If you want to change your behavior but find yourself struggling to do so, get professional help. "It may mean that you have developed some destructive habits or an addiction, and the sooner you deal with it, the better," says Dr. Chopp. "Facing and dealing with your difficulties will ultimately make you stronger."

Index

Underscored page references indicate boxed text. **Boldface** terms and references indicate primary discussions. *Italic* references indicate illustrations.

A

Abdominal crunches, *366*
Abdominal fat, health hazard presented by, 361–62
Abuse, physical and emotional
  divorce as result of, <u>401</u>
  self-esteem and, 421
Academy of Family Mediators, 404
Acidic foods
  avoiding, and urinary tract infections, 136
  canker sores related to, 37–38
  dry mouth and, 67
Acidic sprays, for dry mouth, 66
Acidophilus milk, for bad breath, 20
Acidophilus suppositories, for yeast infections, 149–50
Acne. *See* Blemishes
Activated charcoal, for gas, 73–74
Activity. *See* Aerobic exercise; Exercise(s); Inactivity; Strength training; Stretches; Workout(s); *specific activities*
Acupressure, as relief for
  labor pains, 266
  menstrual cramps, 275
  repetitive strain injury, 242–43
Addictions
  drug, divorce as result of, <u>401</u>
  exercise (*see* Exercise(s), addiction to)
  work (*see* Workaholics)
Aerobic exercise. *See also specific activities*
  cellulite, combatting with, 321
  depression, alleviating with, 398
  fibromyalgia, alleviating with, 188, <u>189</u>
  heart disease, preventing with, 201
  high blood pressure, alleviating with, 208
  irritable bowel syndrome, alleviating with, 220
  menopause and, 272
  strength training, balancing with, 464
  trouble zones, combatting with, 363–65
  winter doldrums, combatting with, 444–45
Affirmations, for overcoming negative thinking, 428
Age spots, 311–14
  causes of, 311–12
  fading, 313–14
  prevention of, 312–13
Aging
  forgetfulness and, 404–5
  post-workout soreness and, 94
AHAs. *See* Alpha hydroxy acids
Air conditioners, asthma and, 166, 168
Air currents, dry eyes and, 63
Air filters
  air travel and, 496
  asthma and, <u>167</u>
  bolstering immune system and, 237
  sinusitis prevention with, 111
Air pollution, sinusitis and, 107
Air travel. *See* Travel
Alcohol, limiting consumption of
  cancer prevention and, 171
  caregivers and, 515
  cold sores and, 36

Alcohol, limiting consumption of
    (continued)
  conception and, 253
  heartburn and, 88
  high blood pressure and, 208
  hot flashes and, 261
  irritable bowel syndrome and, 218
  migraine headaches and, 129
  osteoporosis and, 225
  premenstrual syndrome and, 296
  sinusitis and, <u>179</u>
  sleep problems and, 116
  tinnitus and, 133
Alfalfa tea, for bad breath, 21
Allergies
  asthma and, 164
  beauty products and, 195
  canker sores and, 39
  chronic fatigue and, 180
  conjunctivitis and, 39, 40, 41, 43
  food (*see* Food allergies)
  hypoallergenic skin products and, 356
  yeast infections related to, 148
Allicin, for high blood pressure, 205
Alliums. *See also* Garlic
  for cancer prevention, 173
Alpha hydroxy acids (AHAs), as
    treatment for
  age spots, 314
  blemishes, 317
  dark circles, 325–26
  expression lines, 335
  melasma, 347
  wrinkles, 373–74
Alzheimer's Association, 513
American Academy of Matrimonial
    Lawyers, 403
American Association of Naturopathic
    Physicians, <u>193</u>
American Herbalists Guild, <u>193</u>
Anemia, iron-deficiency, 153–57
  prevention of, 156–57
  remedies for, 154–56, <u>155</u>
Anger, 378–83. *See also* Hostility
  causes of, 378–79
  coping tactics for, 379–80
  problem-solving and, 380, <u>381</u>,
    382–83

Anise, as treatment for gum disease, 82
Anorexia, 467, 470
Antacids
  heartburn and, 84
  queasy stomach and, 104
Antidepressants, queasy stomach as result
    of, 103
Antidiarrheals, 57–58
Antioxidants. *See* Beta-carotene; Vitamin
    C; Vitamin E
Anxiety. *See* Computer anxiety; Nervous
    tension
Apis, as treatment for
  conjunctivitis, <u>42</u>
  vaginitis, <u>140</u>
Arch supports, to increase flexibility, 121
Arm stretches, to prevent post-workout
    soreness, *101*
Arnica, as treatment for
  bruises, 53–54
  muscle pain, 8, 95, 102
Aromatherapy, as treatment for
  anger, 380
  dry hair, <u>330</u>, 331
  energy slumps, <u>72</u>
  forgetfulness, 406
  hot flashes, 258
  laryngitis, 50
  menstrual cramps, 275
  oily hair, 349
  premenstrual syndrome, 292
  tension headaches, 127
Arsenicum, as treatment for diarrhea, 58
Arthritis, 157–63
  exercise for, 160, 162–63
  prevention of flare-ups of, 159–60
  remedies for, 158–59, <u>161</u>, 163
Artificial sweeteners
  diarrhea and, 60
  flatulence and, 76
  headaches and, 129
  queasy stomach and, 104
  urinary incontinence and, 301
Artificial tears, for dry eyes, 61
Ascorbic acid. *See* Vitamin C
Asian ginseng. *See* Panax ginseng
Aspartame. *See* Artificial sweeteners
Assertiveness training, for shame, 412

<u>Underscored</u> page references indicate boxed text. **Boldface** terms and
references indicate primary discussions. *Italic* references indicate illustrations.

Association of Labor Assistants and
    Childbirth Educators, 265
Asthma, 164–69
  causes of, 164
  heartburn and, 168
  remedies for, 165–66, <u>167</u>, 168–69
Astragalus
  bolstering immune system and, <u>233</u>
  for colds and flu, 32
Atherosclerosis, 209. *See also* Blood
    cholesterol, high
Attentive listening, memory and, 407
Attitudes
  toward exercise, reshaping, 465–67
  toward self (*see also* Self-esteem, low)
  overeating and, 440–41
Attorneys, for divorce, 403

B

"Baby blues," 286–89
Back curls, post-pregnancy, *18*
Back leg lifts, *370*
Back pain, 9–19
  bras to relieve, 5
  during menstruation (*see* Menstrual
    discomforts)
  position to relieve, 6
  prevention of, 11–12, *12–14*, 14–18
  remedies for, 9–11, <u>16</u>, *16–17*
Back stretches, to prevent post-workout
    soreness, *99*, *101*
Bacterial infections
  conjunctivitis as result of, 39
    remedies for, 42
  queasy stomach and, 103
  vaginosis, 139, 141
Bad breath, 19–21
  causes of, 19, 21
  remedies for, 20–21
Bad moods. *See* Mood(s), bad
Bandages, to speed healing, 53
Bath(s)
  hot
    back pain and, 11
    breast pain and, 25
    chronic fatigue and, 180

    colds and flu and, 32
    energy slumps and, <u>72</u>
    hemorrhoids and, 90
    morning stiffness and, 118
    sleep problems and, 117
    varicose veins and, 147
  sensitive skin and, 357–58
  warm
    arthritis and, 158
    hot flashes and, 258
    during labor, 266
    menstrual cramps and, 275
    tension headaches and, 126
Bath oils, for sensitive skin, 357
Bay essential oil, for dry hair, <u>330</u>
BDD, 441–43
Beans
  chronic fatigue relief and, 177
  reducing flatulence associated with,
    <u>76</u>
Beauty products, allergens in, 195
Bed, limiting activities in, 116
Bedrooms, asthma and, 166, <u>167</u>
Beef. *See* Meats, red
Belladonna, for menstrual cramps, 281
Benzoyl peroxide, for blemishes, 316
Bergamot, oil of, sun sensitivity as result
    of, 312
Berloque dermatitis, 313
Beta-carotene
  bolstering immune system and, 232
  for heart disease prevention, 203
Beta hydroxy acids, as treatment for
    expression lines, 335
  sensitive skin, 357
  wrinkles, 374
Betony tea, for tension headaches, 126
Bilberry, for varicose veins, <u>145</u>
Bills, organizing, 477–78
Binge-purge syndrome, 467, 470
Bioflavonoids, as treatment for
  asthma, 168–69
  varicose veins, 144
Biological clock, 112–13
Birth control methods. *See also specific
    methods*
  for urinary tract infection prevention,
    138

<u>Underscored</u> page references indicate boxed text. **Boldface** terms and
references indicate primary discussions. *Italic* references indicate illustrations.

Black cohosh, as treatment for
  fibromyalgia, _192_
  hot flashes, 258
  menopause, 271
Black currant oil, for painful periods,
    278
Black haw, for menstrual cramps, 274
Black tea, irritable bowel syndrome and,
    218
Bladder retraining, for urinary
    incontinence, 302
Bladder supports, for urinary
    incontinence, 299
Bleaching creams, for dark circles, 325
Bleeding, rectal, 89, 92. _See also_
    Hemorrhoids
Blemishes, 315–20
  causes of, 315–16
  remedies for, 316–20, _328–29_
Blood cholesterol, high, 209–14
  prevention of, 210–14, _212_
Blood pressure, 204–9
  high, 204–9
    oral contraceptives and, _207_
    remedies for, 205–8
    stress reduction to prevent, 208–9
  normal readings for, 204
Blood sugar, 21–24
  control of, exercise for, 185–86
  monitoring and diabetes, 183
  problems with, 21–24
    remedies for, 22–23
Blow-drying
  of dry hair, 331
  of fine hair, 337, _338–39_, _338–39_
Body dysmorphic disorder (BDD). _See_
    Body image, poor
Body fat. _See also_ Body weight; Cellulite;
    Overweight
  abdominal, health hazard presented by,
    361–62
  trouble zones for (_see_ Trouble zones)
Body image, poor, 441–43
  strategies to improve, 442
Body weight. _See also_ Body fat;
    Overweight; Weight control
  arthritis and, 163
  breast pain prevention and, 27

cancer prevention and, 171
  coughing related to, 51
  goal for, 470–71
  ideal, calculating, 51
  following menopause, 361
  set point theory of, 469
  varicose vein prevention and, 143
  waist-to-hip ratio and, 185
Boredom, 387–91
  employment to alleviate, 389–90
  enhancement of home life to alleviate,
    390–91
  health implications of, 387–88
  social ties to alleviate, 388–89
Boric acid suppositories, for yeast
    infections, 149–50
Bowel movements. _See_ Constipation;
    Diarrhea; Hemorrhoids
Bowel transit time, exercise and, 171
Bras
  breast pain relief and, 25
  upper-body aches and, 5
Breakfast, weight loss and, 229
Break(s) for, as stress reliever
  caregivers, _514_
  relaxation, _520_
Breakouts. _See_ Blemishes
Breast cancer, prevention of, 269
Breast discomfort, 24–28
  prevention of, 25–27
  remedies for, 25, 27–28
Breastfeeding, breast pain associated
    with, 24
Breath, bad, 19–21
Breathing
  deep (_see_ Deep breathing)
  during labor, 266
Bromelain, for varicose veins, _145_
Brow furrows. _See_ Expression lines
Bruises, remedies for, 8, 53–54
Brushes
  for dry hair, 329
  for frizzy hair, 344
Bubble baths, vaginitis and, 140
Buchu, for urinary tract infections, _137_
Buffer zones, for anger, 380
Bulimia, 467, 470
Burdock root, for dry hair, _330_

Underscored page references indicate boxed text. **Boldface** terms and references indicate primary discussions. _Italic_ references indicate illustrations.

Burning mouth syndrome, **246–49**
causes of, 248–49
remedies for, 247–48
Business trips. *See* Travel
Butcher's-broom, for varicose veins, <u>145</u>
Butterfly stretch, modified, for menstrual
cramps, *277*
Buttocks, back leg lift for, *370*

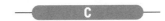

Caffeine
blood sugar problems related to, 23
breast pain related to, 26–27
caregivers and, 515
coffee nerves associated with, 28–30
conception and, 250–51
depression and, 397–98
diarrhea and, 59
energy related to, 70
heartburn and, 86
hectic pace and, 519
hot flashes and, 260
for migraine headaches, 128–29
nervous tension and, 432
osteoporosis and, 225
sleep problems and, 116
tinnitus and, 133
urinary incontinence and, 300
vaginal dryness and, 308
Caladium, for vaginitis, <u>140</u>
Calcium
sources of, <u>198</u>, 206
as treatment for
gum disease, 83
high blood pressure during
pregnancy, 206
osteoporosis, 221–23
painful periods, 278
Calcium supplements, <u>198</u>
calcium carbonate, for osteoporosis, 222
calcium citrate, for osteoporosis, 223
during dieting, <u>473</u>
with iron supplements, 157
osteoporosis and, 222–23
painful periods and, 278
Calculus, gum disease and, 77

Calendula flowers, for dry hair, <u>330</u>
Calendula officinalis, for wound healing,
52
Calf stretch, to prevent post-workout
soreness, *97*
Calories
counting, 466
determining requirement for, 185
healthy intake of, 472–73
Cancer prevention, **170–74**, 269
Candida infections
dry mouth and, 65
vaginal (*see* Yeast infections)
Canker sores, **35**, **37–39**
prevention of, 38–39
remedies for, 37–38
Capsaicin, as treatment for
burning mouth syndrome, 247–48
osteoarthritis, 159
Caraway seed oil, for irritable bowel
syndrome, 219
Carbohydrates. *See also* Sugar; Sweets
energy related to, 70
for nervous tension, 432
Cardamom, for flatulence, 75
Caregivers, **510–16**
breaks for, <u>514</u>
moving elders into one's home and,
512–13
overextended, 516
plan to increase energy, endurance, and
vitality of, 515–16
preparing for future and, 511–13
sleep and, 513–14
Carotenoids, for cancer prevention,
172–73
Carpal tunnel syndrome, 238. *See also*
Repetitive strain injury
acupressure for, 242–43
Carpeting
asthma and, 166
immune system and, 237
Carrot juice, for coughing, 48
Celery, as treatment for
high blood pressure, 205
menopause, 269–70
Cellulite, **320–322**
remedies for, 321–22

<u>Underscored</u> page references indicate boxed text. **Boldface** terms and
references indicate primary discussions. *Italic* references indicate illustrations.

Chair(s)
ergonomically adjustable, 15
for repetitive strain injury prevention,
239
Chair lifts, for back pain prevention,
13
Chamomile essential oil, for hot flashes,
258
Chamomile flowers, for dry hair, <u>330</u>
Chamomile tea, as treatment for
conjunctivitis, 43
gas, 74
puffy eyes, <u>352</u>, <u>501</u>
queasy stomach, 104
tension headaches, 126
travel fatigue, <u>501</u>
Charcoal, activated, for gas, 73–74
Chasteberry, as treatment for
hot flashes, 258
menopause, 271
premenstrual syndrome, 291–92
Cheese
for osteoporosis, 222
urinary incontinence and, 300
Chemical relaxers, for frizzy hair, 345
Chest crossovers, *369*
Chest presses, *369*
Chest stretches, to prevent post-workout
soreness, *101*
Chewing food
for iron-deficiency anemia, 154
limiting flatulence and, 74
Chewing gum
dry mouth and, 65
heartburn and, 84
queasy stomach and, 104
Childbirth education classes, 264–65
Children. *See also* Infants
carrying, 18
lifting, *18*
sick, caring for, <u>487</u>
Children of Aging Parents, 513
Chinese angelica. *See* Dong quai
Chlorinated water, dry hair and, 332
Chocolate, heartburn and, 87
Cholesterol. *See* Blood cholesterol, high
Cigarette smoking. *See* Smoking
cessation

Cinnamon, burning mouth syndrome
and, 249
Circadian rhythms, 112–13
Classes, to dispel boredom, 389
Clothing
compression hose, 143–44, 146
tight
heartburn and, 84
queasy stomach and, 106
sperm count and, 252
yeast infections and, 151
underwear (*see* Underwear)
Clutter, pressure created by, 477
Cod-liver oil, for dry eyes, 62
Coenzyme Q$_{10}$, as treatment for
chronic fatigue, 177
gum disease, 82
Coffee. *See also* Caffeine
decaffeinated, heartburn and, 86–87
irritable bowel syndrome and, 218
Coffee nerves, 28–30
Cognitive restructuring, <u>448</u>
Cold. *See also* Compresses, cold; Ice
cold packs, as treatment for
arthritis, 158
breast pain, 25
Colds and flu, 30–34
prevention of, 33–34
remedies for, 31–33
resistance to, 31
spread of, 30–31
Cold sores, 34, 35–37
prevention of, 36–37
remedies for, 35–36
Collagen production, vitamin C and,
160, 224
Combs
for dry hair, 329–31
for fine hair, 337
Common cold. *See* Colds and flu
Community events/activities, to dispel
boredom, 388–89
Compresses
cold, as treatment for
conjunctivitis, 40, 42, <u>42</u>
dark circle prevention, 324–25
hemorrhoids, 90
puffy eyes, 353

<u>Underscored</u> page references indicate boxed text. **Boldface** terms and references indicate primary discussions. *Italic* references indicate illustrations.

hot, as treatment for
 back pain, 11
 muscle spasms, 11
 sinusitis, 108
warm, as treatment for
 dry eyes, 62
 headaches, 124–25
 morning stiffness, 118
Compression hose, for varicose veins,
 143–44, 146
Computer anxiety, 391–94
 building experience and, 393–94
 strategies for getting started with
  computers and, 392–93
Computer use, repetitive strain injury
 prevention and, 239–40, 241
Concealer, to hide
 dark circles, 326–27, 327
 puffy eyes, 353–54
Conception, difficulty with, 249–54
 health remedies for, 250–51
 remedies for couples and, 253–54
 remedies for male and, 251–52
Conditioners, as treatment for
 dandruff, 56
 dry hair, 328–29, 330, 331
 fine hair, 337
 frizzy hair, 342–43
 oily hair, 351
Condoms
 lubricants used with, 420
 for urinary tract infection prevention, 138
 yeast infections related to, 148
Conflict
 inability of exercise to resolve, 466–67
 minimizing, to bolster immune system,
  236
Conjunctivitis, 39–43
 allergic, 39, 40, 41, 43
 bacterial, 39, 42
 remedies for, 40–43
 viral, 40
Constipation, 43–46
 causes of, 44
 hemorrhoids and, 89
 laxatives for, 43
 prevention of, 46
 remedies for, 44–45, 45

Contact lenses
 during conjunctivitis attacks, 40
 with dry eyes, 61, 62
Corn oil, for dry eyes, 62
Cornstarch, for hemorrhoids, 90
Cosmetics
 for concealing
  blemishes, 317, 319
  dark circles, 326–27, 327
  puffy eyes, 353–54
 conjunctivitis and, 41
 sensitive skin and, 355–56
Coughing
 prevention of, 50–51
 remedies for, 47–48
Counseling
 marital, 400–401
 for shame, 412
Counting, for anger, 380
Cramp(s), menstrual. See Menstrual
 discomforts
Cramp bark, as treatment for
 fibromyalgia, 192
 irritable bowel syndrome, 219
 menstrual cramps, 274
 tension headaches, 126
Cranberry capsules, for urinary tract
 infections, 136
Cranberry juice, as treatment for
 urinary incontinence, 299
 urinary tract infections, 136, 137–38
Cravings, during pregnancy, 284
Crow's-feet. See Expression lines
Crunches, for trouble zones, 365, 366
Crying
 benefits of, 429
 dry eyes and, 61
 puffy eyes as result of (see Eye(s),
  puffy)
 sinusitis and, 111
Cumin, to limit flatulence, 75
Curcumin, for rheumatoid arthritis, 159
Curlups, for back pain prevention, 14
Cuts, 51–54
 stitches for, 54
Cycling
 for arthritis, 163
 increasing flexibility and, 121

Underscored page references indicate boxed text. **Boldface** terms and references indicate primary discussions. *Italic* references indicate illustrations.

D

Dairy foods. *See also* Cheese; Milk;
    Yogurt
  diarrhea and, 59
  flatulence and, 75
  for osteoporosis, 221–22
  reducing, for painful periods, 278
  sinusitis and, 110
Dandelion, for urinary tract infections,
    137
Dandruff, 54–57
  remedies for, 55–56, 350
Dang-quai. *See* Dong quai
Dark circles, 323–27
  concealing, 326–27
  lightening, 325–26
  minimization and prevention of,
    324–25
Dating, by single mothers, 488
Day care, guilt regarding, 409, 410
Decaffeinated coffee, heartburn and,
    86–87
Decision-making, overcoming mental
    blocks and, 425–26
Deep breathing
  bolstering immune system and, 235
  as treatment for
    anger, 380
    bad moods, 386
    fibromyalgia, 189–90
    headaches, 128, 130
    hot flashes, 256–57
    irritable bowel syndrome, 216
    premenstrual syndrome, 291
    queasy stomach, 105–6
    tension headaches, 128
    worrying, 446
Degenerative joint disease. *See*
    Osteoarthritis
Deglycyrrhizinated licorice root. *See*
    Licorice root, deglycyrrhizinated
Dental problems, bad breath related to,
    21
Depression, 394–99
  postpartum, 286–89
    causes of, 286–87
    remedies for, 287–89

  remedies for, 395–98, 396–97
  during winter (*see* Winter doldrums)
Dermatitis, seborrheic, of scalp, 55
Detanglers, for frizzy hair, 342
Detergents, sensitive skin and, 357
Diabetes, 181–87
  blood sugar control and, 185–86
  dietary prescription for, 182–83
  gestational, 181–82
  heart disease prevention and, 202
  self-care for, 182–84
  Type I, 181
  Type II, 181–82, 184
  weight loss and, 184–85
Diaphragms, for urinary incontinence, 298
Diaries
  for depression, 398
  exercise, for chronic fatigue, 176
  food (*see* Food diaries)
  headache, 129
  mood, 385
  time, 477
Diarrhea, 57–60
  chronic, 59–60
  infectious, 57
  with magnesium therapy, 5
  during menstruation (*see* Menstrual
    discomforts)
  remedies for, 57–59
Diet(s). *See also* Meal(s); Nutrition;
    Snacks; *specific foods and nutrients*
  blood sugar control and, 23
  diarrhea and, 58–59
  iron sources in, 155–56, 155
  Ornish, for cholesterol management,
    212
  variety in, for heart disease prevention,
    203
  vegetarian
    iron sources in, 155–56
    for rheumatoid arthritis, 161
Dietary fat
  breast pain related to, 26
  cellulite and, 321
  heartburn and, 86
  limiting
    diabetes and, 185
    fibromyalgia and, 192–93

Underscored page references indicate boxed text. **Boldface** terms and
references indicate primary discussions. *Italic* references indicate illustrations.

heart disease prevention and,
202–3
tinnitus prevention and, 133
proportion of calories consumed as,
473–74
Dietary fiber
breast pain prevention and, 26
cholesterol management and, 211
constipation and, 44–45, 46
diabetes and, 184
flatulence limitation and, 75
hemorrhoid prevention and, 91–92
irritable bowel syndrome and,
217–18
urinary incontinence and, 299
varicose veins and, 144
weight loss and, 228–29
Dieting. *See also* Weight control
anemia as result of, 153–54
chronic, 468–74
healthy eating versus, 472–74
stopping, 470–71
strategies for resolving conflicts
leading to, 471–72
wrinkles and, 376
Dining out, food allergies and, 195
Dishwashing, split nails and, 359
Disinfection, for cold and flu prevention,
33
Divorce, 399–404
amicable parting and, 402–3
grieving and, 399
mediators for, 403–4
prevention of, 400–401
unavoidable, 401
Dong quai
side effects of, 271–72
sunlight exposure and, 280
as treatment for
hot flashes, 258
menopause, 271
painful periods, 280
Douching
vaginal dryness and, 308
vaginitis and, 140
Dressings, to speed healing, 53
Drug addiction, divorce as result of, 401
Dust mites, asthma and, 164, 166

E

Ear(s), ringing in. *See* Tinnitus
Earplugs, for tinnitus prevention, 133–34
Eating disorders, 467, 470
Echinacea
bolstering immune system and, 233
for colds and flu, 32
Eczema, of scalp, 55
Elders, caring for. *See* Caregivers
Electric blankets, for arthritis, 158
Electric toothbrushes, 78
Electrolytes, to prevent post-workout
soreness, 103
Emotion(s). *See also* Mood(s); Winter
doldrums; *specific emotions*
sinusitis and, 111
Emotional abuse. *See* Abuse, physical and
emotional
Employment
addiction to (*see* Workaholics)
balancing personal and professional
lives and, 476, 492–93
dispelling boredom and, 389–90
environment, cancer prevention and,
172
mental blocks related to, 424–25
repetitive strain injury as result of, 238
shift work and (*see* Shift workers)
travel for (*see* Travel)
workload management and, 482–83
Energy slump, 68–72. *See also* Fatigue,
chronic
remedies for, 69–71, 72
Environment
dry eyes and, 61, 63
immune system and, 236–37
sinusitis and, 107
temperature of, hot flashes and, 257
Essential oils. *See* Aromatherapy
Estrogen. *See also* Hormone-replacement
therapy (HRT)
body weight and, 27, 253, 254
dental health and, 81
heart disease and, 199–200
high cholesterol and, 210
isoflavone effects resembling (*see*
Isoflavones)

Underscored page references indicate boxed text. **Boldface** terms and
references indicate primary discussions. *Italic* references indicate illustrations.

Estrogen *(continued)*
  melasma and, 345–46
  pain perception and, 192
  phytoestrogens and, 269–70
  vaginal moisture and, 303–4
Eucalyptus essential oil, for laryngitis, 50
Evening primrose oil, as treatment for
  asthma, 169
  burning mouth syndrome, 248
  dry eyes, 62
  dry mouth prevention, 67
  hot flashes, 258
  painful periods, 278
Exercise(s). *See also* Workout(s); *specific*
    activities
  addiction to, 461–67
    optimum workouts and, <u>463</u>
    rebuilding exercise routine and,
      462–65
  aerobic (*see* Aerobic exercise)
  asthma and, 166
  attitude toward, 440
  blood sugar control with, 23
  bolstering immune system and, 232, 234
  by caregivers, 516
  for cholesterol management, 214
  increasing flexibility and, 121–22
  Kegel (*see* Kegel exercises)
  during labor, 265
  lack of (*see* Inactivity)
  post-workout soreness and (*see*
    Workout(s), soreness following)
  during pregnancy, 262, <u>263</u>, 264
  to prevent
    back pain, 11–12, *12–14,* 15–17,
      16–18
    cancer, 171–72
    constipation, 46
    hot flashes, 260–61
    varicose veins, 143
  for relief of
    arthritis, 160, 162–63
    breast pain, 28
    chronic fatigue, 175–76
    diabetes, 185–86
    energy slumps, 71
    gas, 74
    nervous tension, 430

  osteoporosis, <u>223</u>
  postpartum depression, 289
  premenstrual syndrome, 291
  repetitive strain injury, 240, 243, 244
  urinary incontinence, <u>300–301</u>
  vaginal dryness, 308
  scheduling, 519, 521
  shift work and, 505
  strength training (*see* Strength
    training)
  stretching (*see* Stretches)
  while traveling, 500–502
  voiding before, 298
  weight loss and, 230–31
Exercise diaries, for chronic fatigue, 176
Expression lines, 332–35
  preventing deepening of, 333–34
  smoothing out, 334–35
Eye(s)
  dark circles under (*see* Dark circles)
  dry, 60–64
    causes of, 60–61
    prevention of, 63–64
    remedies for, 61–63, <u>62</u>
  puffy, 351–54
    causes of, 351–52
    concealing, 353–54
    minimizing, 352–53, <u>352</u>
    remedies for, <u>501</u>
  rubbing during conjunctivitis attacks, 41
Eye baths, for conjunctivitis, 42
Eyebright, for conjunctivitis, 43
Eye gel, for puffy eyes, 353
Eye makeup, conjunctivitis and, 41

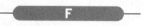

Face washing, for blemishes, 316–17
Facial lines. *See* Expression lines; Wrinkles
Family time, 479, 482
  for shift workers, 507, <u>508</u>, 509
Fast food, healthy choices, 519
Fatigue. *See also* Energy slump
  chronic, 174–80
    allergies and, 180
    exercise for, 175–76
    nutritional remedies for, 176–79

<u>Underscored</u> page references indicate boxed text. **Boldface** terms and references indicate primary discussions. *Italic* references indicate illustrations.

rest and, 180
sinusitis and, 178–79
during menstruation (see Menstrual discomforts)
travel, remedy for, 501
Fatty acids
in flaxseed, 191
omega-3 (see Omega-3 fatty acids)
Feminine hygiene sprays, vaginitis and, 140
Fennel, as treatment for
conjunctivitis, 43
gas, 74
menopause, 269–70
Fenugreek seeds, for cholesterol management, 213
Ferrous sulfate, for iron-deficiency anemia prevention, 156
Fever blisters. See Cold sores
Feverfew, 3–4
for tension headaches, 126
Fibromyalgia, **187–94**
prevention of flare-ups of, 190–94
remedies for, 188–90, 189, 192–93
Filing, of nails, 359–60
Filtering air. See Air filters
Fingernails. See Split nails
Fish, fatty acids in. See Omega-3 fatty acids
Fish oil, as treatment for
asthma, 169
burning mouth syndrome, 248
Fitness, setting goal for, 463
Fitness Connection, 501
Flattening irons, for frizzy hair, 344–45
Flatulence. See Gas
Flaxseed, as treatment for
constipation, 44–45
fibromyalgia, 191–92
irritable bowel syndrome, 218
menopause, 268–69
painful periods, 278
premenstrual syndrome, 296
Flaxseed oil, for burning mouth syndrome, 248
Flexibility, increasing, 120–22
Flossing, 79–80
for bad breath, 20

Flu. See Colds and flu
Fluids
air travel and, 496
heartburn and, 86
hot, for colds and flu, 31–32
during pregnancy, 284
for prevention of
breast pain, 26
constipation, 46
hemorrhoids, 92
post-workout soreness, 102
sinusitis, 110
to reduce appetite before meals, 229
for relief of
bad breath, 20
dandruff, 56
diarrhea, 59
dry mouth, 66
energy slumps, 70–71
irritable bowel syndrome, 219–20
laryngitis, 50
menstrual cramps, 275
urinary incontinence, 299–300
urinary tract infections, 136
vaginal dryness, 308
Folate
for cancer prevention, 172
deficiency of, burning mouth syndrome and, 248
Fold and Hold Method, for muscle pain, 8
Folic acid
aiding conception and, 250
for cancer prevention, 174
for energy slumps, 70
excess of, 174, 250
for postpartum depression, 288
Food allergies, **194–99**
conjunctivitis and, 41
lactose intolerance, 197, 198
prevention of, 195–97, 199
Food Allergy Network, 195
Food diaries, for monitoring
diarrhea, 60
fibromyalgia, 194
food allergies, 197
irritable bowel syndrome, 218
urinary incontinence, 301–2
weight loss, 230

Underscored page references indicate boxed text. **Boldface** terms and references indicate primary discussions. *Italic* references indicate illustrations.

Food poisoning, 103
Foot pain, remedies for, 6–7
Footwear. *See* Shoes
Forgetfulness, 404–8
  causes of, 404–5
  herbal remedies for, 405–6
  reminder services for, 407
  techniques for overcoming, 406–8
Formaldehyde, immune system and, 236
Fragrances
  sensitive skin and, 355, 357
  sun sensitivity as result of, 312
Freckles, 312
Frown lines. *See* Expression lines
Fruit(s)
  chronic fatigue and, 177
  citrus
    hot flashes and, 260
    urinary incontinence and, 300
  constipation and, 44, 46
  flatulence and, 75
  gum disease and, 83
  heart disease prevention and, 203
  irritable bowel syndrome and, 217

G

Game, for iron-deficiency anemia, 154
Gargling, for sore throat, 49
Garlic
  bolstering immune system and, 233
  cancer prevention and, 173
  cholesterol management and, 211
  gum disease and, 82
  high blood pressure and, 205
  hot flashes and, 260
Garlic supplements, for cholesterol
    management, 211
Gas, 73–77
  limiting frequency and severity of,
    74–77, 76
  remedies for, 73–74
Gastroesophageal reflux, 88
Gender, forgetfulness and, 405
Geranium essential oil, for premenstrual
    syndrome, 292
Gestational diabetes, 181–82

Ginger
  hot flashes and, 260
  for relief of
    migraine headaches, 129
    morning sickness, 283
Ginger ale, warm, for queasy stomach, 104
Ginger tea, 3
  as treatment for
    colds and flu, 32
    gas, 74
    menstrual cramps, 274
    rheumatoid arthritis, 159
    sinusitis, 107–8
Gingivitis, 77, 81, 84
  during pregnancy, 80–81
Ginkgo biloba
  for forgetfulness, 406
  side effects and interactions of, 132
  for tinnitus, 132
  for varicose veins, 145
Ginseng
  Asian (*see* Panax ginseng)
  bolstering immune system and, 233
Gloves, for relief of
  sensitive skin, 356
  split nails, 359
  stiff hands, 120
Glucose tolerance, impaired, 181
Glycolic acid, for age spots, 314
Goldenseal, for conjunctivitis, 42, 43
Grains
  for constipation prevention, 46
  for relief of
    chronic fatigue, 177
    irritable bowel syndrome, 217
Grieving, divorce and, 399
Grit/gravel, removing from wounds, 52
Grocery shopping, time-saving ideas for,
    478
Groin stretches, to prevent post-workout
    soreness, *98*
Grooming, time allowed for, body image
    and, 442
Guided imagery. *See* Imagery
Guilt, 408–412
  about day care, 409, 410
  remedies for, 411
  sources of, 409

Underscored page references indicate boxed text. **Boldface** terms and references indicate primary discussions. *Italic* references indicate illustrations.

Gum chewing. *See* Chewing gum
Gum disease, 77–84
nutrition to prevent, 83–84
oral hygiene to prevent, <u>78–80</u>
remedies for, 81–83

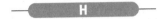

Hair
dandruff remedies for, <u>350</u>
dry, 327–32
causes of, 327–28
remedies for, 328–29, <u>330</u>, 331–32
styling, 329–31
fine, 335–40
cuts for, 340
hygiene for, 336–37
styling, 337, <u>338–39</u>, *338–39*
frizzy, 341–45
causes of, 341
hygiene for, 341–43
styling, 343–45
oily, 348–51
grooming of, 351
hygiene for, 348–51
washing (*see* Shampooing)
Hair brushes. *See* Brushes
Halitosis. *See* Bad breath
Hamstring stretches, to prevent post-
workout soreness, *98*
Hands
arthritis in, exercises for, 163
stiff, remedies for, 119–20
washing
bolstering immune system and,
237
for cold and flu prevention, 33
during conjunctivitis attacks, 41
Hat wearing
dandruff and, 56
expression lines and, 334
Hazardous materials, cancer prevention
and, 172
Headache(s). *See* Menstrual discomforts;
Migraine headaches; Tension
headaches
Headache diaries, 129

Head elevation, for relief of
colds and flu, 32
coughing, 48
heartburn, 88
puffy eyes, 352
Headsets. *See* Phone use
Head-to-knee stretches, modified, for
menstrual cramps, *276*
Heartburn, 84–88
asthma and, 168
prevention of, 85–88
remedies for, 85, <u>87</u>
Heart disease, 199–204
exercise to prevent, <u>202</u>
lifestyle changes to prevent, 200–202
magnesium therapy with, 5
nutrition to prevent, 202–3
Heart rate, for monitoring workouts, 464
Heat. *See also* Bath(s); Compresses;
Showers
hot packs for repetitive strain injury
and, 242
hot soaks for headaches and, 124
as treatment for
menstrual cramps, 275
repetitive strain injury, 242
stiff hands, 119
varicose veins and, 147
Heavy objects, moving, 15
Hemorrhoids, 88–93
factors contributing to, 89
pain relief with, 90–91
prevention of, 91–92
remedies for, 89–90
thrombosed, 90, 93
Herbalists, finding, <u>193</u>
Herbal remedies. *See also specific herbs*
bolstering immune system and, <u>233</u>
cholesterol management and, 213
conjunctivitis and, 41–43
constipation and, <u>45</u>
dry eyes and, <u>62</u>
fibromyalgia and, <u>192–93</u>
forgetfulness and, 404–6
heartburn and, <u>87</u>
hot flashes and, 258
irritable bowel syndrome and, 218–19
menopause and, 271–72

<u>Underscored</u> page references indicate boxed text. **Boldface** terms and
references indicate primary discussions. *Italic* references indicate illustrations.

Herbal remedies *(continued)*
  during pregnancy, 262
  puffy eyes and, <u>352</u>, <u>501</u>
  tension headaches and, 126
  urinary tract infections and, <u>137</u>
  vaginal dryness and, 306–7
  varicose veins and, <u>145</u>
Herpes simplex virus, cold sores as result
    of. *See* Cold sores
Hip abduction, *367*
Hip stretches, to prevent post-workout
    soreness, *99*
Homeopathic remedies
  bruises and, 53–54
  conjunctivitis and, <u>42</u>
  painful periods and, 280–81
  post-workout soreness and, 95, 102
  potency of medicines used in, 53
  vaginitis and, <u>140</u>
  yeast infections and, <u>150</u>
Honey, for laryngitis, 49
Honeybee. *See* Apis
Hormone-replacement therapy (HRT)
  melasma and, 345
  as treatment for
    hot flashes, 257
    vaginal dryness, 304–5
Hose, compression, 143–44, 146
Hostility, 413–15
  addressing cause of, 414–15
  strategies for reducing, 414
Hotels, 502
Hot flashes, 254–61
  prevention of, 257–61
  remedies for, 256–57
  sleep problems and, 113, 114
Hot-oil treatments, for dry hair, 329
Hot packs, for repetitive strain injury, 242
Hot peppers. *See* Red peppers
Hot soaks, for headaches, 124
Household chores
  asthma and, 166
  mental blocks about, 425
  time required for, <u>480–81</u>
HRT. *See* Hormone-replacement therapy
Humidity, as relief for
  colds and flu, 32
  dandruff, 56

dry eyes, 63
sensitive skin, 358
sinusitis prevention, 111
Humor, to bolster immune system,
    235–36
Hydrocortisone, as treatment for
  hemorrhoids, 89
  itching, 357–58
Hydrogen peroxide
  gum disease and, 81
  for removing grit from wounds, 52
Hydroquinone, as treatment for
  age spots, 314
  dark circles, 325–26
  melasma, 347
Hyperglycemia, 181
Hypericum perforatum, to soothe nerves,
    54
Hypertension. *See* Blood pressure, high
Hypoallergenic products, for sensitive
    skin, 356
Hypoglycemia. *See* Blood sugar, problems
    with

IBS. *See* Irritable bowel syndrome
Ibuprofen, for menstrual discomforts, 273
Ice, as treatment for
  back pain, 11
  bruises, 53
  cold sores, 35
  migraine headaches, 128
  muscle strain, 7–8
  post-workout soreness, 94–95
  repetitive strain injury, 242
Iliopsoas muscles, resting, 6
Imagery. *See also* Visualization
  during labor, 266–67
  for relief of
    canker sores, 38
    headaches, 125–26
    irritable bowel syndrome, <u>216</u>
    worrying, 447
Immune system
  boosting, 32, 110
  cold and flu prevention and, 31

<u>Underscored</u> page references indicate boxed text. **Boldface** terms and references indicate primary discussions. *Italic* references indicate illustrations.

weakened, 231–37
    bolstering, 232, <u>233</u>, 234–37
    environmental changes to support,
        236–37
    stress reduction for, 235–36
Impaired glucose tolerance, 181
Inactivity, 452–60
    declining physical abilities and, <u>456–57</u>
    establishing manageable exercise
        routine and, 455–60
    maintaining motivation for exercise
        and, 460
    modifying mindset about exercise and,
        454–55
    music to set pace for exercise and,
        <u>458–59</u>
Incontinence, urinary, 297–303
    minimizing, 298–99
    prevention of, 299–303
    stress, 297, 298
    urge, 297–98
Infants
    breastfeeding, breast pain associated
        with, 24
    carrying, 18
Infections
    bacterial (*see* Bacterial infections)
    Candida
        dry mouth and, 65
        vaginal (*see* Yeast infections)
    herpes (*see* Cold sores)
    prevention of, with cuts and scrapes, 52
    urinary tract (*see* Urinary tract infections)
Infectious diarrhea, 57
Infertility. *See* Conception, difficulty with
Insecurity, 421
Insomnia, 112. *See also* Sleep problems
Insulin
    diabetes and, 181 (*see also* Diabetes)
    exercise and, 172
    phase I insulin release and, 22
Introl, for urinary incontinence, 299
Ipecacuanha (Ipecac), for queasy
        stomach, 104
Iron
    bolstering immune system and, 235
    deficiency of (*see* Anemia, iron-
        deficiency)

Iron supplements, 156–57
    calcium supplements with, 157
    for painful periods, 279
    side effects of, 285
Irritable bowel syndrome (IBS), 59,
    215–20
    prevention of, 215, <u>216</u>, 217–18
    remedies for, 218–20
Isoflavones
    for hot flash prevention, 259–60
    for menopause, 268, <u>270</u>
    for osteoporosis, 224
    for vaginal dryness, 307
Isolation, of single mothers, 484–85
Itching
    of skin, remedies for, 357–58
    vaginal (*see* Vaginitis; Yeast
        infections)

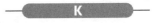

Jet lag, managing, 497–99
Jitters, caffeine-associated, 28–30
Jobs. *See* Employment
Joints. *See* Osteoarthritis; Rheumatoid
        arthritis; Stiffness, of joints;
        specific joints
Juniper berry, for urinary tract infections,
    <u>137</u>

K

Kava kava root, for sleep problems,
    114–15
Kefir, for bad breath, 20
Kegel exercises
    during pregnancy, 262, 264
    for relief of
        urinary incontinence, <u>300–301</u>
        vaginal dryness, 308
Kidney problems, magnesium therapy
        with, 5
Kreosotum, as treatment for
    vaginitis, <u>140</u>
    yeast infections, <u>150</u>

<u>Underscored</u> page references indicate boxed text. **Boldface** terms and
references indicate primary discussions. *Italic* references indicate illustrations.

L

Labels, on packaged foods and beverages, 195–96
Labor, 261–67
  preparation for, 262, _263_, 264–65
  strategies for easy delivery and, 265–67
Labor assistants, 265
Lactase supplements, 75, _198_
Lactobacillus acidophilus, for urinary incontinence, 299
Lactose, diarrhea and, 59
Lactose intolerance, 197, _198_
  flatulence and, 75
Laryngitis
  prevention of, 50–51
  remedies for, 49–50
Laugh lines. _See_ Expression lines
Lavender essential oil, for relief of
  dry hair, _330_
  energy slumps, _72_
  menstrual cramps, 275
  oily hair, 349
  tension headaches, 127
Lavender flowers, for dry hair, _330_
Lavender tea, for tension headaches, 126
Lazy bowel, 43
Ledum palustre, for puncture wounds, 53
Leg(s), elevating, for varicose veins, 146
Leg lifts, _367_
Lemon balm, as treatment for
  sleep problems, 115
  tension headaches, 126
Lemon drops, for dry mouth, 66
Lemon essential oil, for hot flashes, 258
Lemon juice, as treatment for
  bad breath, 20
  dry mouth, 66
  laryngitis, 49
Lemon scent, for morning sickness, 285
Licorice root
  deglycyrrhizinated, as treatment for
    heartburn, _87_
    vaginal dryness, 306
  side effects of, 258, 272
  as treatment for
    hot flashes, 258
    menopause, 271

Life expectancy, 152
Lifting, 15
Light. _See also_ Sunlight
  exposure to
    bad moods and, 387
    jet lag and, 499
    shift workers and, 505–6
    winter doldrums and, 444
Lignans, as treatment for
  fibromyalgia, 191
  menopause, 268–69
Lime juice, for bad breath, 20
Lip balm, for cold sore prevention, 37
Lip lines. _See_ Expression lines
Liquids. _See_ Fluids
Listening, attentive, 407
Liver spots. _See_ Age spots
Lower back stretches, to prevent post-workout soreness, _99_
Lubricants, vaginal, for relief of
  intercourse pain, 305
  vaginal dryness, 420
  vaginal itching and irritation, 305
Lumbar rolls, 15
Lunch, weight loss and, 229
Lunges, _372_
Lycopene, for cancer prevention, 173
Lying position
  avoiding morning stiffness and, 120
  for hemorrhoids, 90
  during labor, 266
  for wrinkle prevention, 376
Lysine, for cold sore prevention, 37

M

Magnesia phosphate, for menstrual cramps, 281
Magnesium
  side effects of, 169
  for tinnitus prevention, 133
  as treatment for
    asthma, 169
    caregivers under stress, 516
    chronic fatigue, 177, 178
    energy slumps, 70
    fibromyalgia, 190–91

Underscored page references indicate boxed text. **Boldface** terms and references indicate primary discussions. _Italic_ references indicate illustrations.

gum disease, 83
high blood pressure, 205–6
menstrual migraines, 125
osteoporosis, 224
painful periods, 278–79
premenstrual syndrome, 296
Magnesium ascorbyl phosphate, for dark
circles, 326
Magnesium glyconate
for migraines, 5
side effects of, 5
Makeup. See Cosmetics
Malic acid, as treatment for
chronic fatigue, 177
fibromyalgia, 190–91
Mannitol. See Artificial sweeteners
Mantras, for relieving hostility, 414
Marriage. See also Divorce
spending time with spouse and,
521–22
Marriage counselors, 400–401
Marsh mallow root, as treatment for
heartburn, 87
sore throat, 49
Masking noise, for tinnitus, 132
Mask of pregnancy. See Melasma
Massage, for relief of
dry hair, 332
fibromyalgia, 188–89
foot pain, 6–7
post-workout soreness, 94
tension headaches, 127–28
Meal(s). See also Diet(s); Nutrition;
specific foods
pace of eating and, heartburn and,
85–86
preparation of
fast food and, 518–19
for single mothers, 486, 488
serving sizes and
assessing, 472
controlling overeating and, 439–40
for trouble zone management, 362
weight loss and, 228
small
for depression, 396–97
for menopause, 271
for nervous tension, 431

for premenstrual syndrome, 296
for weight loss, 229
timing of
coughing related to, 51
energy related to, 69
heartburn and, 86
for irritable bowel syndrome, 217
for nervous tension, 432
for sleep problems, 115
weight loss and, 229–30
Meats
cured, avoiding for headache
prevention, 129
red
cancer and, 173
fibromyalgia and, 193
for iron-deficiency anemia, 154
osteoporosis and, 224–25
Meat tenderizer, for cold sores, 35–36
Mediators, for divorce, 403–4
Medications. See also specific medications
and types of medications
dry mouth with, 66–67
for menstrual discomforts, 273
photosensitizing, 312
queasy stomach as result of, 103
tinnitus as result of, 131–32
urinary incontinence and, 302–3
for yeast infections, 148
Meditation, for arthritis, 163
Melasma, 345–48
prevention of, 346–47
remedies for, 347–48
Melatonin
jet lag and, 498–99
shift workers and, 506
sleep and, 113
sunlight and, 176
Memorization, of sequential information,
408
Memory lapses. See Forgetfulness
Memory paths, 408
Menopause, 267–72
burning mouth syndrome and, 246–47
conjunctivitis following, 39
dry eyes and, 60, 62
dry mouth and, 65
early or surgical, 268

Menopause *(continued)*
  heart disease and, 200
  high cholesterol and, 210
  hot flashes and (*see* Hot flashes)
  perimenopausal symptoms and, 268
  protecting health during and after,
      268–72, 269, 270
  sleep problems during, 113
  vaginal dryness and (*see* Vaginal
      dryness)
  weight gain following, 361
Menstrual discomforts, 273–81
  dietary changes for, 278–80
  remedies for cramps and, 274–75
  yoga for, 276, 276–77
Menstruation
  asthma during, 164, *165*, 169
  bad breath during, 19
  breast pain associated with, 24
  canker sores associated with, 37
  cessation of (*see* Menopause)
  constipation and, 44
  energy during, 70
  iron loss during, 153
  irregular periods and, 272
  irritable bowel syndrome and, 215
  migraine headaches and, 123, 124–25
  migraines associated with, 5
  post-workout soreness during, 93
  premenstrual syndrome and (*see*
      Premenstrual syndrome)
  smoking cessation and, 171
Mental blocks, 423–26
  about household chores, 425
  in workplace, 424–25
Mental illness, divorce as result of, 401
Mentholated ointments, for sinusitis, 108
Mercurius solubilis, for vaginitis, 140
Mercurius vivus, for vaginitis, 140
Methylcellulose, for hemorrhoid
    prevention, 92
Migraine headaches, 123
  prevention of, 129–30
  remedies for, 5, 124–26, 124–25,
      128–29
Milk
  acidophilus, for bad breath, 20
  for osteoporosis, 221, 222

sinusitis and, 179
  for sleep problems, 115
Minerals. *See also specific minerals*
  energy related to, 69
Mineral supplements. *See also specific
    minerals*
  bolstering immune system and, 235
  for caregivers, 515–16
  heart disease prevention and, 203
  for relief of
    energy slumps, 70
    fibromyalgia, 191
Mint, heartburn and, 87
Moisture. *See also* Fluids; Humidity;
    Steam
  for dandruff, 56
Moisturizers
  for relief of
    blemishes, 317
    expression lines, 334, 335
    fine hair, 337
    sensitive skin, 358
    wrinkles, 375
  for split nail prevention, 359
Molding gels, for frizzy hair, 343
Moles, 312
Monosodium glutamate, headaches and,
    129
Mood(s). *See also* Anger; Depression;
    Winter doldrums
  bad, 383–87
    remedies for, 385–87
  setting, for sexual encounters, 417
Mood diaries, 385
Morning sickness, 282–85
  nutrition and, 284–85
  remedies for, 282–84
Mothers, single. *See* Single mothers
Motivation, for exercise, maintaining, 460
Mouse use, for repetitive strain injury
    prevention, 239
Mouth. *See also* Gum disease; Tooth
    brushing; Toothpastes; Tooth
    problems
  dry, 64–68
    bad breath related to, 19
    prevention of, 66–67
    remedies for, 20, 65–66

Underscored page references indicate boxed text. **Boldface** terms and references indicate primary discussions. *Italic* references indicate illustrations.

Mouthwashes, for relief of
  bad breath, 19
  gum disease, 82
Movement
  following meals, during pregnancy, 285
  for varicose vein prevention, 143
Multivitamin supplements. *See also specific vitamins*
  bolstering immune system and, 235
  for caregivers, 515–16
  during dieting, 473
  fibromyalgia and, 191
  heart disease prevention and, 203
Muscle relaxation. *See* Progressive muscle relaxation
Muscle soreness
  remedies for, 7–8
  working through, 460
Muscle spasms, remedy for, 11
Music
  during labor, 267
  to set pace for exercise, 458–59

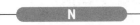

Nails. *See* Split nails
Naps, for sleep problems, 117
Nasal sprays, for sinusitis, 107, 179
National Association of Professional Geriatric Care Managers, 513
National Organization of Single Mothers, 486
Naturopathic doctors, finding, 193
Nausea, 103–6
  causes of, 103
  during menstruation (*see* Menstrual discomforts)
  during pregnancy (*see* Morning sickness)
  prevention of, 105–6
  remedies for, 104
Neck
  pain in, bras to relieve, 5
  stiff, remedies for, 120
Neck stretches, to prevent post-workout soreness, *100*
Negative-ion generators, for winter doldrums, 444

Negative thinking, 426–29
  dealing with negative people and, 428
  unlearning, 427–29
Neroli essential oil, for premenstrual syndrome, 292
Nerves, soothing, 54
Nervous tension, 429–34. *See also* Computer anxiety
  caffeine-associated, 28–30
  medical problems and, 431
  nutritional approaches for, 430–32
  public speaking and, 433
  situational, 432–34
  strategies for overcoming, 430
Neti, for sinusitis, 109
Nettles, for sleep problems, 115
Night sweats, sleep problems and, 113, 114
Nitrites, avoiding for headache prevention, 129
Noise
  masking, for tinnitus, 132
  protection from, for tinnitus prevention, 133–34
Nose cleaning, sinusitis and, 111
Nutrition. *See also* Diet(s); Meal(s); Snacks; *specific foods; specific nutrients*
  arthritis and, 159–60
  bad moods and, 386
  blemishes and, 318, 318–19
  bolstering immune system and, 232, 234–35
  breast pain prevention and, 25–27
  burning mouth syndrome and, 247–48
  cancer prevention and, 172–74
  canker sores related to, 37–38
  for caregivers, 515–16
  cholesterol management and, 210–12, 212
  chronic fatigue and, 176–79
  cold sore prevention and, 36
  constipation relief and, 44–45
  diabetes and, 182–83
  energy related to, 69–71
  fast food and, 518–19
  fibromyalgia and, 190–94
  gum disease and, 82–83
  healthy eating versus dieting and, 472–74

Underscored page references indicate boxed text. **Boldface** terms and references indicate primary discussions. *Italic* references indicate illustrations.

Nutrition *(continued)*
  heart disease prevention and, 202–3
  hemorrhoid prevention and, 91–92
  hot flash prevention and, 259–60
  iron-deficiency anemia and, 154–56, _155_
  irritable bowel syndrome and, 215, 217–18
  menstrual migraines and, _124–25_
  nervous tension and, 430–32
  painful periods and, 278–80
  postpartum depression and, 288
  premenstrual syndrome and, 292, 294–97, _294–95_
  queasy stomach and, 105
  for shift workers, 506–7
  trouble zones and, 362–63
  urinary incontinence and, 299–302
  varicose veins and, 144
  weight loss and, 228–30
  while traveling, 499–500
Nuts, for painful periods, 278

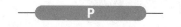

Oat bran, for diabetes, 184
Oatstraw, for sleep problems, 115
Obsessive-Compulsive Foundation, 443
Occupations. *See* Employment
Oil(s). *See also specific oils*
  for dry eyes, 62
Oil of bergamot, sun sensitivity as result of, 312
Olive oil
  cancer prevention and, 174
  dry eyes and, 62
  split nail prevention and, 359
Omega-3 fatty acids
  arthritis and, 160
  cancer prevention and, 173
  cholesterol management and, 211
  dry hair and, 331–32
  dry mouth prevention and, 67
  fibromyalgia and, 192
  heart disease prevention and, 203
  joint stiffness and, 122
  painful periods and, 278

Onions, hot flashes and, 260
Opening flower exercise, during labor, 266–67
Oral contraceptives
  high blood pressure and, _207_
  melasma and, 345
Oral hygiene, _78–80_
Orange blossom essential oil, for premenstrual syndrome, 292
Oregon grapes, for urinary tract infections, _137_
Orgasms, conception and, 251
Ornish diet, for cholesterol management, _212_
Osteoarthritis, 157–163
  exercise with, 160, 162–63
  prevention of flare-ups of, 159–60
  remedies for, 158–59, 163
Osteoporosis, 220–26
  prevention and treatment of, 221–25, _223_
Overcontrolling, 434–36
  tactics for overcoming, 435–36
Overeating, 436–41
  attitude change for controlling, 440–41
  binge-proofing your home and, 438–40
  heartburn and, 86
  method of eating and, 438, _439_
  overcoming urge to binge and, 437–38
Overweight, 226–31. *See also* Body weight
  effects of, 226
  hemorrhoids and, 89
  during pregnancy, _227_
  weight loss and (*see* Dieting; Weight control)
Ovulation, conception and, 254

Pain, 4–9. *See also specific types and sites of pain*
  of childbirth, acceptance of, 267
  estrogen and, 192
  with hemorrhoids, remedies for, 90–91
  menstrual (*see* Menstrual discomforts)

Underscored page references indicate boxed text. **Boldface** terms and references indicate primary discussions. *Italic* references indicate illustrations.

post-workout (*see* Workout(s), soreness following)
relaxation to reduce, <u>6</u>
significance of, 9–10
substance P and, 159, 188
Panax ginseng
for hot flashes, 258
for menopause, 271
for vaginal dryness, 306–7
Panty liners, vaginitis and, 140
Parent(s), caring for. *See* Caregivers
Parenting, by single mothers, 488–89
Parsley, for relief of
bad breath, 21
menopause, 269–70
Parsley root, for urinary tract infections, <u>137</u>
Partners, for exercise, 455
Party girls, 523–27
personal goals and, 524–26
strategies for change and, 526–27
Passionflower, for sleep problems, 114–15
Peak flow monitors, for asthma, 165–66
Pelvic tilts, for back pain prevention, *13*
Peony, for fibromyalgia, <u>193</u>
Pepper(s), red. *See* Capsaicin; Red peppers
Peppermint essential oil, as treatment for
irritable bowel syndrome, 219
laryngitis, 50
tension headaches, 127
Peppermint tea
gas and, 74
during pregnancy, 104
queasy stomach and, 104
Perfumes. *See* Fragrances
Period(s). *See* Menstruation
Periodontitis, 81
Personal relationships, to bolster immune system, 236
Personal trainers, 455
Pet(s), conjunctivitis and, 41
Petroleum jelly, for relief of
dry eyes, 62
dry mouth, 66
Phase I insulin release, 22

Phone use
flexibility and, 121
repetitive strain injury prevention and, 240
Photosensitizers, 312
Physical abuse. *See* Abuse, physical and emotional
Physical activity. *See* Aerobic exercise; Exercise(s); Inactivity; Strength training; Stretches; Workout(s); *specific activities*
Phytochemicals, to bolster immune system, 232
Phytoestrogens, for menopause, 269–70
Pill. *See* Oral contraceptives
Pillows, for air travel, 496
Pimples. *See* Blemishes
Pineal gland
sleep and, 113
sunlight and, 176
Pineapples, urinary incontinence and, 300
Pinkeye. *See* Conjunctivitis
Pipsissewa, for urinary tract infections, <u>137</u>
Plantain, for heartburn, <u>87</u>
Plaque, on teeth, 77
PMS. *See* Premenstrual syndrome
Polish, for fingernails, split nails and, 360
Pollen
asthma and, 166, 168
conjunctivitis and, 41
Pollution, sinusitis and, 107
Portions. *See* Meal(s), serving sizes and
Positions
increasing flexibility and, 121
lying (*see* Lying position)
for queasy stomach prevention, 106
sitting (*see* Sitting posture)
Postpartum depression. *See* Depression, postpartum
Posture
improving, 14–15
sitting (*see* Sitting posture)
Potassium
for high blood pressure, 205–6
preventing post-workout soreness, 103
Potency, of homeopathic medicines, 53

Underscored page references indicate boxed text. **Boldface** terms and references indicate primary discussions. *Italic* references indicate illustrations.

Powders, for hemorrhoids, 90
Pregnancy. *See also* Labor
  anemia during, 153
  asthma during, 164–65
  back strengthening after, 15–19, *18*
  blood sugar control during, 23
  conception and (*see* Conception,
    difficulty with)
  constipation during, 44
  diabetes during, 181–82
  dry eyes during, 62
  heartburn during, 84
  hemorrhoids during, 89
  high blood pressure during, 206
  mask of (*see* Melasma)
  morning sickness during (*see* Morning
    sickness)
  nails during, 358
  oral health during, 80–81
  overweight during, <u>227</u>
  peppermint tea and, 104
  repetitive strain injury and, 238
  sleep problems during, 113
  stretch mark prevention during, 323
  varicose veins during (*see* Varicose
    veins)
  vitamin A during, 84
Premenstrual syndrome (PMS), 290–97
  causes of, 290
  insomnia with, 113
  prevention of, 292, <u>293–95</u>, 294–97
  remedies for, 290–92, 387
Pressure equalization, for air travel, 497
Problem-solving, productive, 380, <u>381</u>,
  382–83
Prodrome, of cold sores, 35
Professional goals, for boredom relief,
  389
Progesterone, as treatment for
  hot flashes, 258–59
  premenstrual syndrome, <u>293</u>
Progressive muscle relaxation
  during labor, 264
  for relief of
    fibromyalgia, 190
    irritable bowel syndrome, <u>216</u>
    nervous tension, 430
    worrying, 447

Protein(s)
  energy related to, 69
  for flatulence, 75–76
  for nervous tension, 432
Psoralens, sun sensitivity as result of, 312
Psoriasis, of scalp, 55
Psyllium seed
  for constipation relief, 45
  hemorrhoid prevention and, 92
  for irritable bowel syndrome, 218
Public speaking, anxiety about, <u>433</u>
Puffy eyes. *See* Eye(s), puffy
Pulsatilla, for menstrual cramps, 281
Pumpkin seed, for painful periods, 278
Puncture wounds, remedies for, 53
Purple cornflower, for colds and flu, 32
Pyrophosphate, burning mouth
  syndrome and, 249

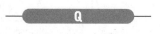

Quadriceps stretches, to prevent post-
  workout soreness, *97*
Queasy stomach. *See* Nausea
Quercetin, for asthma, 168–69

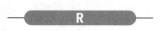

Radiant breath exercise, during labor,
  267
Raspberry leaf tea
  for diarrhea, 58
  during pregnancy, 262
Reaching, repetitive strain injury
  prevention and, 240
Rectal bleeding, 89, 92. *See also*
  Hemorrhoids
Red clover blossoms, for sleep problems,
  115
Red meats. *See* Meats, red
Red peppers. *See also* Capsaicin
  for burning mouth syndrome relief,
    247–48
  hot flashes and, 260
  for laryngitis relief, 49
  for sinusitis relief, 108

<u>Underscored</u> page references indicate boxed text. **Boldface** terms and references indicate primary discussions. *Italic* references indicate illustrations.

Reflexology, for tension headaches, 127
Refrigerator stretches, 16, *16–17*
Relaxation
    deep, 6–7
        for arthritis, 163
    during labor, 264
    of muscles (*see* Progressive muscle
        relaxation)
    for relief of
        bad moods, 386
        canker sores, 38
        dandruff, 56
        high blood pressure, 209
        irritable bowel syndrome, 216
        worrying, 446–47
    stress breaks for, 520
Relaxin, back muscles and, 16
Reminder services, 407
Renal problems, magnesium therapy
    with, 5
Repetition, for forgetfulness, 407
Repetitive strain injury, **237–44**
    prevention of, 238–40, 241
    remedies for, 240, 242–44
Resistance, poor. *See* Immune system,
    weakened
Resistance training. *See* Strength training
Rest. *See also* Sleep
    back pain and, 11
    chronic fatigue and, 180
    colds and flu and, 31
    cold sore prevention and, 36
    increasing flexibility and, 121
    postpartum depression and, 288–89
    repetitive strain injury and, 244
    of voice, for laryngitis, 50
Restaurants, food allergies and, 195
RETHINK technique, for controlling
    anger, 381
Retin A, for dark circles, 325
Rheumatoid arthritis, **157–63**
    exercise with, 160, 162–63
    prevention of flare-ups of, 159–60
    remedies for, 158, 159, 161, 163
Riboflavin, for menstrual migraines, 124
Rocking, during pregnancy, 163
Room temperature, hot flashes and, 257
Rose essential oil, for anger, 380

Rosemary essential oil, as treatment for
    dry hair, 331
    forgetfulness, 406
    oily hair, 349
Rosemary leaves, for dry hair, 330
Rotating oblique crunch, *366*
Routine, for sleep problems, 117
Rugs. *See* Carpeting

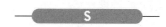

Sacroiliac belts, for back pain relief, 15
SAD. *See* Winter doldrums
Sage tea
    for gum disease, 82
    as oily hair rinse, 350–51
St.-John's-wort, as treatment for
    depression, 395–96
    sleep problems, 114–15
Salicylic acid, for blemishes, 316
Saline solutions, for conjunctivitis, 40
Saliva
    absence of (*see* Mouth, dry)
    artificial, for dry mouth, 66
    bad breath and, 19
    heartburn and, 84
    queasy stomach and, 104
    stimulating production of, 65–66
Salmon bones, for osteoporosis, 222
Salt. *See* Sodium
Saltwater gargles, for sore throat, 49
Saltwater rinses, for sinusitis, 109
Sandalwood essential oil, as treatment for
    dry hair, 330, 331
    premenstrual syndrome, 292
Satchidananda Ashram-Yogaville, 202
Scalp problems, **54–57**
    remedies for, 55–56
Scheduling workouts, 455–57
Scrapes, **51–53**
Seafood. *See* Omega-3 fatty acids
Seasonal affective disorder (SAD). *See*
    Winter doldrums
Seated stretches, for back pain
    prevention, *12*
Seborrheic dermatitis, 55
    remedies for, 55–56

Underscored page references indicate boxed text. **Boldface** terms and references indicate primary discussions. *Italic* references indicate illustrations.

Selenium
  for blemishes, 319
  for dandruff, 55
  sinusitis prevention and, 110
  sperm health and, 252
  tinnitus prevention and, 133
Self-esteem, low, 421–23
  remedies for, 422–23
Self-talk
  for getting into exercise habit,
    454–55
  guilt and, 411
  for overcoming negative thinking,
    427–28
  for postpartum depression, 287
  to raise self-esteem, 422–23
Semivegetarian diets, for rheumatoid
    arthritis, 161
Serotonin, energy related to, 70
Serving sizes. See Meal(s), serving sizes
    and
Sesame oil, for dry hair, 330
Sesame seed, for painful periods, 278
Set point theory of body weight, 469
Sexual activity
  for arthritis, 163
  vaginal dryness and, 308
Sexual desire, inhibition of, 415–21
  setting mood and, 417
  strategies to increase anticipation and,
    417–20, 418–19
Shame, 409–10
  remedies for, 412
Shampooing
  blemishes and, 317
  dandruff and, 55–56, 350
  hair types and
    dry, 328
    fine, 336–37
    frizzy, 341–43
    oily, 349–51
Shift workers, 503–9
  family ties and, 507, 508, 509
  nutrition for, 506–7
  sleep and, 504–6
Shoes
  increasing flexibility and, 121
  for varicose veins, 146

Shoulders
  pain in, bras to relieve, 5
  repetitive strain injury of, 240
Shoulder stretches, to prevent post-
    workout soreness, 100
Showers
  hot
    colds and flu and, 32
    morning stiffness and, 118
    sinusitis and, 108
    varicose veins and, 147
  warm
    arthritis and, 158
    during labor, 266
Silicone, for frizzy hair, 343–44
Single mothers, 484–89
  caring for sick children and, 487
  conflicting demands on, 485–86
  isolation felt by, 484–85
  meal preparation and, 486, 488
  parenting by, 488–89
Sinusitis, 106–12
  chronic fatigue and, 178–79
  prevention of, 110–11
  remedies for, 107–8, 109, 110
Sitting posture, 15
  repetitive strain injury prevention and,
    239–40, 241
  for varicose veins, 146
Sitz baths, for hemorrhoids, 90
Sjögren's syndrome, dry mouth in, 65
Skin
  scalp disorders and, 55
  sensitive, 354–58
    hygiene and, 357–58
    prevention of irritations and,
      355–57
    during winter, remedies for, 358
Skullcap
  for fibromyalgia, 192
  for sleep problems, 114–15
Skunk cabbage, for fibromyalgia, 192
Sleep. See also Rest
  bolstering immune system and, 234
  for caregivers, 513–14
  dark circle prevention and, 324
  excessive, chronic fatigue and, 180
  fibromyalgia and, 187

Underscored page references indicate boxed text. **Boldface** terms and references indicate primary discussions. *Italic* references indicate illustrations.

interruption by hot flashes, 255, 256
jet lag and, 497–99
position during, to avoid morning
    stiffness, 120
postpartum depression and, 288
puffy eyes and, 352
saliva flow during, 19
shift work and, 504–6
Sleep problems, 112–17
factors contributing to, 112–13
prevention of, 114–17
remedies for, 114, <u>115</u>
Slippery elm, as treatment for
diarrhea, 58
heartburn, <u>87</u>
irritable bowel syndrome, 218
Smoking cessation
bad breath and, 21
cancer prevention and, 170–71
cold and flu prevention and, 34
conception and, 253
coughing and, 50–51
dry eyes and, 63
expression lines and, 334
heartburn and, 88
heart disease prevention and, 200–201
hot flash prevention and, 261
osteoporosis and, 225
sleep problems and, 116
tinnitus prevention and, 133
urinary incontinence and, 303
wrinkle prevention and, 376
Smooth Move tea, for constipation relief,
    <u>45</u>
Snacks
exercise and, for people with diabetes,
    186
weight loss and, 229
Sneezing, 111
covering mouth during, 33
Soaks, warm, for stiff hands, 119
Soaps
sensitive skin and, 356
yeast infections and, 151
Social activities
dispelling boredom and, 388–89
for elders, 512
excessive (*see* Party girls)

Social support networks
depression and, 398
    postpartum, 288
for single mothers, 486
Society for Light Treatment and
    Biological Rhythms, 506
Sodium
breast pain related to, 26
high blood pressure and, 205
osteoporosis and, 225
during pregnancy, 284–85
Sodium lauryl sulfate, canker sores and,
    38
Solar lentigines. *See* Age spots
Sorbitol. *See* Artificial sweeteners
Soreness. *See* Pain; Workout(s), soreness
    following; *specific sites and types of
    pain*
Sore throats
prevention of, 50–51
remedies for, 48–49
Soups, for chronic fatigue, 177
Soy foods
hot flash prevention and, 259–60
menopause and, 268
soybeans, for osteoporosis, 224
soy protein, for heart disease
    prevention, 203
vaginal dryness and, 307
Soy oil, for dry hair, <u>330</u>
Sperm, 251–52
body weight and, 253–54
maximizing concentration of, 254
Spicy foods
canker sores related to, 37–38
dry mouth and, 67
gum disease and, 81
irritable bowel syndrome and, 218
urinary incontinence and, 300
Spinach, for iron-deficiency anemia, 154
Spiritual support, for single mothers, 486
Splints, for repetitive strain injury, 243
Split nails, 358–60
minimizing, 359–60
Sportenine, for post-workout soreness, 95
Sports bras, 5
Squats, *371*
during pregnancy, <u>163</u>

Underscored page references indicate boxed text. **Boldface** terms and
references indicate primary discussions. *Italic* references indicate illustrations.

Steam
  for laryngitis, 50
  for sinusitis, 110, _179_
Stiffness
  in back (_see_ Back pain)
  in hands, remedies for, 119–20
  of joints, 118–22
    remedies for morning stiffness and,
      118–20, _119_
    remedies for stiff neck and, 120
    strategies to increase flexibility and,
      120–22
  morning, remedies for, 118–20, _119_
  post-workout (_see_ Workout(s), soreness
    following)
Stitches, for cuts, 54
Stockings, compression, 143–44, 146
Stomach upset. _See_ Nausea
Straightening irons, for frizzy hair,
  344–45
Strain, repetitive. _See_ Repetitive strain
  injury
Strawberries, urinary incontinence and,
  300
Strength training
  aerobic exercise and, 464
  cellulite, alleviating with, 322
  menopause and, 272
  trouble zones, combatting with, 365,
    _366–72_
Stress. _See also_ Computer anxiety;
    Nervous tension
  canker sores associated with, 37
  of caregivers, magnesium for, 516
  forgetfulness and, 405
  high blood pressure and, 204
  irritable bowel syndrome and, 215
  queasy stomach and, 103
  reduction of
    bolstering immune system and,
      235–36
    canker sores and, 38
    cold sores and, 36, 37
    conception and, 251
    dandruff and, 56
    heart disease prevention and, 201–2
    high blood pressure and, 208–9
    hostility and, 414–15

  relaxation for (_see_ Relaxation)
  repetitive strain injury and, 243
  vaginitis and, 140
  of single mothers, 485
Stress incontinence, 297, 298
Stretches
  arthritis and, 162–63
  back pain and, _10_, 12, _12_, _16_, _16–17_
  menstrual cramps and, _276_, _276–77_
  morning stiffness and, 118, _119_
  post-workout soreness and, 94, _96_,
    _96–101_, 102
  repetitive strain injury prevention and,
    240
  stiff neck and, 120
  trouble zones and, 364
  varicose vein prevention and, 143
Stretch marks, 320–23
  prevention of, 322
  remedies for, 322–23
Substance abuse, divorce as result of, _401_
Substance P, pain sensation and, 159, 188
Sugar. _See also_ Blood sugar; Sweets
  depression and, 397–98
  for diarrhea, 59
Sunflower seed, for painful periods, 278
Sunlight
  age spots and, 311, 312–13
  blemishes and, 316
  for chronic fatigue, 176
  dry hair and, 332
  protection from
    age spot prevention and, 312
    blemishes and, 317
    cold sore prevention and, 37
    dark circle prevention and, 325
    expression lines and, 333–34
    melasma prevention and, 346–47,
      348
    varicose veins and, 146–47
    wrinkle prevention and, 375–76
  sleep problems and, 115, 116, 117
  stretch marks and, 323
  winter doldrums and (_see_ Winter
    doldrums)
  wrinkles and, 372–73
Support networks. _See_ Social support
  networks

Underscored page references indicate boxed text. **Boldface** terms and references indicate primary discussions. _Italic_ references indicate illustrations.

Sweets. *See also* Sugar
  caregivers and reduction of, 515
  gum disease and, 82
  nervous tension and, 431–32
  sleep problems and, 116
  winter doldrums and, <u>445</u>
  yeast infections and, 151
Swimming
  arthritis and, 163
  back pain prevention and, 12
  increasing flexibility and, 122

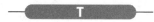

Tai chi, for arthritis, 163
Tailor sitting, during pregnancy, <u>163</u>
Tampons, for urinary incontinence, 298
Tannin, for canker sores, 37
Tanning beds, wrinkles and, 376
Tar, for dandruff, 55
Tartar, 77
Tea bags, for canker sores, 37
Tears, artificial, for dry eyes, 61
Telephone use. *See* Phone use
Temperature. *See* Bath(s); Cold;
    Compresses; Heat; Ice; Room
    temperature; Showers
Tension. *See* Computer anxiety; Nervous
    tension; Stress
Tension headaches, 122–23
  prevention of, 129, 130
  remedies for, 124, 126–28
Tetanus shots, 54
Thighs
  lunges for, *372*
  squats for, *371*
Thinking
  negative (*see* Negative thinking)
  sleep problems and, 117
Throat. *See* Sore throats
Thumb walk, for arthritis, 163
Thyme, for coughing, 47–48
Thymus vulgaris, for coughing, 47
Time diaries, 477
Time management, **475–83**
  balancing personal and professional
    lives and, 476, 492–93

family time and, 479, 482
  finding lost time and, 477
  simplifying life and, 477–78
  time required for household chores
    and, <u>480–81</u>
  workload management and, 482–83
Timing
  effectiveness of remedies related to, 4
  of meals (*see* Meal(s), timing of)
Tinnitus, **130–34**
  prevention of, 132–34
  remedies for, 131–32
Tobacco use. *See* Smoking cessation
Toddlers, carrying, 18
Tomatoes
  for cancer prevention, 173
  hot flashes and, 260
  urinary incontinence and, 300
Tongue, brushing, 20
Tooth brushing, <u>78–79</u>, *78*
  bad breath and, 20
  canker sore prevention and, 38
Toothpastes
  burning mouth syndrome and, 249
  canker sore prevention and, 38
  gum disease and, 82
Toothpicks, for bad breath prevention, 20
Tooth problems, bad breath related to, 21
Towels, changing
  during cold sore attacks, 36
  during conjunctivitis attacks, 41
Travel, **495–502**
  accommodations and, 502
  by air
    comfort during, 496–97
    managing jet lag and, 497–99, <u>498–99</u>
  exercise and, 500–502
  nutrition and, 499–500
  puffy eyes and, <u>501</u>
Triceps extensions, *368*
Triceps kickbacks, *368*
Trips. *See* Travel
Trouble zones, **360–72**
  aerobic exercise for, 363–65
  permanent lifestyle changes for
    managing, 362–63
  resistance training for toning, 365,
    366–72

<u>Underscored</u> page references indicate boxed text. **Boldface** terms and references indicate primary discussions. *Italic* references indicate illustrations.

Tryptophan, for sleep problems, 115
Turkey, for sleep problems, 115
Turmeric
    for cholesterol management, 213
    to limit flatulence, 75
Tyramine, avoiding for headache
        prevention, 129
Tyrosine, energy related to, 69

U

Umbelliferae, for menopause, 269–70
Underwear
    hot flashes and, 257
    urinary tract infections and, 136, 138
    yeast infection prevention and, 151
Upper arm stretches, to prevent post-
        workout soreness, *101*
Upper back stretches, to prevent post-
        workout soreness, *101*
Urge incontinence, 297–98
Urinary incontinence. *See* Incontinence,
    urinary
Urinary tract infections (UTIs), 134–39
    prevention of, 137–39
    remedies for, 134–36, <u>137</u>
Urinating. *See* Voiding
UTIs. *See* Urinary tract infections
Uva ursi, for urinary tract infections, <u>137</u>

V

Vaginal dryness, 303–9
    remedies for, 304–7
    vaginal health and, 307–9
Vaginal secretions, conception and, 251
Vaginal suppositories, for vaginal dryness,
    305–6
Vaginitis, 139–41. *See also* Yeast
    infections
    remedies for, <u>140</u>, 141
Vaginosis, bacterial, 139, 141
Valerian, as treatment for
    fibromyalgia, <u>193</u>
    sleep problems, 115
Vaporizers, for dandruff, 56

Varicose veins, 142–47
    prevention of, 143–44
    remedies for, 144, <u>145</u>, 146–47
Vegetables. *See also* Diet(s), vegetarian;
        specific vegetables
    cancer prevention and, 172–73
    constipation and, 44, 46
    flatulence and, 75–76
    gum disease and, 83
    heart disease prevention and, 203
    irritable bowel syndrome and, 217
    osteoporosis and, 222
Veins, varicose. *See* Varicose veins
Vervain tea, for tension headaches,
        126
Vinegar, for oily hair rinse, 350
Visualization. *See also* Imagery
    caregivers and, 514
    for relief of
        bad moods, 386
        depression, <u>396–97</u>
        forgetfulness, 407
        hot flashes, 257
        shame, 412
        sleep problems, <u>115</u>
Vitamin(s). *See also* Multivitamin
        supplements; *specific vitamins*
    energy related to, 69
    for energy slumps, 70
Vitamin A
    blemishes and, <u>318</u>
    coughing and, 48
    dry eyes and, 62
    dry mouth prevention and, 67
    gum disease and, 82–83
    painful periods and, 279–80
    during pregnancy, 84
    tinnitus prevention and, 133
Vitamin B-complex
    chronic fatigue and, 178
    dry mouth prevention and, 67
    energy slumps and, 70
    menopause and, 270–71
    painful periods and, 279
    premenstrual syndrome and, 296
Vitamin B_6
    asthma and, 169
    blemishes and, <u>319</u>

Underscored page references indicate boxed text. **Boldface** terms and references indicate primary discussions. *Italic* references indicate illustrations.

deficiency of, burning mouth
    syndrome and, 248
morning sickness and, 283–84
postpartum depression and, 288
premenstrual syndrome and, 387
side effects of, 67
Vitamin B₁₂
deficiency of, burning mouth
    syndrome and, 248
postpartum depression and, 288
tinnitus prevention and, 133
Vitamin C
arthritis and, 160
asthma and, 168
blemishes and, 319
bolstering immune system and, 232,
    234–35
cancer prevention and, 174
cholesterol management and, 212
colds and flu and, 32–33
coughing and, 50
dark circles and, 325
excess of, 252
flatulence and, 76–77
gum disease and, 83
heart disease prevention and, 203
iron-deficiency anemia and, 154, 156
menopause and, 270–71
osteoporosis and, 224
sinusitis prevention and, 110
sore throats and, 50
sperm problems and, 252
tinnitus prevention and, 133
urinary incontinence and, 301
urinary tract infections and, 136
varicose veins and, 144
wrinkles and, 374–75
Vitamin D
menstrual migraines and, 124–25
osteoporosis and, 223–24
Vitamin E
blemishes and, 319
bolstering immune system and,
    234–35
breast pain prevention and, 25–26
cancer prevention and, 174
diabetes and, 184
heart disease prevention and, 203

hot flash prevention and, 260
menopause and, 271
menstrual migraines and, 125
painful periods and, 279
side effects of, 271
sinusitis prevention and, 110
sperm problems and, 252
tinnitus prevention and, 133
vaginal dryness and, 307
Vitex. See Chasteberry
Voiding
before exercise, 298
for urinary tract infection prevention,
    138
Vomiting, during pregnancy. See
    Morning sickness

W

Waist-to-hip ratio, body weight and, 185
Walking
anger and, 380
back pain prevention and, 11–12
bad moods and, 386
bolstering immune system and, 232
cancer prevention and, 171
constipation prevention and, 46
diabetes and, 186
energy slumps and, 71
headache prevention and, 130
heartburn and, 84
increasing flexibility and, 121
menstrual cramps and, 275
trouble zones and, 363–64
Water. See also Bath(s); Fluids; Humidity;
    Showers; Steam
chlorinated, dry hair and, 332
Weight control. See also Dieting
for cholesterol management, 213–14
conception and, 253–54
for diabetes, 184–85
dietary strategies for, 228–30
exercise for, 230–31
heart disease prevention and, 201
high blood pressure and, 206, 208
increasing flexibility and, 121
pace of, 227

Underscored page references indicate boxed text. **Boldface** terms and references indicate primary discussions. *Italic* references indicate illustrations.

Weight control *(continued)*
  programs for lasting weight loss and,
    227–28
  stretch mark prevention and, 322–23
Wheat, sinusitis and, <u>179</u>
Winter doldrums, **443–45**
  remedies for, 71
  in shift workers, 505–6
  strategies to lighten mood and,
    444–45, <u>445</u>
Wintergreen essential oil, for menstrual
    cramps, 275
Work. *See* Employment
Workaholics, **490–94**
  balancing professional and personal life
    and, 492–93
  recognizing, 491–92
  strengthening family ties and, 493–94
Work environment, cancer prevention
    and, 172
Workout(s). *See also* Aerobic exercise;
    Exercise(s); Strength training;
    Stretches; *specific activities*
  building routine for, 462–65
  optimum, <u>463</u>
  soreness following, **93–103**
    prevention of, <u>96</u>, *96–101*, 102–3
    remedies for, 94–95, 402
Workout machines, post-workout
    soreness and, 93
Worry, **445–49**
  relaxation to control, 446–47
  sleep problems and, 117
  strategies for dealing with, 447–49, <u>448</u>
Wounds. *See specific types of wounds*
Wrinkles, **372–76**
  prevention of, 375–76
  remedies for, 373–75
Wrist(s), exercise for arthritis affecting,
    163
Wrist bands, for morning sickness, 282–83

Y

Yard work, asthma and, 166
Yeast infections, 139, **147–51**
  diagnosis of, 148
  prevention of, 149–51
  remedies for, 148–49
Ylang-ylang essential oil, for
    premenstrual syndrome, 292
Yoga
  arthritis and, 163
  finding instructors for, <u>202</u>
  heart disease prevention and, <u>202</u>
  menstrual cramps and, <u>276</u>, *276–77*
  repetitive strain injury and, 243
  sinusitis and, <u>109</u>
Yogurt
  bad breath and, 20
  flatulence and, 75
  osteoporosis and, 222
  urinary incontinence and, 299
  yeast infections and, 148

Z

Zinc, 4
  blemishes and, <u>319</u>
  bolstering immune system and,
    235
  chronic fatigue and, 177
  cold sores and, 36
  dry eyes and, 62
  energy slumps and, 70
  gum disease and, 83
  sperm count and, 252
  tinnitus prevention and, 133
Zinc gluconate
  colds and flu and, 33
  sore throat and, 48–49
Zinc pyrithione, for dandruff, 55

<u>Underscored</u> page references indicate boxed text. **Boldface** terms and references indicate primary discussions. *Italic* references indicate illustrations.